T0190209

DOCUMENTATION AND REIMBURSEMENT FOR SPEECH-LANGUAGE PATHOLOGISTS

PRINCIPLES AND PRACTICE

DOCUMENTATION AND REIMBURSEMENT FOR SPEECH-LANGUAGE PATHOLOGISTS

PRINCIPLES AND PRACTICE

Nancy B. Swigert, MA, CCC-SLP, BCS-S
Swigert & Associates, Inc.
Biltmore Lake, North Carolina

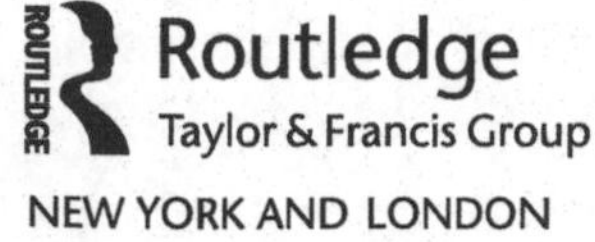

NEW YORK AND LONDON

Documentation and Reimbursement for Speech-Language Pathologists: Principles and Practice includes ancillary materials specifically available for faculty use. Included are PowerPoint slides. Please visit www.routledge.com/9781630913809

First published 2018 by SLACK Incorporated

Published in 2024 by Routledge
605 Third Avenue, New York, NY 10158

and by Routledge
4 Park Square, Milton Park, Abingdon, Oxon, OX14 4RN

Routledge is an imprint of the Taylor & Francis Group, an informa business

Cover Artist: Anita Santiago

Library of Congress Cataloging-in-Publication Data

Names: Swigert, Nancy B., author.
Title: Documentation and reimbursement for speech-language pathologists : principles and practice / Nancy B. Swigert.
Description: Thorofare, NJ : Slack Incorporated, [2018] | Includes bibliographical references and index.
Identifiers: LCCN 2018008392 (print)
ISBN 9781630913809 (pbk.)
Subjects: | MESH: Speech-Language Pathology | Documentation | Reimbursement Mechanisms
Classification: LCC RC428.5 (print) | NLM WL 21 | DDC 616.85/5--dc23
LC record available at https://lccn.loc.gov/2018008392

ISBN: 9781630913809 (pbk)
ISBN: 9781003523864 (ebk)

DOI: 10.4324/9781003523864

Dedication

This book is dedicated to my husband of 43 years, Keith, who graciously allows me solitude to concentrate on writing when he would much rather I get up from the desk and share time with him.

Contents

Documentation and Reimbursement for Speech-Language Pathologists: Principles and Practice includes ancillary materials specifically available for faculty use. Included are PowerPoint slides. Please visit http://www.efacultylounge.com to obtain access.

Acknowledgements

I would like to extend thanks to:

- My colleagues at Swigert & Associates, Inc. and Baptist Health Lexington who over the years participated in developing, revising, and using the various forms shared in the book.
- Luis Riquelme and Jill Kobak for significant contributions to Chapter 4 concerning electronic health records.
- Renee Kinder, Barbara Moore, Karyn Searcy, Rebecca Skrine, and Lynne Brady-Wagner and her co-authors, Denise Ambrosi and Daniel Meninger for agreeing to take on the major task of writing a chapter.
- My fellow ASHA volunteer leaders who are also passionate about coding, reimbursement, and documentation and with whom I had the pleasure of serving on the Health Care Economics Committee for 9 years: Ken Bouchard, Kyle Dennis, Bernard Henri, Tom Rees, Gwen Reeves, Martin Robinette, Neil Shepard, Walt Smoski, Stu Trembeth, and Robert Woods; with very special appreciation to Becky Cornett, Bob Fifer, Wayne Holland, and Dee Nikjeh, who have shared not only their knowledge but close friendship as well.
- ASHA staff who shared their incredible expertise in all things coding and reimbursement: Steve White, Mark Kander, and Janet McCarty; and Neela Swanson and Lisa Satterfield, who also authored a most excellent resource on all things Medicare.
- ASHA staff in the practice areas who are always ready to answer questions and advise: Janet Brown and Lisa Rai Mabry-Price.

About the Author

Nancy B. Swigert, MA, CCC-SLP, BCS-S, speech-language pathologist, is the former director of Speech-Language Pathology and Respiratory Care at Baptist Health Lexington, an acute care facility in Lexington, Kentucky. Prior to that, her private practice, Swigert & Associates, Inc., provided services to children and adults for 26 years. In 2016-2017 she served as the Process Excellence Coordinator and a Certified Green Belt in Lean/Six Sigma in the Quality Outcomes Department at Baptist, where she coached teams to use data and Lean/Six Sigma process improvement methodologies. As president of Swigert & Associates., Inc., now a consulting company, she continues to teach and write in the areas of dysphagia, coding and reimbursement, and documentation.

Her main clinical interests are in the areas of pediatric and adult dysphagia. She has authored seven publications with Pro-Ed (Linguisystems): *The Source for Dysphagia* (4th Edition), *The Source for Dysarthria* (2nd Edition), *The Source for Pediatric Dysphagia* (2nd Edition), *The Source for Reading Fluency*, *The Source for Early Intervention*, *The Source for Children's Voice Disorders*, and *Reading Fluency and Comprehension*. She lectures extensively in the areas of dysphagia and motor speech disorders. She has authored numerous book chapters and articles focusing on documentation and reimbursement.

She received her master's degree from the University of Tennessee—Knoxville. She is a former President of the Kentucky Speech-Language-Hearing Association and the Council of State Association Presidents. She was President of the American Speech-Language-Hearing Foundation in 2004-2005. She chaired the American Board of Swallowing and Swallowing Disorders from 2012-2014.

She has served in numerous volunteer capacities for the American Speech-Language-Hearing Association (ASHA). In the mid-1990s, she co-chaired the ASHA Task Force on Treatment Outcomes, which initially developed the National Outcomes Measurement System (NOMS). She served on the Health Care Economics Committee for 9 years and chaired it for 6. It was during that tenure that she gained invaluable knowledge about reimbursement and documentation requirements. She served on the ASHA Executive Board for 6 years, 3 as Vice President for Governmental and Social Policies and then as President-Elect, President (1998), and Past President. She is an ASHA Fellow and received the Honors of ASHA in 2015.

Contributing Authors

Denise M. Ambrosi, MS, CCC-SLP (Chapter 11)
Spaulding Rehabilitation Hospital
MGH Institute of Health Professions
Charlestown, Massachusetts

Lynne C. Brady Wagner, MA, CCC-SLP (Chapter 11)
Chief Learning Officer, SRN
Associate Director, Spaulding Stroke Research and Recovery Institute
Director, Clinical Scholars Program
Chair, Ethics Advisory Committee
Spaulding Rehabilitation Hospital
Charlestown, Massachusetts

Renee Kinder, MS, CCC-SLP, RAC-CT (Chapter 12)
Encore Rehabilitation
Lexington, Kentucky

Daniel Meninger, MSPT (Chapter 11)
Spaulding Rehabilitation Hospital
Charlestown, Massachusetts

Barbara J. Moore, EdD, CCC-SLP, BCS-CL (Chapter 16)
East Side Union High School District
San Jose, California

Karyn Lewis Searcy, MA, CCC-SLP (Chapter 15)
Clinical Director
TERI Crimson Center for Speech & Language
Clinical Faculty
San Diego State University
San Diego, California

Rebecca Skrine, MS, CCC-SLP, CHCE, COS-C (Chapter 13)
Baptist Health
Louisville, Kentucky

Introduction

If It Wasn't Documented, It Wasn't Done

I have often heard that statement quoted, written, and referenced. I do not know to whom it should be attributed, but I do know that regarding documentation, it is the most important thing you will learn. The work you will do with clients, students, and their caregivers and the collaborative efforts in which you will participate with your colleagues is the reason you have selected a career in speech-language pathology. But that work exists in the moment. Of course, it is important that you know how to perform evaluations, establish evidence-based treatment plans, conduct treatment activities, measure progress, talk to caregivers and colleagues about the treatment, determine when discharge is indicated, and establish home programs.

However, each of those activities has to be documented. Once the session is over, the conversation with the colleague completed, and the home program explained to the caregivers, the only evidence that those things ever happened lies in the accurate documentation of the events. Many times, the speech-language pathologist feels as if she spends more time documenting than doing. Therefore, it is important to learn not only how to document, but how to do so efficiently.

How This Book Is Organized: Sections and Chapters

This book is divided into sections, with chapters related to each section's topic. The book begins with a section on the basics of documentation and includes chapters on the reasons we document and the basic rules of documentation, particularly for health care settings; different documentation formats you will encounter depending on where you work; how coding and documentation relate to reimbursement in health care settings; and why our documentation, regardless of setting, should focus on function.

The next section covers the different types of services speech-language pathologists provide and how to document each of those. The chapters address evaluation, treatment plans, progress notes, and discharge summaries.

The next two sections are organized around the different settings in which speech-language pathologists work, and I have invited some esteemed colleagues who work in different settings to contribute. There is a section on health care settings for adults. Each chapter will address documentation and reimbursement in that setting: acute care, inpatient rehabilitation facilities, skilled nursing facilities, home health, and outpatient. As this book covers both health care and educational settings, the terms *client*, *patient*, and *student* will be used in different chapters, depending on the focus of the chapter.

There is also a section on documentation and reimbursement for pediatrics. This section has chapters on settings that are much like the health care settings for adults: early intervention and outpatient pediatric clinics (including private practices). It also has a chapter that will be very different from the other settings and will addresses reimbursement, processes, and how to document for services provided to students in school settings.

The final section of the book has only one chapter and will cover other types of writing you will do that might not be considered client documentation. Speech-language pathologists write letters to caregivers and other professionals. They construct fax cover sheets and memos. These must be done professionally because the recipients of that correspondence make judgments about the quality of your services based on your writing skills. The chapter also addresses oral presentations and writing for job search.

What You Will Find in Each Chapter

Each chapter will include helpful learning materials. The opening will give you an idea of what you will find in the chapter. At the end of each chapter, you will find some review questions that will help you recall what you've just read. There are also activities that will help you practice applying what you've learned.

Helpful Materials at the End of the Book

The glossary is a quick and easy place to look when you forget what a certain term means. There is also a list of abbreviations culled from chapters throughout the book.

Using the Book Now and After You Graduate

During graduate school, you will have limited opportunities to see clients in different settings and thus to practice documentation in those settings. I hope the book helps you hone your documentation skills in those clinic and extern settings. However, I also hope it prepares you for whatever setting in which you begin your career and throughout your career as you change settings.

Keep in mind that documentation and reimbursement requirements change; therefore, you should always check to make sure the information in this book, particularly as it relates to reimbursement regulations, is still current. The website of the American Speech-Language-Hearing Association is a wonderful resource for up-to-date information on documentation and reimbursement.

I

Basics of Documentation

This section addresses the basics of documentation necessary to understand before delving into the chapters more directly related to documentation of client services. These basics will be important regardless of work setting or type of client being seen. For example, the basic rules of documentation and the reasons for documenting lay groundwork for the development of more specific skills of documenting covered in Section II. Similarly, the fundamental principles of coding and payment are the stepping stones to understanding the detailed specifics of coding and reimbursement rules in different health care and education settings described in Sections III (adult settings) and IV (pediatric settings).

This section also introduces the topic of focusing on function, applicable in any work setting with any type of client. Chapter 4 in this section is a compilation of information on different formats for documenting as well as examples of different kinds of forms.

1

Basic Rules of Documentation

Nancy B. Swigert, MA, CCC-SLP, BCS-S

Who Makes the Rules?

Speech-language pathologists work in a variety of health care and educational settings, and their services are reimbursed by a number of different third-party payers, both private and public. In health care settings, the gold standard for what should or should not be included in documentation is prescribed by the Centers for Medicare & Medicaid Services (CMS). Whether the services are being provided to an infant in a neonatal intensive care unit, a preschooler in a speech-language pathologist's office, an elderly patient in his or her home, or a working-age adult in a clinic, if the stringent guidelines established by CMS are followed, the documentation will generally meet the standards of any other payer. Specifics of documentation in public school settings are described in Chapter 16, but the CMS guidelines are helpful in that setting as well. Although the same stringent rules are not required in school settings, the guidelines can serve as a model.

The rules established by CMS are intended to ensure that the services being reimbursed are those that are covered by Medicare or Medicaid. For example, the specific elements required in a treatment note help to support that the treatment rendered is skilled and that the client is making progress. These rules of documentation support reimbursement, which is described in more detail in Chapter 4.

Of course, there are many other rules to guide documentation. Some are truly legal rules or requirements, such as the confidentiality rules described. Others are not legally binding but are good guidelines to follow when documenting, such as being concise and recording information in a logical order.

Confidentiality

The speech-language pathologist should first and foremost ensure that any documentation protects the client's right to privacy. This is required both in written/electronic documentation and also in any conversations. Doing what is right for the client should always be the guiding principle for documentation.

The American Speech-Language-Hearing Association Code of Ethics

The American Speech-Language-Hearing Association (ASHA) Code of Ethics addresses the importance of confidentiality in Principle 1: "Individuals shall honor their responsibility to hold paramount the welfare of persons they serve professionally or who are participants in research and scholarly activities, and they shall treat animals involved in

Swigert, N. B.
Documentation and Reimbursement for Speech-Language Pathologists: Principles and Practice (pp. 3-15).

research in a humane manner." Two specific rules provide more detail:

O. Individuals shall protect the confidentiality and security of records of professional services provided, research and scholarly activities conducted, and products dispensed. Access to these records shall be allowed only when doing so is necessary to protect the welfare of the person or of the community, is legally authorized, or is otherwise required by law.

P. Individuals shall protect the confidentiality of any professional or personal information about persons served professionally or participants involved in research and scholarly activities and may disclose confidential information only when doing so is necessary to protect the welfare of the person or of the community, is legally authorized, or is otherwise required by law. (ASHA, 2016)

Health Insurance Portability and Accountability Act of 1996

As more and more medical record documentation became electronic, and thus more easily breached, the federal government addressed the importance of protecting clients' rights to confidentiality as part of a law called the Health Insurance Portability and Accountability Act (HIPAA) of 1996. Title I of HIPAA allows workers to keep their insurance coverage when they change jobs. It also prohibits discrimination against employees and their dependents based on any health factors, including prior medical conditions. Title II targeted the prevention of fraud and abuse and required the U.S. Department of Health and Human Services (HSS) to establish rules to protect the privacy of clients' personal health information (U.S. Department of Labor, 2015).

The Privacy Rule set standards for health care plans, clearinghouses, and health care providers who hold health information or conduct health care transactions electronically. This would include, for example, saving client documentation in an electronic format, billing electronically, sending an email with information about a client, sending a record as an attachment to an email, or even faxing some client information. Compliance with this rule was required as of April 2003.

Clients have specific rights delineated in the regulations, including the following:

- Getting a copy of their medical record in written or electronic format (The client may have to pay to have the copies made.)
- Correcting any incorrect information in the record
- Knowing who has access to the information in the record
- Asking that the information not be shared with certain groups or individuals (U.S. Department of Health & Human Services [HHS], n.d.)

The Privacy Rule also establishes the conditions under which protected health information may be used or disclosed by covered entities for research purposes (HHS, 2013).

The Security Rule went into effect in 2005 and operationalized the Privacy Rule by setting national standards for protecting the confidentiality, integrity, and availability of electronic protected health information. The Security Rule required health care entities to put in place safeguards to keep electronic records safe. These safeguards could include the following:

- Access control tools like passwords and personal identification numbers
- Encrypting the stored information
- Setting up an audit trail to track who has accessed the records (HHS, 2014)

The health care entity is also required to notify the client if the security has been breached. For example, if a fax containing a client's information was sent to the wrong physician, this would be considered a breach. If the client believes his or her health information privacy rights, or someone else's rights, have been breached, he or she can file a complaint with the Office of Civil Rights (HHS, 2016).

Complying With Health Insurance Portability and Accountability Act

Most health care facilities have a compliance officer who is responsible for educating staff concerning the privacy and security requirements and for monitoring compliance with these regulations. If a speech-language pathologist inadvertently breaches a client's security, he or she should immediately talk to the compliance officer at that facility. For example, perhaps the speech-language pathologist used the wrong fax cover sheet when sending a report to the referring physician and mistakenly sends Client A's report to a physician who has never seen Client A. The compliance officer will help determine the next steps to take regarding reporting the breach.

Clinicians may be tempted to share information when they have treated clients who have some notoriety, whether locally or nationally. There are many examples of employees at health care facilities being disciplined, fined, and sometimes fired for accessing the records of celebrities (Ornstein, 2015). It is also easy to inadvertently share information about a friend, neighbor, coworker, or family member. A well-meaning acquaintance, knowing that the speech-language pathologist works at a facility, might inquire about a friend who is hospitalized. The speech-language pathologist must be careful not to divulge any information, even though the client in question is a friend. He or she should not even confirm the person is a patient at that facility because the patient may have requested not to have his or her name shared when individuals call to inquire about his or her status.

The speech-language pathologist should not leave a client's record where someone else can see it. For example, in a nursing station in a long-term care facility, the client's chart should be turned face-down if the speech-language pathologist is walking away from the chart and it is on a counter where a visitor might see it. With electronic charting, the clinician should not leave client information up on the computer screen unattended. In certain situations where there is not much visitor foot traffic, the facility may consider it acceptable to just turn the monitor off. Still other facilities may require the clinician to log off if leaving the workstation only temporarily. Clinicians must also be cognizant of when and where they discuss patient information so they are not overheard by others who have no reason to hear the discussion.

Family Educational Rights and Privacy Act

Just as HIPAA provides statutory and regulatory guidelines about privacy of health records, the Family Educational Rights and Privacy Act (FERPA) delineates students' rights and privacy regarding educational records (U.S. Department of Education, 2015). FERPA gives parents certain rights with respect to their children's education records, and these rights transfer to students when they turn 18 years old. These rights are very similar to those outlined in HIPAA for health records. Parents have the right to do the following:

- Inspect and review the student's records
- Request that the school correct records they believe to be inaccurate
- Determine to whom records will be released and give written permission

ACCURATE DOCUMENTATION

Sometimes the acronym ACUTE is used as a reminder of rules for documenting: It should be Accurate, Codeable, Understandable, Timely, and Error free (ASHA, n.d.). But there are more than five things to keep in mind when documenting, so let's expand that acronym to $AC^3C^3URA^2TE$ (Table 1-1) and use some of those letters multiple times.

Accurate

The documentation of client encounters must contain a description of what actually happened during the evaluation, treatment session, telephone call, etc. The clinician must record things like test scores and percent of accuracy on a treatment task. Statements by the client and caregivers should be recorded as stated. Behaviors must be correctly described. For example, if a child has been late for two appointments over the past 6 months, the clinician would not describe the client as chronically late for appointments. Not only must the factual information be precise, but the clinician's interpretation must also be accurate. For instance, if test scores on a standardized test are all within one standard deviation of mean scores, the clinician should not document a severe disorder.

Table 1-1

$AC^3C^3URA^2TE$ Rules for Documenting

A	Accurate
C	Client centered
	Confidential
	Clear
C	Complete
	Concise
	Codeable
U	Unbiased
R	Readable/legible
A	Authenticated
	Abbreviations used correctly
T	Timely
E	Error free

In addition to the content of the documentation, the *what*, accuracy is also required in the *who*, *when*, and *where* of the documentation. The clinician who conducted the session or had the conversation must be the one to document the session or encounter. The date and time of the encounter must be accurate, including the length of the session. The clinician should get in the habit of noting the time an encounter starts and when it stops. Sometimes charting cannot be done during or immediately after a session and the clinician should not rely on memory to note what time earlier in the day the encounter occurred. Some payers require that the service be rendered in a particular setting, and in those instances the location must be accurately represented. For instance, home health services are reimbursed only if rendered in the home. If one day the patient instead visits the outpatient center, it would not be accurate to document this as a home health visit (and it would not be reimbursable).

It should go without saying, but documentation should not contain any spelling, grammatical, or punctuation errors. If using a word processing program, pay close attention to any errors highlighted for your attention and fix them. If handwriting, stop and carefully proofread your entry. The quality of your clinical work is being judged by others largely based on the quality of your documentation.

Client Centered

If the clinician always keeps in mind that the most important reason for documenting is to serve the client, any other questions that arise about how to document are more easily answered. Client-centered documentation can mean several things. Document as if each client was the person most important to you. If that client were, for instance, your best friend, mother, or uncle, what would you want the documentation to be? It also means the client and caregivers should be able to understand the documentation. Client centered also means using people-first language. You are not treating "the aphasic outpatient" or evaluating "the 4-year-old phonological disorder." You are seeing the individual who has aphasia and the 4-year-old with a phonological disorder. People-first language emphasizes the person and not the disability ("What is people first language?" n.d.). Additionally, client-centered means that you should be describing what the client did more than what the clinician did, although in the discussion of documenting skilled services in Chapter 4, you will see that documenting the role of the clinician is important too in order to demonstrate skilled care.

Confidential

This chapter has described confidentiality and privacy rules. Keeping records confidential also means they have to be stored securely. Paper charts should be kept in locked, fireproof file. Although individual states generally establish laws for how long medical records are to be retained, HIPAA rules require a provider who serves Medicare patients to retain required documentation for 6 years from the date of its creation or the date when it last was in effect, whichever is later (Centers for Medicare & Medicaid Services [CMS], 2010).

Electronic records should be password protected and stored securely. If laptops and tablets are used, they should also be password protected and stored securely. If the clinician is using flash drives, these should be secure drives with password protection as well.

Clear

Documentation should not require the reader to guess at what is meant or try to read between the lines. There is a balance to be obtained between using professional language and terminology and writing so that everyone can understand what was written. This is a skill that comes with practice. Consider this example of a summary paragraph of a reading evaluation that is factual but likely not clear to non–speech-language pathologists who read it:

The client achieved a standard score of 90 on a subtest of single word reading placing him in the 26th percentile, standard score of 92 on word attack (percentile 30) and standard score of 82 on decoding (percentile 19). His reading rate, accuracy, and fluency are in the 9th, 32nd, and 16th percentiles.

What is not clear about this paragraph? There are no references for the lay reader. What is a standard score? What does the percentile mean? Is this client having a problem? This is not to say that a report should not include standard scores and percentiles. The clinician can explain terms like percentile for the reader.

The same information might be more clearly communicated as the following:

The client demonstrates some skills in the low average range: the ability to read single words; the ability to sound out words; and his ability to accurately and smoothly read a passage. On the other hand, his reading rate is below average, with 91% of students his age reading more quickly than he does.

Complete

A medical or educational record should include all information relevant to the care of the client, whether this is a paper or electronic chart. Records should include the following important identifying information about the client:

- Name
- Date of birth
- Age
- Address
- Phone numbers
- Parents/significant other/partner/spouse
- Health insurance information
- Emergency information
- Attending physician
- Referring physician

On documentation that is more than one page in length, such as a diagnostic report, the identifying information should appear on each page. Not all information is needed, but at least the client's name and date of the report and page number should appear on each page (Figure 1-1). In facilities using a unique patient identifier, like a medical record number or encounter number, that information should also be included on each page. It is also a good idea, particularly in handwritten entries that will continue on a second page, to indicate "continued" at the bottom of the first page.

The record should include all forms of documentation created by the clinician and information received about the client (Table 1-2). Generally, handwritten notes that are then entered into a typed or electronic format are not considered a part of the permanent record and can be discarded securely. This typically means those documents should be shredded. Each facility may have its own policy regarding whether test forms are to be kept in the record. If all of the information from the test forms has been captured in the written report, most facilities determine that these forms can be shredded.

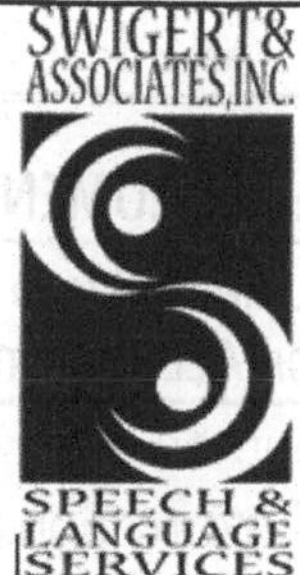

REPORT OF EVALUATION

Name:	Arthur Articulation	**Telephone:**	(555) 555-5555
B.D.: 3-24-13	**Age:** 3-11	**Physician:**	Dirk Developmental MD
Parents:	Amy and Arnold Articulation	**Referral Source:**	Preschool teacher
Address:	1066 Speech Lane Communicate, KY 44444	**Date of Evaluation:**	02-23-17

Background and Related Information:
Arthur Articulation, age 3-11, was seen for re-evaluation of his articulation skills at his mother's request.

Arthur Articulation 2-23-2017 Evaluation Page 2

Diagnosis: Mild articulation disorder

Recommendations:

1. Individual therapy to address the errors described above.
2. Therapy should also stimulate accurate production of sibilants.

Frequency of Visits: 2x week ½ hour sessions

Figure 1-1. Enter identifying information on each page of documentation.

Concise

Do you have an acquaintance you dread running into when you are pressed for time because you know it won't be a quick exchange? That person whose stories are so long, you keep wondering when he or she will get to the point? Documentation can be like that too. It can be poorly organized or contain irrelevant information or too much information. Students and clinicians new to documentation typically err on the side of writing too much. As clinicians gain experience, it becomes easier to ascertain what is and is not important to include. Clinicians with experience also learn how to organize reports and notes in logical order and use headers and paragraphs, making the documentation more concise.

Other health care and education personnel to whom the speech-language pathologist sends a report are busy and do not have time to wade through pages and pages of a long report to get the necessary information. They want to read a paragraph or two at most of a concise summary of the speech-language pathologist's findings, interpretation, and recommendations.

Consider an analogy between makes of cars and reports generated by speech-language pathologists. In graduate school, the student is taught to be thorough and include every piece of information about the client. This type of report might be considered a Mercedes-Benz. Third-party payers are not paying for the luxury model. They are paying for, let's say, a Hyundai. A Hyundai provides all the basics needed for transportation but no extra bells and whistles. The third-party payer is willing to pay for the Hyundai report, but not the Mercedes-Benz report. Clinicians have to learn to provide everything that is necessary but not superfluous.

Table 1-2

Examples of Internal and External Documents to Include in a Client's Record

Internal Documents Generated by the Clinician	Internal Documents Used at the Facility for All Clients	External Documents Sent/Brought to the Facility
• Intake form • Interview form • Test forms • Evaluation reports • Treatment plans • Progress notes • Discharge summaries • Letters (e.g., to referral sources) • Fax cover sheets	• Consent/authorization form • Release of information form • Insurance forms • Signed HIPAA forms • Attendance tracking forms	• Physician's order • Medical records from physician • Media (e.g., picture from endoscopic exam by ENT) • Educational records • List of medications

Abbreviations: ENT=ear, nose, throat doctor

Table 1-3

Examples of Biased and Unbiased Statements

Objective, Unbiased Statements	Statements That Could Be Perceived as Being Biased
Child accompanied by mother, who stated they had not had time to practice the homework.	Once again, the child's mother had not bothered to practice the homework with her.
Client able to complete only 5 of the 10 swallowing exercises.	Client appears lazy today as he only completed half of the exercises.
Patient did not initiate any conversation but responded when presented with specific questions.	Patient seems depressed today.
Client's daughter sat in on the session today but declined to participate.	Client's daughter continues to show no interest in her father's therapy.
Child's receptive language skills are at least 2 years behind same-age peers.	Given child's very sad home situation, it is not surprising that his language is so delayed.

The term *elevator speech* is used in marketing and public relations. This means condensing your message to the length that it can be delivered in the course a short elevator ride. Clinicians should seek to condense summaries of evaluation reports, progress notes, letters, etc., to that same concise format.

Codeable

Documentation of client encounters (e.g., evaluations, therapy) should contain enough information that a third party could determine both the appropriate diagnostic code(s) and the correct procedural codes. Chapter 4 provides in-depth information about coding and documentation.

Unbiased

Clinicians should use objective language in their documentation. State facts and summarize observations, and do not make judgments or comments that are not backed by the facts. Progress notes always include an analysis of the client's performance, but these should be factual as well, and should not include comments about the client's personality or emotional state. The speech-language pathologist's comments should not indicate that he or she is favoring one party or the other. For example, perhaps a child comes to therapy on alternate weeks with her mother and then her father. You notice that the child's homework is never done on the week she is with her mother. Avoid comments that indicate you are making a judgment about how supportive either parent is of the child's therapy goals (Table 1-3).

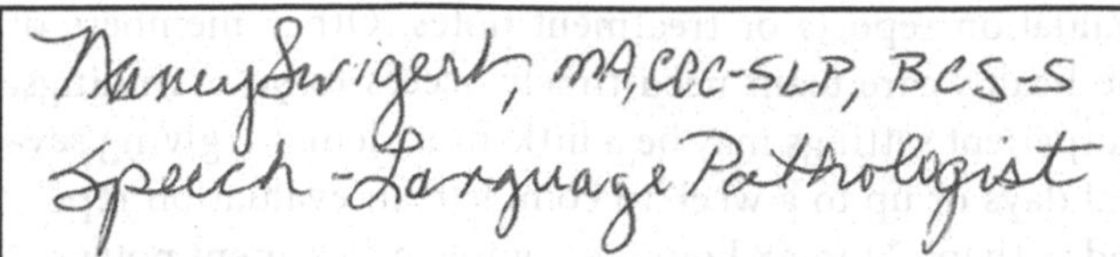

Figure 1-2. Signature to authenticate entry.

Readable/Legible

As large health care institutions move more toward fully electronic medical records, the dilemma of illegible entries decreases. However, in many health and education settings, entries are still handwritten. There is no excuse for penmanship that is unreadable. If the clinician does not have good handwriting, he or she can print instead. Although more time consuming, it is crucial that a handwritten entry be read easily. In any medical setting in which physician orders are still handwritten, you can observe a familiar scene in the nursing station: One clinician will take a chart to another clinician for help deciphering a physician's order or even the signature.

An illegible entry might even result in the service not being reimbursed. If a third-party payer requests a record to review, they will match documentation to dates of service billed. If they cannot read the documentation well enough to determine whether it supports a covered service, they may deny payment.

When making handwritten entries in a chart, it is generally accepted that black ink should be used, although blue ink is used as well. This is a long-standing practice, probably because those colors photocopy more clearly than other colors of ink. Never make entries with pencil because those can be erased and changed, calling into question the legitimacy of the record. Avoid felt-tip pens because these entries can easily smudge and make them difficult to read (Cameron & Turtle-Song, 2002).

Authenticated

Every entry in a chart should include the clinician's first initial (or full first name) and last name, degree, and credentials. It is also a good idea in a chart used by many different professionals to include the profession (Figure 1-2). Do not leave a space between the last line of the entry and the signature. This might be interpreted by a lawyer as something missing. An empty line or two also means someone else could enter information in that space unknown to the author of the note (Cameron & Turtle-Song, 2002). Entries in the chart should be dated and timed. The time should be the time that the encounter started. For instance, if the speech-language pathologist was with the client from 10:00 a.m. until 11:00 a.m. and then wrote or entered the note at 12:00 p.m., the time should be 10:00 a.m.

In an electronic medical record, the clinician has nothing to sign. In some programs, a PDF of the clinician's signature may be imported into the report. In others, the clinician making the entry authenticates it by saving the information. Often, there is a screen that will cue the clinician before a final save, such as "Ready to save?" or "Entry complete?" If a printout of the record is required (for example, to send to another facility), the entry will say something like "Electronically verified by" with the clinician's name.

Notes by graduate students should be cosigned by the supervising speech-language pathologist. Depending on state licensure laws, the notes by a clinical fellow may need to be cosigned. In states where the clinical fellow operates under a provisional license, that is usually not necessary.

> The client was seen for a clinical swallow exam (CSE), which revealed mild oral dysphagia with slowed mastication and bolus preparation. Thin liquids presented during the CSE were given via cup and straw and the client exhibited delayed throat clearing. Although the reason for the throat clearing cannot be determined on a CSE, this sign of pharyngeal dysphagia warrants a videofluorscopic swallow study (VFSS). A full assessment of the pharyngeal phase can be done on the VFSS, which is scheduled for this afternoon.

Figure 1-3. How to abbreviate.

Abbreviations Used Correctly

An organization may have a list of approved abbreviations. The clinician should always check to see what the facility's policy is on abbreviations. Each profession tends to develop abbreviations, such as SLP (speech-language pathologist), CSE (clinical swallow exam), and GFTA-3 (Goldman-Fristoe Test of Articulation-3). The problem with such profession-specific abbreviations is that only others within the profession know what they mean. When using an abbreviation, it should be spelled out the first time it is used. Then, for the remainder of the report or note, the abbreviation can be used (Figure 1-3). A list of abbreviations that the speech-language pathologist might encounter and use in a medical setting are included at the end of this book.

The Joint Commission, an accreditation body for health care facilities, has taken the approach of developing a list of unapproved abbreviations. In 2001, the Joint Commission issued a Sentinel Event Alert on the subject of medical abbreviations and a year later approved a National Patient Safety Goal requiring accredited organizations to develop and implement a list of abbreviations not to use. This was based on medical errors that occurred because an abbreviation was misunderstood. It does not apply to electronic medical records, but to handwritten entries.

As an example, the Joint Commission indicates that the abbreviations QD (every day) and QOD (every other day) should not be used because they are easily mistaken for

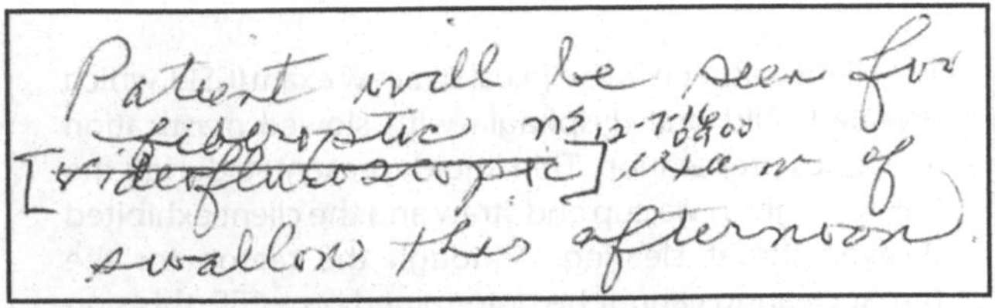

Figure 1-4. Correcting an error in handwritten entry.

each other. Instead, the provider should write out "daily" or "every other day" (The Joint Commission, 2016).

Timely

Documentation should ideally occur at the time the service is provided. If you have been to your physician lately, it is likely that the medical assistant sat at the computer while he or she asked you questions about your reason for seeing the physician and entered this information as you answered the questions. When the physician came in, he or she probably also sat at the computer reading the information and entering findings from his or her exam. The contemporaneous charting is not only more efficient (when you leave the office, all of the physician's charting is done), it is more accurate. There is no remembering what was said or trying to decipher a scribbled note.

The same holds true for speech-language pathologists as they see clients. However, trying to chart while keeping a 3-year-old engaged or during a swallowing therapy session requiring hands-on activities with the client are just two examples of why such contemporaneous charting remains challenging for clinicians. Evaluation reports also require time for scoring and analysis before they can be written.

If the charting cannot be done while the clinician is with the client, then the next best alternative is to chart each session immediately after it is completed and before seeing the next client. The speech-language pathologist's schedule, whether in an inpatient or outpatient setting, should be structured to allow this to happen. In an outpatient setting in which clients typically receive a half-hour session, the session should conclude at 25 minutes, with the remaining 5 minutes used for charting. Schedules in inpatient settings should also accommodate charting at the end of the session. This allows the clinician to engage the client and caregivers in the documentation process and keeps the documentation focused on function (see Chapter 10).

Realistically speaking, there are days that just do not go as planned, and at the end of the day, there is patient documentation that has not been completed. Facilities have guidelines about the timeliness in which things must be done. For example, in many in-patient settings, documentation must be done before the end of the day, whether evaluation reports or treatment notes. Other members of the health care team need timely access to your findings. Outpatient settings may be a little more lenient, giving several days or up to a week to complete an evaluation report and perhaps 24 to 48 hours to complete treatment notes.

Discharge summaries on outpatients are often viewed as a low priority. This is unfortunate. If the clinician finds him- or herself with a stack of charts of patients discharged several months ago, it is not likely that the discharge summary will be very accurate. Additionally, sending a copy of the discharge summary to the referral source after such a delay is certainly not a good reflection on the facility or on the clinician.

It is not just client documentation that needs to be completed in a timely way. Related billing and productivity forms should also be filled out after each session. The accuracy and timeliness of these records help assure the facility will be reimbursed correctly and in a timely way.

Error Free

We have already described the importance of accuracy in documentation. Proofreading your entry before authenticating should be a rule of thumb. If you realize you have made an error, correct it. In electronic documentation, this is easy to do if you have discovered your error before you save your entry. In handwritten documentation, correct an error by enclosing the section in brackets and drawing a single line through the entry so that the person reading the record can still read what was there. Then initial, date, and time by the line you drew through the entry. Do not use correction fluid, do not erase, and do not scratch through the entry so much that it cannot be read (Cameron & Turtle-Song, 2002) (Figure 1-4).

Sometimes you realize immediately after you have authenticated your entry that you omitted some important information. The information can be added and marked as an addendum. Sometimes, however, it is later in the day or even the next day that the clinician realizes important information was left out. This information can be added but is considered a late entry, not an addendum. It should be dated, timed, and reauthenticated. Another way to think about the difference in an addendum and a late entry is when you are handwriting a note in a medical chart. If another provider has written in the chart since your original note, your additional information is a late entry. If you start a new page for that note, it should be kept in chronological order (not put back where your original handwritten entry is) and labeled as a late entry with a short explanation. For example: LATE ENTRY Additional information obtained from patient's daughter after dysphagia evaluation.

ASHA Code of Ethics and Documentation Rules

The ASHA Code of Ethics mentions the speech-language pathologist's responsibility regarding documentation in Rule I, Principle Q:

> Individuals shall maintain timely records and accurately record and bill for services provided and products dispensed and shall not misrepresent services provided, products dispensed, or research and scholarly activities conducted. (ASHA, 2016)

ASHA Preferred Practice Patterns

Although not rules, the ASHA Preferred Practice Patterns for Speech-Language Pathology provide the following guidance about documentation:

- "Speech-language pathologists prepare, sign, and maintain, within an established time frame, documentation that reflects the nature of the professional service.
- Results of assessment and treatment are reported to the patient/client and family/caregivers, as appropriate. Reports are distributed to the referral source and other professionals when appropriate and with written consent.
- The privacy and security of documentation are maintained in compliance with the regulations of the Health Insurance Portability and Accountability Act (HIPAA), Family Educational Rights and Privacy Act (FERPA), and other state and federal laws.
- Except for screenings, documentation addresses the type and severity of the communication or related disorder or difference, associated conditions (e.g., medical or educational diagnoses) and impact on activity and participation (e.g., educational, vocational, social).
- Documentation includes summaries of previous services in accordance with all relevant legal and agency guidelines." (ASHA, 2004, p. 6)

More specific guidance about documentation of assessments and treatment are found in the Preferred Practice Patterns related to different types of services provided.

References

American Speech-Language-Hearing Association. (n.d.). Module 3: Documentation of SLP services in different settings. Retrieved from http://www.asha.org/Practice/reimbursement/Module-Three-Transcript/

American Speech-Language-Hearing Association. (2004). Preferred practice patterns for the profession of speech-language pathology. Retrieved from https://www.asha.org/policy/PP2004-00191/

American Speech-Language-Hearing Association. (2016). *Code of Ethics*. Retrieved from http://www.asha.org/Code-of-Ethics/

Cameron, S., & Turtle-Song, I. (2002). Learning to write case notes using the SOAP format. *Journal of Counseling and Development, 80*(3), 286.

Centers for Medicare & Medicaid Services. (2010). Medical record retention and media format for medical records. Retrieved from https://www.cms.gov/Outreach-and-Education/Medicare-Learning-Network-MLN/MLNMattersArticles/downloads/SE1022.pdf

The Joint Commission. (2016). Facts about the official "Do Not Use" list of abbreviations. Retrieved from https://www.jointcommission.org/facts_about_do_not_use_list/

Ornstein, C. (2015). Celebrities' medical records tempt hospital workers to snoop. *National Public Radio*. Retrieved from http://www.npr.org/sections/health-shots/2015/12/10/458939656/celebrities-medical-records-tempt-hospital-workers-to-snoop

U.S. Department of Education. (2015). Family Educational Rights and Privacy Act. Retrieved from http://www2.ed.gov/policy/gen/guid/fpco/ferpa/index.html

U.S. Department of Health & Human Services. (n.d.). Your rights under HIPAA. Retrieved from http://www.hhs.gov/hipaa/for-individuals/guidance-materials-for-consumers/

U.S. Department of Health & Human Services. (2013). Research. Retrieved from http://www.hhs.gov/hipaa/for-professionals/special-topics/research/index.html

U.S. Department of Health & Human Services. (2014). Protecting the privacy and security of your health information. Retrieved from https://www.healthit.gov/patients-families/protecting-your-privacy-security

U.S. Department of Health & Human Services. (2016). How to file a health information privacy or security complaint. Retrieved from http://www.hhs.gov/hipaa/filing-a-complaint/complaint-process/index.html

U.S. Department of Labor. (2015). The Health Insurance Portability and Accountability Act. Retrieved from https://www.dol.gov/ebsa/newsroom/fshipaa.html

What is people first language? (n.d.). *The Arc*. Retrieved from https://www.thearc.org/who-we-are/media-center/people-first-language

Review Questions

1. What does ASHA's Code of Ethics say about confidentiality?
2. What does HIPAA stand for?
3. What are some patients' rights regarding privacy assured by HIPAA?
4. Which part of HIPAA requires facilities to put safeguards in place to keep health information secure?
5. What is the law called that provides privacy and security rights for students in school?
6. What does it mean to authenticate an entry in a chart?
7. Explain the difference between a late entry and an addendum.

Activity A

Rewriting a Note Using Abbreviations

Using abbreviations found at the end of this book (see appendix beginning on p. 361), rewrite the following notes. Use as many abbreviations as possible for practice, but keep in mind that abbreviations should not be overused in charting.

Client #1

This patient is status post-coronary artery bypass graft with a history of coronary artery disease and hypertension. Patient is currently eating nothing by mouth, but prior to surgery was on the American Diabetes Association diet. If he does not pass his clinical swallow exam, the physician is eager to insert a nasogastric tube for nutrition because he does not consider the patient stable enough to undergo a videofluoroscopic swallow exam at this time.

Client #2

This 75-year-old patient has a complicated medical history, including multiple sclerosis, status post-ST elevated myocardial infarction 3 weeks ago, and yesterday suffered a left middle cerebral artery wake-up stroke, so she did not qualify for tissue plasminogen activator. She presents with right-sided weakness and significant aphasia. She failed the nursing swallow screening, and the physician assistant provided a telephone order for a dysphagia consult by speech-language pathology.

Client #3

Pediatrician referred a 4-year-old boy who is reportedly unintelligible for an evaluation. In addition to the usual childhood diseases, the child reportedly had a tonsillectomy and adenoidectomy 6 months ago. His gross motor skills are reported to be within normal limits, and his cognitive skills are reported to be within functional limits. Unfortunately, the family did not keep the appointment.

ACTIVITY B

You have been asked to see a child because his regular speech-language pathologist is out sick. Read this handwritten note and mark all the words you cannot read. Discuss how this might impact your ability to provide service to the child.

Pt can hold his head up when in sitting for
several moments. He munches on SLP's gloved
fingers + tolerates touch to the gums, tongue and
roof of mouth. No gagging observed. Presented
bottle c̄ slow flow nipple c̄ apple-prune
juice in semi-reclined position. Tried more
upright position, but s̄ an angle-neck bottle
it's more difficult. He got choked 2-3x @
end of the feeding. Controlled jaw support
reduces excess jaw excursion. Positioned him
upright and he coughs + clears. Mom presented
small amounts of pureed peaches on spoon. He does
not clean spoon c̄ lips but exhibits munching + then
suckle to move food backwards. No anterior loss.
Parents to continue to advance diet to include
other Stage 1 baby foods.
• use spoon that fits comfortably
• place food on tongue + encourage him
to close lips to clean spoon.

Activity C

Mark the statements might be perceived as biased and not objective. Then rewrite those statements to be more objective.

____________ Child achieved 75% accuracy at word level on target sound after model.
____________ Patient accompanied by his daughter to this session.
____________ As expected, child did not perform as well with Dad as he did with Mom.
____________ Patient's responses delayed by up to 3 seconds after stimulus presented.
____________ Patient stated, "I was too busy with work this week to complete the voice exercises."
____________ Patient seemed depressed today, with delayed responses.
____________ Child's mother forced spoon into the child's mouth despite his turning away.
____________ Client's performance on Mendelsohn maneuver improved when provided with tactile cues.
____________ Child sat down on the floor in the hall. His mother picked him up and carried him into the exam room.
____________ Client seems to purposely antagonize this clinician by refusing to respond in a timely way.

Activity D

These entries are part of an intradepartmental update, which is not a part of the medical record. It is used to share pertinent information between the different speech-language pathologists. Using a highlighter, mark which words, phrases, and sentences you think could be deleted or changed to make the entry more concise while maintaining the essential information. Each note should contain only significant information or change in patient status.

Patient #1

77 y/o M admit from Facility Z w/ PNA. Transferred here 2' c/o AMS, s/p fall and head injury (minor). Apparently he had CVA a few mos ago and was living in SNF w/ PEG and severe aphasia. He was then transferred to the Facility Z due to aggressive bx. PMH: COPD, dementia, depression, GERD, HTN, mult falls. CXR: RLL infiltrate (PNA). CT of head shows chronic subdural hemorrhage Ⓛ parietal lobe. Limited hx about dysphagia, pt w/ PEG but RN states that Facility Z was giving him mech soft diet but his wife reports that he "can't swallow." BS: pt sleeping soundly when entered room able to wake him up and sit him up in bed. Gave ice chip and sip of h_20—oral holding and ant. Loss w/ thins. Pt then scooted all the way down in his bed covered his head w/ blanket and went to sleep. Not appropriate for further PO trials or MBS. REC: con't NPO w/ meds via PEG, RD is putting in tube feeding rec's now, re-assess daily to determine readiness for MBS (3-4-17). Attempted BS again today, pt much the same as yesterday. Allowed oral care, though stated he didn't like the bristles on the toothbrush, that they were rough. Took ice and tsp of h_20. s/s of asp noted today—wet vocal quality and delayed coughing. Explained these s/s to the patient's wife. Pt again laid down in bed covered head w. blanket. REC: con't NPO w/ PEG and check on again tomorrow. Chatted with the nurse after the visit and he said it looks like they may be consulting neuro surg 2' chronic hematoma/hemorrhage? (3-5-17).

Patient #2

78yo M adm with acute on chronic hypoxic respiratory failure, severe aortic stenosis, B infiltrates, NSTEMI, acute mixed heart failure, B CAD. PMH: CHF, aortic stenosis, dyslipidemia, HTN, skin cancer, UTI, type 5 hereditary sensorimotor neuropathy. CXR: B patchy infiltrates, Ⓡ>Ⓛ. Nsg reports pna vs CHF not yet determined. B/S: OME WFL. Pt and wife report h/o dysphagia (coughing with intake of liquids and food) for the past several months since a heart procedure he had (stents), also approximately when dysphonia began per pt/wife. Wife reports they have discussed multiple times with primary care physician and were thinking about seeing an ENT about the voice. However, they have not pursued making an appointment. PO trials of thin via cup and straw presented inconsistent coughing and t/c, however this did take "pushing" larger sips at b/s to achieve s/sx. No s/sx observed with mixed or regular at b/s, although they report it does sometime happen with food. Rec: FEES. (02-17-17) FEES: Severe pharyngeal dysphagia characterized by dec BOT retraction, dec PPW contraction, dec pharyngo-laryngeal sensation, with severe hypopharyngeal residue and vallecular residue and aspiration post-swallow across consistencies. Dec vestibular closure also visualized with thin via straw resulting in aspiration during the swallow. All aspiration events during FEES were silent. Anatomically, the Ⓡ VF appeared to have less mass than Ⓛ, pt is dysphonic with weak voice; however this did not affect movement or swallow function and head turn was not successful. For future studies, MBS may be more appropriate d/t tightness in hypopharynx limiting view, pt discomfort, as well as to allow for trials of compensations as indicated. Rec: NPO with alternate nutrition, meds alternate route, dysphagia tx QD. May recommend to RN/family for pt to consult ENT upon d/c to address voice/VF issue further. (2-18-17) RN called pt very anxious to get tx started or re-eval. Think it may be that the nurse is tired of hearing from the patient. Provided extensive educ to this nurse about FEES results and that we will do MBS in few days to allow time for improvement. Initiated tx and left exercises w/ pt and 2 dtrs who are very supportive and will help pt complete. Pt family very motivated, high priority tx (2-19-17). NG fell out overnight. Pt refusing to have replaced until we repeat—deferred to MBS: No improvement. Mild, ? mod oral (DNT solids), severe pharyngeal dysphagia. Prolonged oral with tongue pumping. Severe residue—same story as above—min BOT retraction, PPW stripping (turned oblique—no asymmetry), min hyoid excursion. Almost no bolus passing into esophagus. Use of chin tuck + head turn (either way) + effortful resulted in min more passing into esophagus. Eventual aspiration after the swallow with thinner materials, will eventually aspirate all as thins with secretions—has nowhere else to go. I looked up neuropathy the wife mentioned he presents—affects LE and leads to pain/temp insensitivity. He seemed bit confused when discussing abstract info, little increased agitation when didn't follow the convo. Seems very much like a Parkinson's to me (weak voice, flat affect, conf) but has no known neuro dx. Relayed info to MD Rec: Cont NPO, consider PEG (getting heart valve replacement in couple weeks so seems palliative discussion is off the table for now), aggressive oral care. Consider neuro w/u, dys tx (2-20-17).

Patient #3

82yo M adm with myocardial infarction/STEMI. Mediastinal hemorrhage, CAD, cardiac catheterization, paroxysmal Afib, renal insufficiency, Ⓛ renal stent, HTN, GERD, hyperlipidemia, cholecystectomy, coronary artery bypass surgery, abdominal aortic aneurysm repair, anxiety. B/S: Pt failed RN dysphagia screen. OME remarkable only for decreased mandibular opening for PO trials. Overt clinical s/sx suspected aspiration with ice chips and NTL via tsp characterized by inconsistent coughing, wet v/q, and multiple swallows. Pt voice is hoarse. Has been intubated for five days and it took two attempts to get the patient intubated. Suspect poor secretion management. Recommend: NPO, f/u for FEES readiness and dysphagia tx. (6/21/17). BS: Garbled speech noted. Positioned patient upright for b/s exam. His daughter from Ohio was present. She's not the primary caregiver but does take him to her house once a month for a few days. Pt given trials of thin and ice chip. Delay coughing noted with large sips of thin via straw; no overt s/s with tsp trials. Pt appropriate for FEES today REC: cont NPO until FEES (6/22/17). FEES: severe pharyngeal dysphagia. Mild blood noted in left pyriform likely due to placement of NG. Unable to assess breath hold due to impaired comprehension. Delay to pyrifom with thins. Moderate vallecular and pyrform sinuses with thin and pudding (only consistencies tested in this study). Sensate aspiration after the swallow from posterior commissure and lateral channels residue with all consistencies. Pudding consistency thinned out and was aspirated. REC: NPO, dysphagia Tx QD, s/l eval when pt appropriate (6/22/17). Pt has been begging for water. RN and even the unit clerk are desperate for re-assessment. Pt with immediate cough following ice chips, tsp of water and tsp of applesauce. Secretions and voice improving, but otherwise, pt just not ready. Pt also reports feeling like pureed texture is sticking. I was able to successfully use teach back for pt to repeat back why he is NPO, asp risk, etc. even after a delay. As pt is showing great improvements, check with family next time—none present for my tx) to determine baseline status before S/L eval (No garbled speech today and comprehension was good). . . . (6/23/17). Little change from yesterday immediate coughing after all trials. Pt's voice is strong and no wet vocal quality, per RN pt is coughing secretions to mouth today. Not ready for FEES today though given overt s/s of asp after all p.o trials. Con't to monitor for readiness. Still some confusion today, pt is also HOH, wearing H.A's con't to monitor mental status, no family present (6/24/17). FEES: Patient is so pleasant. He doesn't mind at all as scope is placed, though the daughter observing seemed pretty squeamish. Unfortunately, this gentleman still has severe pharyngeal dysphagia. Delay to PS and diffuse residue, resulting in spill over post-commissure post-swallow resulting in aspiration across consistencies (thin, ntl, pudding all via tsp). Cued cough did not clear. Sometimes silent aspiration, inconsistent sensation. Rec: cont npo with alt nutrition, dys tx QD. Re: S/L, consider ICU delirium, RN states s/sx consistent with delirium-RN knew him outside hospital. They attended the same church. Monitor for S/L eval indication. (6/25/17) Participated in tx. Still confused and easily distracted (6/26/17). RN called twice a MD ok'd pt for ice chips, but per RN he was unaware of severe dysphagia. Educ pt, son and the daughter from Ohio and RN on ice chip protocol. Pt has been begging for water. Trialed w/ thins and puree- swishing w/ thins and suspect delayed initiation, mult swallows w/ all. Priority tx. Left exercises for practice w/ son and RN (6/27/17). Dys tx: still confused,interfering with ability to perform exercises this date. RN reports pt had to be NT suctioned x4 overnight. Cont tx. (6/28/17)

2

Reasons for Documenting

Nancy B. Swigert, MA, CCC-SLP, BCS-S

Purposes of Documentation

Graduate students learn how to evaluate and treat a variety of communication and swallowing disorders, both in the classroom and in clinic and practicum settings. At each step of the way, they also learn how to document the services they are providing. The American Speech-Language-Hearing Association's (ASHA's) Scope of Practice for Speech-Language Pathology specifically lists documenting as an important part of the eight service delivery domains of speech-language pathology. For example, the domain of assessment includes the following:

- "*Document* assessment and trial results for selecting AAC interventions and technology, including speech-generating devices (SGDs)"
- "*Document* assessment results, including discharge"

The domain of treatment includes the following:

- "Design, implement, and *document* delivery of service in accordance with best available practice appropriate to the practice setting" (ASHA, 2016, p. 12)

There are many reasons to document client care, including the following (Table 2-1):

- Client management
    - Accurately record the client's performance at specific points in time in order to plan and implement the client's care
        - Intake information
        - Evaluation results
        - Treatment notes
        - Progress updates
        - Re-evaluations
    - Determine when the client is ready for discharge
        - Discharge status
- Share information with other health care and educational professionals about the client's communication and swallowing disorder
    - This might include another speech-language pathologist who has to take over the client's care on a short-term basis, or when the client moves to another facility or setting or changes schools.
- Serve as the basis for review of medical/educational record by any number of individuals, third-party payers, or regulatory agencies:
    - To assess quality of care
    - To make decisions about utilization of services
    - To obtain data for research
    - To determine whether regulatory requirements were met

Swigert, N. B.
Documentation and Reimbursement for Speech-Language Pathologists: Principles and Practice (pp. 17-22).

TABLE 2-1
REASONS FOR DOCUMENTING

• Client management
  ◦ Record client's performance
  ◦ Plan and implement care
  ◦ Determine readiness for discharge
• Share information with others
• Serve as basis for review of records
  ◦ Quality
  ◦ Utilization review
  ◦ Research
  ◦ Regulatory
• Business document
  ◦ Reimbursement
  ◦ Productivity
• Legal document

- Serve as a business document
  - Support reimbursement of the services rendered
  - Evaluate productivity
- Serve as a legal document

LEGAL DOCUMENT

Every piece of documentation generated by the speech-language pathologist serves as a legal document. During an evaluation or treatment session, the last thing on the speech-language pathologist's mind is that the documentation completed that day may at some point in the future be used in a legal proceeding.

The work performed (and documented) by the speech-language pathologist might be used in a malpractice suit. The suit might not even be related to the client's communication or swallowing disorder, and the work done by the speech-language pathologist might not even be relevant to the case. That does not mean the records won't be subpoenaed.

Records from speech-language pathologists have been used in custody battles. Documentation, for example, that one parent failed to bring the child to scheduled therapy sessions might be used by the other parent to gain more visitation rights. Other examples of legal uses of documentation include a client who sought to receive workers' compensation for the injury that caused the communication or swallowing disorder. Although this is more common with clients receiving physical or occupational therapy, clients with cognitive deficits after a concussion at work or a communication deficit related to noise-induced hearing loss from the work environment might seek such compensation. Speech-language pathologists also evaluate, and document the evaluation, for clients seeking to be declared disabled, and thus be eligible to receive government financial assistance, called *Supplemental Social Security Income* (Social Security Association, 2017).

DOCUMENTATION AS A BUSINESS DOCUMENT

Each speech-language pathologist works for someone. It might be a large employer, like a rehabilitation agency, a small community hospital, a public or private school, or a small-group private practice. The speech-language pathologist might work for him- or herself, but even in that case, the employer has to be concerned about the business of clinical services.

Support Reimbursement

The documentation of clinical services is used by employers to support the services that were provided if a third-party payer questions the charges. For example, Medicare, Medicaid, or an early intervention funding Agency can audit the records of clients if they think the facility or private practitioner has overbilled or billed for services not rendered. These audits often take place months or even years after the services were rendered. The clinician is not going to remember what was done, when it was done, or how often it was done. The medical (or school) record is the only way the business can substantiate the billing claim. More information about reimbursement is found in Chapter 4.

Productivity

The employer of speech-language pathologists has to be able to pay their bills in order to keep the doors to the facility open. One of the biggest expenses an employer has is the employee. The salary and benefit costs for employees are typically 50% or more of their operating costs. That means that the employees have to be as productive as possible (i.e., generating revenue for most of the time they are at work). Employers use documentation to assess productivity.

Although we typically think of the client's chart as the documentation, any piece of paper or electronic entry that the speech-language pathologist generates related to client care is documentation. That means the billing slips filled out at the end of each day or the time entered into a time clock is part of the speech-language pathologist's documentation, and thus are also legal documents. The employer can monitor how productive an individual speech-language pathologist is by seeing how much billed time, or time with clients, the clinician worked each day (Swigert, 2015).

Documentation as a Basis for Review of Records

There are many reasons that medical and educational records are reviewed, sometimes long after the documentation was completed. Health care facilities often have departments that review records to assess the quality of care that has been rendered. The outcomes department of an acute care hospital, for example, might review records to determine whether quality indicators were met. Quality indicators are typically established by regulatory or accrediting agencies or third-party payers. For example, an accrediting agency like the Joint Commission determined that any patient arriving at the hospital with signs of an acute myocardial infarction should receive an aspirin on admission and be prescribed an aspirin on discharge (The Joint Commission, 2016). The Quality Department would review all records of patients discharged who had an acute myocardial infarction to see how many times the care of these patients met the standard.

Funding agencies also review records to assess the quality of care and to ensure that regulatory requirements are being met. A state agency for early intervention could request the records from a speech-language pathology clinic or practice of all children seen through the early intervention program. The reviewers would check things like completeness of progress notes, accuracy of time in and time out of the session, and whether a re-evaluation was completed at the specified intervals.

Government agencies might review records to determine the utilization of services. For example, they might want to determine how many patients covered by Medicaid in a state saw their primary care provider or how often a certain type of surgery was performed. Utilization data like this is used to determine such things as cost of care and changes in coverage. Utilization review by a health insurance company might be done before they give approval for other services. For example, a health insurance company might reimburse for a speech-language evaluation but request a copy of the evaluation report before determining whether they will approve therapy services.

Records are also used for educational and medical research. Epidemiological studies in particular often gather information from medical records. Such studies analyze certain health conditions and the factors related to those conditions (World Health Organization, 2016). Retrospective studies in communication sciences and disorders also rely on information in medical and educational records (Abbott, Barton, Terhorst, & Shembel, 2016).

Documentation to Share Information With Others

The speech-language pathologist's records are often shared with other educational and health professionals. In health care settings, the records are shared with medical professionals treating the individual. This can include the referring physician or any other physician specialties involved in the individual's care. Other therapists and allied health professionals may need to review the records.

In education settings, classroom teachers and directors of special education need to know what is happening with the student. The student's parents need to see the records of the services being provided. Public schools have a myriad of required paperwork to facilitate sharing of information.

Clients and students often receive services at different facilities across the continuum of care. For example, the patient is discharged from the acute care hospital and is transferred to a rehabilitation facility. The speech-language pathologist at the rehabilitation hospital needs to read the evaluation and progress notes from the speech-language pathologist at the hospital. After a stay at the rehabilitation hospital, the patient might go home and receive further services through a home health agency. Each of the speech-language pathologists involved in the patient's care will gain valuable information from the records sent from the previous facility.

A student receiving services in elementary school moves on to middle school. The speech-language pathologist at the middle school will use the records from the elementary school to help him or her make decisions about the current needs of the student.

In health care and education settings, there is sometimes a change in staff in the middle of the client's care. One speech-language pathologist might go out on leave or even just be sick for a few days. Another speech-language pathologist must pick up the care for the client. Clear and understandable records are necessary to facilitate a seamless transition.

Documentation for Client Management

The most familiar reason for documenting is to manage the care of the client from evaluation to discharge. From the moment the speech-language pathologist receives the referral, documentation begins. Intake information serves as the basis for the speech-language pathologist to determine what kind of evaluation will be needed. Notations might be made on an intake form in an outpatient setting, the school-based speech-language pathologist might make notes when observing a child in the classroom, and the speech-language pathologist in an inpatient setting might make notes as the medical record is reviewed.

Once the speech-language pathologist has contact with the client, the results of the evaluation and the interpretation of those results are documented. The plan of care is documented to guide the treatment the client will receive. Progress notes and re-evaluations document the client's performance throughout care. Home programs are documented so that the client and caregivers can address any continuing needs. A discharge note summarizes the care the client has received.

Much more detailed information about documentation for client management will be found in subsequent chapters in this book. Examples of documentation in various settings is provided.

References

Abbott, K. V., Barton, F. B., Terhorst, L., & Shembel, A. (2016). Retrospective studies: A fresh look. *American Journal of Speech-Language Pathology, 25*(2), 157–163. doi:10.1044/2016_AJSLP-16-0025

American Speech-Language-Hearing Association. (2016). Scope of practice in speech-language pathology. Retrieved from https://www.asha.org/policy/SP2016-00343/

The Joint Commission. (2016). Acute myocardial infarction. Retrieved from https://www.jointcommission.org/acute_myocardial_infarction/

Swigert, N. (2015). Current healthcare climate: What does it mean for SLPs managing patients with dysphagia? *SIG 13 Perspectives on Swallowing and Swallowing Disorders (Dysphagia), 24*(1), 5–11. doi:10.1044/sasd24.1.5

Social Security Association. (2017). Understanding supplemental security income SSI eligibility requirements—2017 edition. Retrieved from https://www.ssa.gov/ssi/text-eligibility-ussi.htm

World Health Organization. (2016). Epidemiology. Retrieved from http://www.who.int/topics/epidemiology/en/

REVIEW QUESTIONS

1. What kind of information is gained through review of medical and educational records?
2. At what points during a client's care is his or her performance documented?
3. Describe examples of times when one speech-language pathologist might need to read the records of another speech-language pathologist.
4. Give an example of a legal situation in which the speech-language pathologist's records might be subpoenaed.
5. Why is documentation of client care considered to start with the intake form rather than the evaluation?

ACTIVITY A

Review of Utilization of Services

You work at an outpatient facility, and your supervisor has asked you to help with a utilization review of records. You are to review the billing records, progress notes, and authorization for services for these clients. Which of these records indicate that services were *not* provided according to what was authorized? Note what does not appear to be in compliance.

Client #1

A 53-year-old with muscle tension dysphonia, authorized for eight therapy sessions after the evaluation date.

PROGRESS NOTES DATED:
July 1
July 5
July 8
July 12
July 14
July 16

BILLED FOR THERAPY ON:
July 1
July 7
July 8
July 12
July 15
July 16
July 18

Client #2

A 4-year-old with moderate articulation disorder related to repaired cleft. Insurance indicates it pays for therapy after surgery or injury. Limit of 10/calendar year.

PROGRESS NOTES DATED:
September 6
September 8
September 13
September 15
September 20
September 22
September 29
October 1

BILLED FOR THERAPY ON:
September 6
September 8
September 13
September 15
September 20
September 22
September 29
October 1

Client #3

After the evaluation on August 1, an authorization was received on August 10 for five therapy sessions.

Progress Notes Dated:	Billed for Therapy On:
August 6	August 6
August 8	August 8
August 10	August 10
August 15	August 15
August 17	August 17

Activity B

Match each of the reasons for documentation to indicate whether that is a business or legal use of the documentation. Mark business reasons with a B and legal reasons with an L.

___________ To see whether the speech-language pathologist is seeing enough clients in 1 day.

___________ To determine whether the patient died as a result of the aspiration that occurred during an instrumental swallowing evaluation.

___________ To see whether there is documentation in the record to support each service billed.

___________ To determine whether a client should receive disability payments related to the communication disorder.

___________ To compare the work produced by one employed speech-language pathologist to the others at that practice.

3

Forms and Formats

Nancy B. Swigert, MA, CCC-SLP, BCS-S

Formats for Documenting

When we visualize a medical record, the first image that comes to mind is some form of chart, such as a thick manila folder, three-ring binder, or notebook bulging with papers if the client has been seen by that provider for a long time. The chart contains all of the documentation related to that client's care. Documentation can occur by writing something down on paper or by typing something into a document on a computer (e.g., a Microsoft Word document) that is transferred to the physical chart by printing and inserting or scanning as an attachment. In some settings, such as private practices, clinics not associated with a large health care system, and university clinics, this is likely how documentation is still occurring, and the physical charts still contain all the information. In most settings, there is still some semblance of a physical chart. However, in health care settings, the more predominant method for documenting is using a fully electronic medical record or electronic health record (EHR). All the data are entered directly into the software. The only thing in a temporary physical chart is something that needs to be scanned into the record. Some health care systems are in a transition period, where some documentation is done electronically but others may still be done on paper. These are referred to as *hybrid systems* and present particular challenges because the users of the chart may not be sure where to look for the information they need.

Incentive Programs to Use Electronic Health Records: Meaningful Use

Like many changes in health care, the use of EHRs was jumpstarted by legislation. The American Recovery and Reinvestment Act of 2009 (P.L. 111-5) was enacted on February 17, 2009. This law established incentive payments to eligible professionals (EPs), eligible hospitals, critical access hospitals, and Medicare Advantage Organizations to promote the adoption and meaningful use of health information technology and qualified EHRs. These incentive payments are part of a broader effort under the HITECH Act to accelerate the adoption of health information technology and utilization of qualified EHRs.

Beginning in 2011, the Medicare and Medicaid Electronic Health Record Incentive Programs were established to encourage eligible professionals and hospitals to adopt, implement, and upgrade to demonstrate meaningful use of certified EHR technology. This was rolled out in stages, with specific targets that health care organizations had to meet in order to avoid financial penalties. The stages and incentive programs are commonly referred to as *meaningful use* (Centers for Medicare & Medicaid Services [CMS], 2017).

Swigert, N. B.
Documentation and Reimbursement for Speech-Language Pathologists: Principles and Practice (pp. 23-34).

Electronic Health Records

An EHR is an electronic version of a patient's medical history. The EHR may include all of the key administrative clinical data relevant to that person's care by that provider, including demographics, progress notes, problems, medications, vital signs, past medical history, immunizations, laboratory data, and radiology reports. The provider (eg, physician, hospital, speech-language pathologist) maintains the record over time. The EHR automates access to information and has the potential to streamline the clinician's workflow (CMS, 2012).

Electronic Health Record Advantages

Documentation in the EHR is timely, with most information immediately available to other providers. Imagine this scenario: A patient is taken to the emergency department of the hospital after a car accident and has a concussion, and thus is not able to provide a full medical history. The ED physician logs into the EHR and can read the patient's medical history in the documentation from the primary care physician's office. Or this scenario: The patient sees his or her primary care physician and reports abdominal pain. The physician enters all the background information in the record and sends the patient to the outpatient radiology department of the hospital for a computed tomography scan of the abdomen. The radiology department can get all pertinent history from the record and does not have to ask the patient all the same questions he or she just answered at the physician's office. The computed tomography is performed, and the films immediately interface into the record. The radiologist dictates an interpretation, which does not have to be transcribed, printed, and scanned, but instead goes directly into the record. The patient sees the physician for a follow-up appointment the next day, and all pertinent findings are available on the computer in the physician's office. In fact, there is likely a patient portal with the findings available for the patient to see. The data, and the timeliness and availability of it, will enable providers to make better decisions and provide better care.

The EHR has the ability to support the following other care-related activities directly or indirectly through different interfaces:

- Evidence-based decision support: Most EHRs link to evidence-based literature. If the patient presents with symptoms of disease with which the physician is not familiar, he or she can interface to articles about the latest treatment options.
- Patient education: The EHR can link to materials written for the patient about the disease or disorder. If the patient has been given a new diagnosis—diabetes—the EHR may interface to specific patient education information about diet and lifestyle changes needed.
- Quality management/performance improvement: Facilities can more easily collect, synthesize, and analyze information about patient care and use this information to improve the quality of care. Imagine that a facility without an EHR wants to know how it is doing with meeting certain quality standards (e.g., getting a patient presenting with signs of a heart attack into the catheterization lab in a timely way). The facility would have to manually look through hundreds of charts and calculate the time from admission to time of catheterization. For the speech-language pathology team, data from the EHR can facilitate generating timely and complete performance improvement reports that address timeliness, completeness, diagnoses, outcomes, or other patient care factors. With a properly built EHR, this information can be found with a few clicks in the system.
- Outcomes reporting: The EHR can be built to interface with multiple outcomes-reporting systems. Speech-language pathology departments that collect and submit data to the American Speech-Language-Hearing Association (ASHA) National Outcomes Measurement System (NOMS) would not have to enter the data into the ASHA web-based program. Instead, the EHR can interface and upload the data to NOMS automatically.

The EHR can also improve patient care in the following ways:

- Reducing the incidence of medical error by improving the accuracy and clarity of medical records. Handwritten entries are ripe for misinterpretation. One has only to stand in a nursing station for a few minutes before one observes a clinician asking another health care provider to interpret what has been written or decipher a physician's signature.
- Reducing duplication of tests because the results are immediately available to any other provider with access to the electronic record. For example, if all the physicians within a network are using the same EHR, one physician can see the tests ordered by other physicians and can see the results of those tests.
- Reducing delays in treatment because there is no waiting on dictation to be transcribed or an x-ray to be hand-carried from the hospital to the physician' office.
- Less risk in the case of disaster, like a fire or flood, because the files are backed up and stored securely. (CMS, 2012; U.S. Department of Health & Human Services [HHS], 2014a)

Disadvantages and Challenges to Electronic Health Records in Speech-Language Pathology

Disadvantages can be due to the EHR not being built in an integrated manner, issues with limited functionality, and/or poor multidisciplinary infrastructure to support the system on the hospital side ensuring that decisions related to the EHR take into consideration the needs of all who will be using it as a practice tool and documentation system. This can happen for several reasons and can be vendor/implementation team–specific. If you have a vendor with solution architects who are knowledgeable in the rehabilitation space, the collaboration between software builders and clinical designers works well and is evident in the end product. They will impress upon the organization the need for integration and ensure a change control process is in place, understood, and followed before handing implementation over to maintenance. However, some vendors' approach is to train lay people to be the analysts who will then build and maintain the system. However, these lay people are often lacking a full understanding of the capability of the system and how best to leverage it for integration, efficiency, patient safety, adequate reimbursement, and regulatory compliance. When the vendor uses this approach, it will leave the system with a poor understanding of integration and how best to utilize the very expensive and powerful tool they have just purchased. One question to ask when undergoing this building process is how accessible the speech-language pathology notes will be to physicians and other health care providers. This is relevant because some vendors present an architecture where physician notes are separate from other providers' notes. One can see the difficulty that arises when needing the physician to place orders after a dysphagia assessment, for example.

Although vendors are making strides to focus teams on rehabilitation content, until recently these systems were designed mostly for physicians' and nurses' documentation. Allied health documentation is much further down on the list, and rehabilitation services are lower on the list of priorities than, for example, pharmacy or radiology. This is clearly problematic for speech-language pathology and clinical nutrition services, where attention by the physician or nurse may be required in a timely manner. One might think that when a health care system buys an EHR documentation system, it would be presented with examples of how other health care systems have built and are using the software. Then one could pick and choose from those examples and construct the software to meet their needs. With only about five major vendors in the United States at the time of this writing, it is interesting to see that very few offer add-on packages that include speech-language pathology documentation. Those that do are often expensive and require additional fees for customization. What seems more typical is that each health care system has to start from scratch building templates and models. Pairing that with the knowledge that rehabilitation services are a fairly low priority when a large system is transitioning to an EHR or switching to a new software, one can imagine the product physical and occupational therapists, and speech-language pathologists end up with is less than desirable. Due to the immediacy of communication required by speech-language pathology, specifically for work in the area of dysphagia services, it is possible to request different routing of documentation than that of other rehabilitation services at the facility. An example may be that the speech-language pathology documentation may not be combined in a package with the rehabilitation documentation. It may not be intuitive to a physician who is awaiting completion of a dysphagia consult by the speech-language pathologist to search in the rehabilitation section of the EHR.

The options during the build process vary by vendor, with some being more collaborative than others and some being more rigid and cookie-cutter in their approach. Some vendors offer social media–type options, where systems with their content can post questions, participate in solution-specific calls, and play an active role in prioritizing the roadmap related to the engineering of new functionality. They offer options of staff, called *engagement leaders*, who will work on-site to facilitate meetings related to the EHR and act as a liaison between the software engineers and clinical users. They will even partner with systems to build needed content and then push the updated content to the subscribers when developed. Unfortunately, this is not the case with all vendors.

The larger vendors start their builds with foundation content. This is content that has been developed at the most basic level. It is up to each facility to customize the content and make changes to fit their system best. How this content is approached is very different during the implementation phase. As mentioned previously, some vendors require an implementation team of clinical users—subject matter experts (SMEs). These SMEs are usually representative of various hospital departments and disciplines. The vendor works with the SMEs to increase their familiarity with the foundation content and the functionality of the system. The SMEs then work with paired architects who will execute the build designed by the clinical users. Other vendors approach the implementation phase very differently and may reveal limited glimpses of the foundation content only to ask general questions from appointed SMEs. Some of the challenges encountered by speech-language pathology departments are the following:

- The evidence base to which the software links may not be up-to-date and accurate. It may contain information, for example, about a diagnostic technique that is no longer supported in the literature. However, the charting screens may still have those options built in. This may well be the case in packages that offer pre-established documentation templates/programs. It is incumbent on the end user to request the appropriate edits to meet the needs of the facility.
- The system may have been built for nursing-related goals and not structured to use measurable goals specific to the rehabilitation professional.
- Electronic documentation is not always faster and easier than paper charting. If it is not well designed, it may take longer to click through various screens to find where the data should be entered than it would simply jotting a few sentences on paper.

- Although the software can interface with outcomes systems, it may be a low priority to build the interface with ASHA NOMS.
- Quality management only works if the system is built so that the necessary data elements can be extracted. For example, if the speech-language pathology department would like to track how many patients have a diet upgrade after an instrumental examination of swallowing, a discrete data field needs to be built. Although it can be done, it's very difficult to pull data from narrative documentation for analysis.

The challenges to using the EHR, once built, relate to lack of organization and flow. The way the charting screens are organized might make sense for how nursing care is provided, for example, but not at all for how a communication or dysphagia evaluation and treatment are completed. There are also challenges to using point-of-care documentation (i.e., documentation in real time) with a software program, particularly as clinicians learn the system. It takes skill and practice to be able to keep the client engaged in the session while the clinician hunts for where the documentation of that task is entered. Although completing notes on the EHR while at bedside is challenging, doing so in the outpatient setting is increasingly advisable. In the same manner in which physicians are writing notes while examining the patient, speech-language pathologist can complete sections of the evaluation report in real time. This poses greater challenges for clinicians working with children but may be less difficult for clinicians working with adult patients/clients.

Table 3-1 **Tips on Building an Electronic Health Record**
• Work with rehabilitation and other ancillary counterparts • Build in an integrated manner • Build to address reimbursement and regulatory components • Utilize functionality to increase efficiency and patient safety • Carefully consider organization of screens • Reduce the amount of typing and scrolling needed • Educate end users • Include a revision period • Listen to end users

Tips for the Speech-Language Pathologist Involved in the Build of the Electronic Health Record

For a speech-language pathologist involved in the implementation of an EHR, it is imperative to keep the following in mind (Table 3-1):

- Work with your rehabilitation counterparts to ensure the rehabilitation build is formatted in the same manner. Another potential ally in this process is clinical nutrition. Ensuring physicians are able to easily access the speech-language pathology and clinical nutrition notes is essential in the management of the patient with dysphagia. Doing so will reduce maintenance needs moving forward and ensure you are all speaking the same language when communicating regarding patients and the system.
- Get the most bang for your buck and build in an integrated manner. You want to take into consideration how to utilize the EHR to reduce/eliminate double documentation at every turn across the team and not just within your discipline. For example, when the admitting nurse completes an assessment, information is gathered that is important for the entire team to know, such as living environment, premorbid levels of functioning, temperature, weight, dentition status, and discharge goals. If the record is built correctly, this information should flow throughout the record for the team to see. Depending on the vendor, this shared information may be available on a separate screen or may be imported into the speech-language pathologist's documentation. This will keep each team member from having to ask the patient the same questions when initiating his or her evaluations. They can verify the information instead of asking. For example, during an outpatient evaluation, time may be saved by simply reviewing the past medical history and focusing on the major etiologies relevant to the complaints at hand. This gives the patient the sense that the team already knows about him or her and keeps him or her from repeating, which is a common patient complaint.
- Build with the end in mind. Make sure that any reimbursement and/or regulatory components that need to be included in documentation are built in with hard stops in place to keep users from bypassing. If done right, necessary information is documented in real time, and the bill is ready to drop soon after discharge with a clean/compliant record.
- Utilize functionality to increase efficiency and patient safety. Create rules and pop-ups to ensure that actions that always occur are taken care of through the system. For example, if a speech-language pathology consult is always generated for a swallowing evaluation when a patient fails the nursing dysphagia screen, build a rule that when certain values that would indicate a fail are documented by the nurse, a proposed order is

generated and sent to the physician for cosignature. You can also create protocols that can go before the medical staff governing body for approval supporting the automatic placement of such orders without physician signature when a fail has been documented, which would ensure care in a timely manner, increasing efficiency and improving patient safety. It is likely that regulatory guidelines will require a cosignature by the physician, but the procedure (e.g., instrumental swallowing evaluation) can be performed before the cosignature is obtained.

- Consider how you want the screens for speech-language pathology to be organized. There are different architectures, or ways that the forms can be grouped, that can be used to group the forms the speech-language pathologists will use with patients with communication and/or swallowing disorders. (See Appendix 3-A, "Example Structures for Building Reports Into an Electronic Health Record" at the end of this chapter.)
- Reduce/eliminate typing and scrolling as much as possible. Point-and-click is better. This increases the ability to data-mine information that may be needed for reporting. There are systems that will run reports on how many key strokes are required and how much scrolling occurs, and this can serve as an indicator of whether the system is used efficiently. These reports help to set goals to reduce key strokes and scrolling in an attempt to improve efficiency for end users. This is often difficult for new users. If necessary, include an *Other* field after each major section to allow the clinician to add information not readily available in that section. For example, when completing the speech section of the evaluation report, clickable information may be available; however, if the clinician wishes to add something different to the report, he or she should be able to select *Other* and write freely.
- Create workflow and educate end users on how best to utilize the system. EHRs are powerful tools, but if clinical end users do not know how to utilize them as designed, inefficiencies and frustrations occur.
- Ensure that while building the documentation, a revision period is established. Once end-users start using the formats provided, it is relevant to meet with the team and discuss changes that may enhance use and efficiency. This may be an ongoing process for several months after the original go-live date.
- Listen to your end users. They will be the ones using the EHR most and can present with excellent ideas to maximize the system.

Selecting an Electronic Health Record Specifically for Speech-Language Pathology

If the speech-language pathologist is in a private practice or at a small clinic, EHR designed just for speech-language pathologists, rather than a multidisciplinary program for a large health system, may be used. Multiple options for software exist for rehabilitation outpatient settings that incorporate not only the health record, but also other features for practice management (ASHA, n.d.).

Considerations When Using an Electronic Health Record

EHRs present some challenges, particularly related to confidentiality of the information. The Health Insurance Portability and Accountability Act of 1996 (HIPAA) Security Rule (see Chapter 1) established standards for the security of EHRs. Any staff member with access to the record has to take precautions to prevent unauthorized access, alteration, or disclosure of the client's health information (Scott, 2006). The speech-language pathologist should keep the following points in mind:

- The speech-language pathologist will be given a user name and password.
  - If the clinician can establish his or her own password, carefully follow the guidelines for a secure password.
  - It is likely the password will need to be changed on a periodic basis.
  - Do not share the user name or password with anyone.
- Your user name will be affixed to any documentation once you save the information. This is akin to writing your signature at the bottom of a hand-written note. The affixing of your user name is the authentication of that entry.
- If you are leaving the workstation, log out. Some software has a feature that will take you back to the place you were charting when you log back in.
  - If the workstation is in a secure area where unauthorized people are not going to see the screen, it may be acceptable to simply turn off the screen when you walk away for a brief time.
  - If you use a computer or laptop where you are the only user, there may be a feature that does not require you to log out but to simply lock the computer.

- Do not access any EHR that you do not have direct need to see. There are times one might be tempted to just take a peek at someone's record:
  - A celebrity is admitted
  - A friend or neighbor is admitted and you want to see how serious the problem is
  - A coworker was seen in the ED and you wonder what is wrong
  - You are the caregiver for an elderly relative who is admitted and weren't at bedside when the physician arrived and you want to read her documentation
  - You want to look at your own medical record because your physician hasn't called you yet with the results of a test

  Although you may have what you think is a valid reason to open the EHR, unauthorized access can be traced back to your user name and may be grounds for disciplinary action, termination of employment, and even legal action. Consult the health information department or risk department to learn the appropriate way to access your own record or that of a loved one for whom you have legal responsibility.
- Electronic work stations are often in high-traffic areas (e.g., outside the patient's room). Be aware of this to ensure unauthorized people are not looking at the documentation.
- Do not assume that the EHR prevents any errors in the information entered. Some software may have spell checkers that, for example, change *dysphagia* to *dysphasia*. Always proofread what you have entered before saving the documentation.
- Know whether saving the information requires an action, like hitting a Save button, or whether it occurs automatically when logging out (Gateley & Borcherding, 2016).

Other Methods for Communicating

If an EHR is used, and the other providers are all using the same EHR, then there is no need to send health information to anyone. However, unless the speech-language pathologist is practicing within a highly integrated health care system, the need arises to send a report to, for example, a physician outside the network, another speech-language pathologist at the facility to which the patient is transferring, or the speech-language pathologist at a child's school. Health information is still sometimes sent the old-fashioned way through the U.S. Mail. However, it is typical for such records to be faxed or sent by email as an attachment. Sometimes urgent information or a request may be sent to a physician via text.

> CONFIDENTIAL NOTICE: The materials enclosed with this facsimile transmission are private and confidential and are the property of the sender. The information contained in the material is privileged and is intended only for the use of the individual(s) or entity(ies) named above. If you are not the intended recipient, be advised that any unauthorized disclosure, copying, distribution, or the taking of any action in reliance on the contents of this information is strictly prohibited. If you have received this facsimile in error, please immediately notify us by telephone to arrange for the return of the documents

Figure 3-1. Confidentiality statement on fax cover sheet.

Faxing

Reports and other documents that are faxed are considered to be protected health information (PHI) and thus governed by HIPAA. Any document that is faxed should have a cover sheet clearly indicating the intended recipient. Often the fax cover sheet contains a statement of confidentiality (Figure 3-1).

The sender must ensure the fax is going to the right place. The HIPAA Breach Notification Rule requires most doctors, hospitals, other health care providers, and health insurance companies to notify the patient of a breach if unsecured information is seen by someone who is not supposed to see it. This federal law also requires health care providers and insurance companies to promptly notify the Secretary of HHS if there is any breach of unsecured protected health information and notify the media and public if the breach affects more than 500 people (HHS, 2013).

Email

Email, by its very nature, uses an unsecure protocol. There are a number of risks, including the possibility of data interception. However, there are a number of email encryption solutions that make email a secure medium. Whether the email is sent from a desktop or a mobile device, the speech-language pathologist should find out what the facility's requirements are for sending secure emails (HHS, n.d.). If email is an approved medium at the clinician's facility for patient communication and for forwarding reports, it is often best to only use the facility's email system and user account, not a personal email account.

Texting

Secure electronic texting can be an efficient way to communicate to your clients. It can be used to provide information about appointments, answer questions, and handle coordination between visits. Secure texting is also used from provider to provider. For example, perhaps the speech-language pathologist wants to communicate the results of an evaluation swiftly to the physician, or request an order from the physician (HHS, 2014b).

Texting from cell phone to cell phone is not secure texting. Just encrypting the message is not enough to make it secure. Security goes beyond the encryption of the message in transit. True security means the following:

- Protecting the data while it's on the device
- Requiring a personal identification number to access messages with PHI
- Wiping that PHI in the event a device is lost or stolen
- Being able to identify the sender and understand the context around a critical message
- Being able to track the status of a message: When it was received, opened, etc. (Shallo, 2014)

Encrypted Portable Devices

Sometimes PHI is stored and transported on thumb (flash) drives. Perhaps the clinician works in several different settings, and the system for which he or she works does not have the capacity for information to be viewed remotely from a central storage drive. If information is stored on a portable device, it must also be protected (Kangas, 2012).

Voice and Video Recordings

Voice and video recordings are sometimes made as part of the treatment. For example, clients working on voice or speech production might have video recordings made by the speech-language pathologist to provide valuable feedback. These recordings are considered PHI.

Increasing Efficiency in Paper Charting

If the speech-language pathologist works in a setting that is not using electronic documentation, it is essential to streamline documentation and reduce the amount of time spent in documentation. The use of templates in Word or Excel can be time-consuming to develop but, once developed, can save clinicians a great deal of time. Templates can do the following:

- Facilitate the clinician remembering to capture all necessary information to be compliant with documentation rules and regulations
- Improve speed of documentation
- Improve productivity
- Minimize writing and maximize readability by others
- Improve consistency

Headers and subheaders can be used to guide the reader to the part of the report that is important to that reader. For example, the physician receiving the report may want to skip right to the summary, whereas the coder will want to easily find the diagnosis and diagnostic codes.

Templates can be generic. There can be one for an evaluation, one for the treatment plan, one for progress notes, and one for the discharge summary. However, although it takes more time to develop, generating templates for different disorders and populations served can be even more beneficial. Templates need to be flexible, however, so that the clinician can document any unique aspects of the session. Examples of generic and more defined templates are provided in later chapters.

Other Forms Used in Health Care Settings

The speech-language pathologist in health care settings will be exposed to other documentation requirements not specific to the practice of speech-language pathology. These documentation requirements will be followed by many other disciplines. Some of the documentation is interdisciplinary, like the clinical (or critical) pathways.

Clinical or Critical Pathways

Pathways are typically multidisciplinary documents developed at facilities for certain patient types. They might also be called *care pathways, integrated care pathways*, or *care maps*. For example, a hospital may have a clinical pathway for any patient admitted with stroke or undergoing total knee replacement. Pathways, in use since the 1980s, are to be evidence based and are designed to guide the care of a certain patient population. The pathway typically defines what should happen at specified times on each day of the patient's stay. They usually focus on nursing care and medications, but some pathways include services provided by speech-language pathology. For example, a pathway for a patient with cerebrovascular accident will likely have information about the communication and swallowing interventions needed (Kinsman, Rotter, James, Snow, & Willis, 2010). These pathways may appear in different formats, such as a decision tree, a flow diagram, or columns reflecting what is to happen each day. Sometimes the clinical staff have to document on the pathway to indicate when certain tasks were completed or patient goals met.

Incident Reports

Incident reports are used to document and report adverse events that may have legal or quality management implications. This can be an event involving a patient, visitor, staff, or other person. The incident report serves the following two purposes:

1. By reporting suspected or actual injury or pointing out a safety concern, the incident report alerts management to potential problems that need attention. Facilities are particularly looking for any trends or patterns in the types of events that are occurring.
2. The report also captures all pertinent information for further investigation in case legal action results from the event.

Incident reports are confidential and are not intended to be punitive toward the persons involved in the incident. The point is not to place blame but to understand the safety-related event and make changes to processes and procedures to reduce the likelihood a similar event will occur again (Scott, 2013).

Examples of safety events for which the speech-language pathologist might enter an incident report could include the following:

- Placing a speaking valve without deflating the trach cuff
- Delivering a tray with a regular diet to a patient on a pureed diet
- Nursing staff failing to place the patient in required upright position for oral medication administration

Advance Directives

The Patient Self Determination Act of 1991 specified a patient's right to control health care decisions (Patient Self-Determination Act, 1991). Specifically, health care organizations have to provide patient education about informed consent and the right of the patient to make an advance directive (Koch, 1992; Silverman, Tuma, Schaeffer, & Singh, 1995). Advance directives include legal documents such as living wills and durable power of attorney for health care decision making. The patient has the right to accept or refuse medical or surgical treatment and does not have to follow the recommendations made by the providers. The advance directive would contain information about the patient's wishes regarding resuscitation (Scott, 2013). The speech-language pathologist should know whether the patient has specified wishes regarding things like tube feeding, because it will have an impact on treatment recommendations made.

Informed Consent

Informed consent in speech-language pathology is most often used in research contexts. Obtaining informed consent is meant to protect the subject, or participant, so he or she can understand the risks and benefits of participating in the research and make an independent choice as to whether or not he or she will participate. In research, there is a detailed informed consent form that the patient must sign (Brady Wagner, 2002). However, informed consent also applies to clinical situations. The speech-language pathologist must fully explain procedures and tests and results to the patient so he or she can make an informed choice about whether to undergo the procedure or follow the recommendations based on the results. Most facilities do not require patients to sign a form before a procedure like a videofluoroscopic or fiberoptic endoscopic swallowing evaluation or a videostroboscopy. However, some facilities use consents and waivers when a patient declines to follow recommendations (Horner, Modayil, Chapman, & Dinh, 2016; Sharp, 2015).

Releasing Medical Information

There are specific guidelines about releasing medical information to other health care providers and non–health care providers. HIPAA defines the right of the patient to see, copy, and amend his or her medical records. It also defines how and when the medical facility can share information with others. The facility provides the patient with a copy of a HIPAA privacy notice that specifies all of this information (Scott, 2013). If a patient requests a copy of the speech-language pathologist's records, the best practice is to defer to the health information management department at the facility for the specific requirements, like signed forms, for releasing documents.

Restraints

Patients in inpatient settings are sometimes physically restrained; because patients have been injured, and even died, as a result of restraint use, there are strict guidelines about how and when restraints can be used. Clinical staff, including speech-language pathologists, should be trained in the proper way to apply and release restraints. If the speech-language pathologist is going to see a patient in restraints, he or she should check with the nurse to see if the restraints can be removed. The speech-language pathologist will also need to document the time the restraints were removed and, if reapplied, when that occurred (Scott, 2013).

Pain Scales

Pain scales are more routinely documented by nursing. Of the rehabilitation professionals, physical and occupational therapists likely have more reason to assess and document pain, such as before and after a therapy session requiring the patient to be physically moved. However, if a patient reports to the speech-language pathologist that he or she is in pain, the clinician is obligated to report the pain to the nurse and also to ask the patient to rate the pain and then document that rating (Baker, 2016). There are several formats of pain scales. The most common is an analog scale of 1 to 10, with 1 representing no pain and 10 representing the worst pain imaginable. For children or others not able to understand an analog scale, there is the Wong-Baker FACES pain rating scale. Sometimes a drawing of the front and back of the human body is presented and the patient is asked to point to the area(s) of the pain (Haefeli & Elfering, 2006).

References

American Speech-Language-Hearing Association. (n.d.). Electronic medical records and practice management software for speech-language pathologists. Retrieved from https://www.asha.org/Practice/EMR-and-Practice-Management-Software-for-SLPs/

Baker, D. W. (2016). Joint Commission statement on pain management. Retrieved from https://www.jointcommission.org/joint_commission_statement_on_pain_management/

Brady Wagner, L. C. (2002). Equipoise, informed consent, and clinical research. *SIG 13 Perspectives on Swallowing and Swallowing Disorders (Dysphagia), 11*(2), 22–23. doi:10.1044/sasd11.2.22

Centers for Medicare & Medicaid Services. (2012). Electronic health records. Retrieved from https://www.cms.gov/Medicare/E-Health/EHealthRecords/index.html?redirect=/EhealthRecords/

Centers for Medicare & Medicaid Services. (2017). Electronic health records incentive programs. Retrieved from https://www.cms.gov/Regulations-and-Guidance/Legislation/EHRIncentivePrograms/index.html

Gateley, C. A., & Borcherding, S. (2016). *Documentation manual for occupational therapy: Writing SOAP notes* (4th ed.). Thorofare, NJ: SLACK Incorporated.

Haefeli, M., & Elfering, A. (2006). Pain assessment. *European Spine Journal, 15*(Suppl 1), S17–S24. http://doi.org/10.1007/s00586-005-1044-x

Horner, J., Modayil, M., Chapman, L. R., & Dinh, A. (2016). Consent, refusal, and waivers in patient-centered dysphagia care: Using law, ethics, and evidence to guide clinical practice. *American Journal of Speech-Language Pathology, 25*(4), 453–469. doi:10.1044/2016_AJSLP-15-0041

Kangas, E. (2012). Jump/thumb drives and PHI don't mix. *The LuxSci FYI Blog.* Retrieved from https://luxsci.com/blog/jumpthumb-drives-and-phi-dont-mix.html

Kinsman, L., Rotter, T., James, E., Snow, P., & Willis, J. (2010). What is a clinical pathway? Development of a definition to inform the debate. *BMC Med, 8*(1), 1.

Koch, K. A. (1992). Patient Self-Determination Act. *Journal of the Florida Medical Association, 79*(4), 240–243.

Patient Self-Determination Act. HR 4449. (1991.)

Scott, R. W. (2006). *Legal aspects of documenting patient care for rehabilitation professionals.* Burlington, MA: Jones & Bartlett Learning.

Scott, R. W. (2013). *Legal, ethical and practical aspects of patient care documentation: A guide for rehabilitation professionals* (4th ed.). Burlington, MA: Jones and Bartlett Learning.

Shallo, G. (2014). What does "secure texting" really mean? [Web log post]. Retrieved from http://www.spok.com/blog/what-does-secure-texting-really-mean

Sharp, H. M. (2015). Informed consent in clinical and research settings: What do patients and families need to make informed decisions? *SIG 13 Perspectives on Swallowing and Swallowing Disorders (Dysphagia), 24*(4), 130–139. doi:10.1044/sasd24.4.130

Silverman, H. J., Tuma, P., Schaeffer, M. H., & Singh, B. (1995). Implementation of the patient self-determination act in a hospital setting: an initial evaluation. *Archives of Internal Medicine, 155*(5), 502–510.

U.S. Department of Health & Human Services. (n.d.). Can you use email to send health information using your mobile device? Retrieved from https://www.healthit.gov/providers-professionals/faqs/can-you-use-email-send-health-information-using-your-mobile-device

U.S. Department of Health & Human Services. (2013). Your health information security. Retrieved from https://www.healthit.gov/patients-families/your-health-information-security

U.S. Department of Health & Human Services. (2014a). Protecting the privacy and security of your health information. Retrieved from https://www.healthit.gov/patients-families/protecting-your-privacy-security

U.S. Department of Health & Human Services. (2014b). Use secure electronic messaging. Retrieved from https://www.healthit.gov/providers-professionals/achieve-meaningful-use/core-measures-2/use-secure-electronic-messaging

Review Questions

1. What are the stated advantages to an EHR?
2. What are some of the challenges faced by speech-language pathologists when using an EHR?
3. List three ways the speech-language pathologist can protect the privacy of the EHR in a health care setting.
4. List three tips that can facilitate the build of an EHR.
5. Besides the medical record itself, what are other forms of communication that must also follow guidelines for protecting the privacy and security of the PHI?
6. What is an advance directive, and why might a speech-language pathologist need to know what was in a patient's advance directive?

Activity A

EHRs comprise items with drop-down menus that require the user to click on the pertinent choices. Imagine you are designing an EHR, and sort the drop-down items into the appropriate categories. After each choice, insert A, B, C, D, or E to indicate into which category it best fits.

Reason for referral (A)
Medical history (B)
Social background (C)
Patient characteristics (D)
Nutrition status (E)

Choice in Drop-Down Menu	Goes Best With
NPO (nil per os)	
Impaired ability to communicate	
Difficulty swallowing	
Cooperative	
Percutaneous endoscopic gastrostomy tube	
Alert	
Lives alone	
Pneumonia	
Easily fatigued	
Regular diet	
Cerebrovascular accident	
Combative	
Confused	
Hypertension	
Lives alone with intermittent family support	
Chronic obstructive pulmonary disease	
Resides in skilled nursing facility	
Diabetes mellitus	
Recent-onset altered mental status	
Primary caretaker for spouse	
Difficult to understand	

Appendix 3-A
Example Structures for Building Reports Into an Electronic Health Record

Possible architecture to be instituted in the EHR depending on the facility's and department's needs:

- Structure 1:
    - An evaluation form to cover speech-language and swallowing assessment
    - A treatment note (possibly in SOAP [subjective, objective, assessment, plan] format) to cover speech-language and swallowing
- Structure 2:
    - An evaluation form to cover speech-language and swallowing assessment
    - A treatment note (possibly in SOAP format) to cover speech-language and swallowing
    - A form for instrumental examinations: Videofluoroscopic swallowing study (VFSS) or flexible endoscopic evaluation of swallowing (FEES)
- Structure 3:
    - An evaluation form to cover speech-language assessment
    - An evaluation form to cover swallowing assessment (clinical)
    - A treatment note (possibly in SOAP format) to cover speech-language
    - A treatment note (possibly in SOAP format) to cover swallowing
    - A form for VFSS reporting
    - A form for FEES reporting
- Structure 4:
    - An evaluation form(s) to cover speech-language assessment: Templates for voice, motor speech (adult), motor speech (pediatric), language (adult), language (pediatric), articulation/phonology (pediatric), etc.
    - An evaluation form to cover swallowing assessment (clinical): Pediatric, adult
    - A treatment note (possibly in SOAP format) to cover speech-language
    - A treatment note (possibly in SOAP format) to cover swallowing
    - A form for VFSS reporting
    - A form for FEES reporting

Forms can comprise drop-down menus with point-and-click options to write in additional information. This format seems to be the most widely used at present. Treatment notes may provide drop-down menus with goals that can be edited, or goals may be written in individually. Again, features are based on the capabilities of the system and on preferences of the end users.

4

Coding, Reimbursement, and Documentation

Nancy B. Swigert, MA, CCC-SLP, BCS-S

Why Do We Need Codes?

When submitting a bill for services rendered, it is not enough to list a description of the reason the client was seen and what was done. There needs to be a standard way to do this. Imagine if there were no coding systems and three different speech-language pathologists saw the same client for a voice evaluation in three different clinics. Each submitted a bill using only words to describe the client and the service (Figure 4-1). Now imagine the difficulty the clerk at the insurance company would have when looking at the list of covered services and trying to figure out which of these bills, if any, match what is listed in the policy as covered. Using standard, universally accepted coding systems, one for the diagnosis and another for the procedure(s), eliminates this confusion. Consider the same bills, but now each speech-language pathologist has used codes for the diagnosis and the services provided (Figure 4-2).

Two Coding Systems

Two coding systems are used in health care, and clinicians should be familiar with both. The coding system used to describe the reason the client is being seen is the *International Classification of Diseases, Tenth Revision, Clinical Modification* (ICD-10-CM) (Centers for Medicare & Medicaid Services [CMS], 2016a). Codes to describe the service provided are called Current Procedural Terminology (CPT) codes. The CPT process is owned and managed by the American Medical Association (AMA, 2016a).

International Classification of Diseases, Tenth Revision, Clinical Modification

This coding system is the official system of assigning codes to diagnoses and procedures associated with hospital utilization in the United States. However, ICD-10-CM codes are not used just in hospitals. Almost any health care provider in any setting submitting a bill to a third party uses this diagnostic coding system. The ICD-10-CM is owned by the World Health Organization, but the National Center for Health Statistics and the CMS are the U.S. governmental agencies responsible for overseeing all changes and modifications to ICD-10-CM. The *CM* means Clinical Modification and is the U.S. modification of ICD-10 (CMS, 2016a).

Swigert, N. B.
Documentation and Reimbursement for Speech-Language Pathologists: Principles and Practice (pp. 35-50).

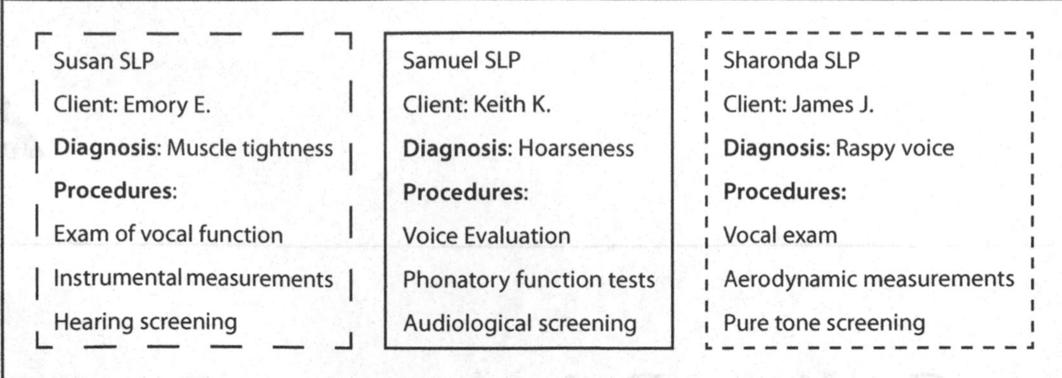

Figure 4-1. Bills by three speech-language pathologists for the same type of patient and same procedures submitted without codes

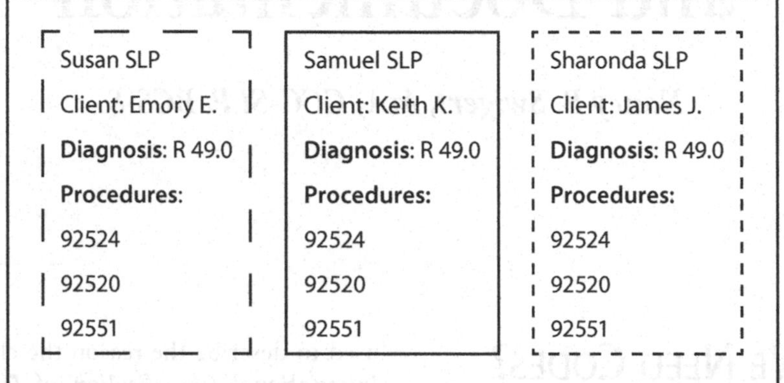

Figure 4-2. Bills by three speech-language pathologists for the same type of patient and same procedures submitted with codes

Uses for *International Classification of Diseases, Tenth Revision, Clinical Modification*

These diagnostic codes have many other uses besides coding for reimbursement. ICD is used around the world to identify health trends and gather statistics. Internationally, it is the standard for reporting diseases and health conditions. For example, when there is an outbreak of a virus, the number of cases in different countries can be tracked because a code is used to report it. ICD is also the standard for research purposes. As it is a standardized system, it allows for the following:

- An easy way to store, retrieve and analyze health information so that evidence-based decisions can be made
- A way for health care facilities, regions, and countries to share and compare health data
- A location to compare data over a period of time (e.g., reporting an increase or decrease in a specific disease, such as an increase in diabetes in a region over time)
- A standardized way to describe a disease or disorder on a health care claim

This classification system has existed since 1948, and, in 1967, the World Health Organization stipulated that member states use the most up-to-date nomenclature to report morbidity and mortality data. ICD-10 was endorsed in May 1990 by the Forty-Third World Health Assembly, but ICD-10 was not implemented in the United States until October 2015, years after other industrialized nations had moved from the older version, ICD-9 (All Things Medical Billing, n.d.). One of the reasons for the delay in implementation was the cost involved for government agencies and health-related businesses to upgrade software and processes from ICD-9 to ICD-10.

ICD-10 uses a seven-character alphanumeric system. The first character is alpha, the second is numeric, and the third through seventh characters are either alpha or numeric. ICD-10 has about 68,000 codes available. This was a large increase in the number of codes, about 13,000, in ICD-9.

Diagnostic Coding of Therapy Services

In order for therapy services to be reimbursed, the client must have a diagnosis that supports the need for services of a speech-language pathologist (Table 4-1). For example, it is logical that a client might need an evaluation by a speech-language pathologist if the client has a diagnosis of stroke, cerebral palsy, Down syndrome, or multiple sclerosis. However, if the only diagnosis on a client's bill was something like broken hip or hypertension, services

Table 4-1

Coding Rules and Guidelines

1	The diagnostic code (ICD-10-CM) has to support the need for services by a speech-language pathologist.
2	The Local Coverage Determination often contains a list of codes that support speech-language pathologist services.
3	The physician applies the medical diagnostic code.
4	The speech-language pathologist can apply the code(s) for the communication and swallowing disorders.
5	The diagnostic code (ICD-10-CM) and the procedural code (CPT) have to make sense together.
6	The speech-language pathologist should code to the highest degree of certainty.
7	Avoid using codes with NOS or NEC.
8	On the claim, list the reason the speech-language pathologist is seeing the client as the primary diagnosis.
9	When the results are normal, use a diagnostic code(s) for the reason the speech-language pathologist was seeing the client.

Abbreviations: NEC = not elsewhere classified; NOS = not otherwise classified.

Data compiled from American Speech-Language-Hearing Association. (2015). 2015 ICD-10-CM diagnosis codes related to speech, language and swallowing. Retrieved from http://www.asha.org/uploadedFiles/ICD-10-Codes-SLP.pdf#search=%22codes%22

of a speech-language pathologist would not seem to be indicated. It is important that all appropriate diagnoses be listed. For example, a client might have suffered a broken hip, a code that does not warrant speech-language services, but might also have Parkinson's disease. If the Parkinson's disease is not coded on the bill along with broken hip, then the charge for speech-language services would likely be denied (American Speech-Language-Hearing Association [ASHA], n.d.-e).

Medicare probably has the most stringent guidelines about which diagnostic codes it considers as logically supporting the need for speech-language services. Medicare Administrative Contractors (MACs) are insurance companies contracted by Medicare to administer the program by region of the country. These MACs can further define Medicare regulations; therefore, there can be different interpretations in different parts of the country. The MACs publish a document called a Local Coverage Determination (LCD), usually one for speech-language services and one for dysphagia services. The LCD usually contains a list of ICD-10 codes that are considered to support speech-language pathology services.

R49	Voice and resonance disorders
	Excludes: Psychogenic voice and resonance disorders (F44.4)
R49.0	Dysphonia
	Hoarseness
R49.1	Aphonia
	Loss of voice
R49.2	Hypernasality and hyponasality
	R49.21 Hypernasality
	R49.22 Hyponasality
R49.8	Other voice and resonance disorders
R49.9	Unspecified voice and resonance disorder
	Change in voice NOS
	Resonance disorder NOS

Figure 4-3. Diagnostic coding to highest degree of certainty. (Data compiled from American Speech-Language-Hearing Association. (2015). 2015 ICD-10-CM diagnosis codes related to speech, language and swallowing. Retrieved from http://www.asha.org/uploadedFiles/ICD-10-Codes-SLP.pdf#search=%22codes%22)

The physician is responsible for determining the code for the medical problem (e.g., concussion), and the speech-language pathologist can apply the code or codes to describe the cognitive, communication, and/or swallowing problem for which the client is being treated. These diagnostic codes should also appear on the order from the physician. Speech-language pathologists can work closely with referring physicians to ensure they are familiar with cognitive-communication and swallowing codes (ASHA, n.d.-a).

The diagnostic code also has to make sense for the particular procedure CPT code(s) reported on the claim. For example, if the diagnostic code is for hoarseness (R 49.0), it wouldn't be logical that the procedure code was for evaluation of speech fluency (92521). It would, however, be logical that a client with hoarseness receive a behavioral and qualitative analysis of voice and resonance (92524) and possibly laryngeal function studies (92520).

Sometimes there appears to be more than one code that might accurately describe the disorder. The guidance is that you should always code to the highest degree of specificity. That means, if there is a code with three characters and one with four characters that could describe the disorder, choose the one with four characters. If there is a four-character code and a five-character code and either describes the disorder, but the code with five characters more specifically describes the problem, choose the code with five characters. Consider that you are evaluating a child with hypernasality (Figure 4-3). R49 (three characters) indicates voice and resonance disorders, and hypernasality is certainly that.

Table 4-2

How to Code Normal Results

Patient Complaint/ Referred for Evaluation of...	International Classification of Diseases, Tenth Revision, Clinical Modification Code (Even When Results Reveal Client's Skills Within Normal Limits)
Hoarse vocal quality	R49.0 Dysphonia, hoarseness
Trouble eating	R63.3 Feeding difficulties
Unintelligible speech	F80.0 Phonological disorder, functional speech articulation disorder
Incoordination of speech after stroke	I69.390 Apraxia following cerebral infarction

Adapted from American Speech-Language-Hearing Association. (n.d.). Coding normal results frequently asked questions. Retrieved from http://www.asha.org/practice/reimbursement/coding/normalresults/

- For **outpatient** services, ICD-10-CM guidelines state, "**Do not code diagnoses documented as 'probable,' 'suspected,' 'questionable,' 'rule out,' or 'working diagnosis' or other similar terms indicating uncertainty.** Rather, code the condition(s) to the highest degree of certainty for that encounter/visit, such as symptoms, signs, abnormal test results, or other **reason for the visit.**"
- For **inpatient** services (including short-term, acute, and long-term care), ICD-10-CM advises "If the diagnosis documented at the time of discharge is qualified as 'probable,' 'suspected,' 'likely,' 'questionable,' 'possible,' or 'still to be ruled out' or other similar terms indicating uncertainty, **code the condition as if it existed or was established.**"

Figure 4-4. Official instructions how to code normal results. (Data compiled from Centers for Disease Control and Prevention. (2017). ICD-10-CM official guidelines for coding and reporting FY 2017 (October 1, 2016 - September 30, 2017). Retrieved from https://www.cdc.gov/nchs/data/icd/10cmguidelines_2017_final.pdf)

However, R49.2 (four characters) is even more specific as hypernasality and hyponasality. But you know this child is presenting with hypernasality, so the five-character code of R49.21, hypernasality, is the most appropriate code to choose.

You will note that some ICD-10 codes use the terms *not otherwise specified* (NOS) and *not elsewhere classified* (NEC). These codes are not very specific and seem to indicate that the clinician does not really know what is wrong with the client. For example, in Figure 4-3, note R49.9, Unspecified voice and resonance disorder, with two NOS examples. Avoid using NOS and NEC unless there simply is no other code to describe the client's problem.

When submitting a claim, the primary diagnosis is the condition (e.g., disease, symptom, injury) that is chiefly responsible for the visit or the reason for the encounter. This primary code is listed on the first line of the list of diagnoses. Secondary diagnoses, which are then listed below the primary diagnosis, are coexisting conditions or symptoms, or things discovered after the evaluation. Let's say a physician has referred a client post-stroke for evaluation of dysarthria. During the course of your assessment, however, you determine that the client has some mild residual expressive aphasia that the physician did not notice. On your claim, and in your report, you would list the dysarthria as primary and the expressive aphasia as secondary. The physician would also have supplied a code for the medical diagnosis of stroke, and that would also be listed as a secondary diagnosis.

ICD-10-CM guidelines indicate that clinicians should not use terms like *rule out*, *probable*, *likely*, *suspected*, or *questionable*. You should not see terms like that on a physician's order, and you should not use terms like that in your report. The physician does not tell a patient, "I think your communication skills are fine. Let's send you to a speech-language pathologist to see if I am correct." Instead, the physician says something like, "I can tell you're having some trouble recalling information to answer my questions. Let's send you to a speech-language pathologist to determine what the problem might be." If you evaluate a client who is referred for a specific reason and determine that no problem exists (e.g., the client's skills are normal or age appropriate), code the signs or symptoms to report the reason the client was referred to you (Table 4-2). Then, in your report, indicate why the client was referred and what your test results found. This information can be found in the ICD-10 Coding Guidelines (Figure 4-4) (ASHA, n.d.-d; Centers for Disease Control and Prevention, 2017).

One of the best resources on diagnostic coding and on many topics related to reimbursement for speech-language pathologists is the ASHA website (ASHA, n.d.-c). You can download a document that lists all the ICD-10-CM codes that a speech-language pathologist might use. The document also includes more information on rules for coding and links to other resources (ASHA, 2018).

Current Procedural Terminology

In addition to coding the diagnosis—the reason the client is being seen—the clinician also uses codes to describe what procedures were performed. These procedural codes are the CPT codes. Unlike the ICD-10-CM process, which is managed by government agencies, the CPT process is owned and maintained by the AMA, which has copyright protection of the codes.

The AMA published the first edition of the CPT manual in 1966, and it was focused mainly on surgical procedures. The goal was to standardize terminology and reporting of these procedures. The fourth edition, released in the 1970s, introduced the system for periodically monitoring and updating CPT. What makes CPT integral to coding in health care is that in 1983, the Health Care Financing Administration, which is now CMS, adopted the CPT as the way all services for Medicare Part B beneficiaries would be reported (University of Texas, n.d.).

Current Procedural Terminology and the Healthcare Common Procedure Coding System

CMS refers to the codes as the Healthcare Common Procedure Coding System (HCPCS), pronounced "hick-picks." The HCPCS includes the AMA CPT codes, but also other codes not covered by CPT. There are three levels of codes in HCPCS:

- Level I: CPT codes
- Level II: Codes for non–physician services not covered by CPT codes like ambulance, supplies, and medical devices. These codes begin with letters (A through V) followed by four numeric digits. Level II codes are updated every year. Speech-language pathologists use these Level II codes for speech generating devices (SGD), voice prosthetics, voice amplifiers, and repair of augmentative and alternative communication systems or devices. A complete list can be found on the ASHA website (ASHA, n.d.-f). Medicare does recognize SGDs as durable medical equipment, which is a covered benefit. However, there are many rules about what kind of devices Medicare will cover. For example, it will not pay for a device (e.g., a computer) that might be useful to someone without a communication disorder. The device has to be used primarily for generating speech (ASHA, n.d.-h).
- Level III: Local codes developed by Medicare contractors, state Medicaid organizations, and private insurance companies. These codes have a similar structure to Level II codes and begin with the letters W through Z, followed by four digits. Level III use was discontinued in 2003 in favor of coding that is consistent regardless of agency or location.

Process to Establish and Revise Current Procedural Terminology Codes

New editions of the updated CPT codes are released each year in October. Codes are added, removed, and revised with each revision. Changes to codes can be initiated by providers, medical societies, or responsible organizations (All Things Medical Billing, n.d.).

ASHA has representatives to the panels that establish and revise the codes. There are two different processes involved in managing the CPT codes. The first step in the process is establishing a new code. There are distinct parameters that must be met before a new code can be created. For example, the code must represent a procedure performed nationally that is not adequately represented by another existing code. In addition, the procedure cannot be experimental. Approval of a new code is done at the CPT panel.

The CPT panel determines not only when a new code can be established, but also when existing codes are reviewed. Once a new code is established or an existing code reviewed, it is sent to another AMA group called the Relative Value Update Committee. Speech-language pathology is also represented in this process. The Relative Value Update Committee determines the value of each code relative to every other code in the book. Adding new codes means the value of some existing codes will be decreased (AMA, 2016b).

The information about the value, which is expressed as a relative numeric value (e.g., 1.24 or .78) is sent to CMS, who ultimately determines the dollar amount that will be reimbursed for a code. Each year, CMS publishes the fees for the upcoming calendar year in the Medicare Physician Fee Schedule (MPFS). ASHA staff analyze the rules and prepare a document on the MPFS with updated information and fees. The fees vary geographically, but the document from ASHA provides the national information (ASHA, n.d.-l).

CMS can also determine that it will not reimburse for certain codes. For example, there is a CPT code for a non-SGD, but CMS has determined it will not reimburse for evaluation and treatment for non–SGD-related services.

CPT codes are used to bill outpatient therapy services. Speech-language pathologists working in inpatient settings may be asked to use CPT codes, but this is for internal tracking and productivity purposes. As all inpatient settings under Medicare are paid through prospective payment systems, it is irrelevant how many and which CPT codes were used.

Evaluation and Treatment Current Procedural Terminology Codes Used by Speech-Language Pathologists

There are approximately 44 CPT codes commonly used by speech-language pathologists. These are reflected on a Model Superbill designed by ASHA (n.d.-j). This superbill categorizes the codes as follows:

- Swallowing related 9
- Speech & language related 20
- Augmentative & alternative 8
- Other 7

More detailed information about the rules for using each of these codes is also found on the ASHA website, including tips on how and when to use certain codes. For example:

- 92597: Evaluation for use and/or fitting of voice prosthetic device to supplement oral speech
  - Under Medicare, applies to tracheoesophageal prostheses (e.g., Passy-Muir valve), artificial larynges, as well as voice amplifiers. Use 92507 for training and modification of voice prostheses. (ASHA, n.d.-i)

These two references on the ASHA website will provide the most updated information on current CPT codes in use by speech-language pathologists and any new rules or limitations on their use. Activities A and B at the end of this chapter provide practice using CPT codes.

Timed and Untimed Current Procedural Terminology Codes

Almost all CPT codes used by speech-language pathologists are not timed. That means, for example, that whether the speech-language pathologist spends 75 minutes or 25 minutes in a therapy session, the same CPT code is billed and the amount of reimbursement will not change based on the length of the session. An untimed code is billed as a session.

Some facilities may pair an artificial unit of time with CPT codes. For example, they might assign 15 minutes to each unit, and the speech-language pathologist might indicate she spent 3 units of therapy time (using CPT code 92507) with a client. This does not mean that three of that CPT codes are being billed. The facility is just using the artificial unit as a measure of productivity. When the bill is sent off to Medicare for those Part B services, they only submit one 92507 CPT code.

Exceptions for Medicare-covered evaluation codes are as follows:

- Evaluation for SGD (92607, first hour; 92608, each additional 30 minutes)
- Evaluation of auditory rehabilitation status (92626, first hour; 92627, each additional 30 minutes).
- Assessment of aphasia (96105, per hour)
- Standardized cognitive performance testing (96125, per hour)

A timed code is billed only if face-to-face time spent in an evaluation is at least 51% of the time designated in the code's descriptor. For example, to bill 1 hour of the code 92607, the speech-language pathologist should have spent 31 minutes face-to-face with the client. In order to bill 92608 for the additional 30 minutes, the speech-language pathologist would have to have spent the full 60 minutes to code 92607, and then at least one-half (16 minutes) of the 30 minutes required to code the 92608. The descriptions of 96105 and 96125 indicate that the hour also includes interpretation and report writing. So, if you spend an hour with the client and at least another 31 minutes analyzing, scoring, and writing the report, you could charge two of the 1-hour codes (e.g., assessment of aphasia, standardized cognitive performance testing). If you spent 25 minutes assessing the client and 20 writing the report (total 45 minutes), you could submit the code once because you spent at least 31 minutes. If you spent less than 31 minutes total with the client and writing the report, you could report the code, but you would have to use the modifier -52 to indicate that the evaluation was shorter than typical (Swanson, 2014).

There are a few timed treatment codes, and typically Medicare covers cognitive skills development but may not cover the other two treatment codes. The speech-language pathologist should check with the MAC. Speech-language pathologists may use sensory integration and self-care/home management codes with payers other than Medicare, although it is always a good idea to check with individual third-party payers to determine whether they will reimburse for the code:

- Cognitive skills development (97532, each 15 minutes)
- Sensory integration (97533, each 15 minutes)
- Self-care/home management training (97535, each 15 minutes)

For CPT codes designated as 15 minutes, follow what is called the *8-minute rule*:

- 1 unit: 8 minutes to <23 minutes
- 2 units: 23 minutes to <38 minutes
- 3 units: 38 minutes to <53 minutes
- 4 units: 53 minutes to <68 minutes
- 5 units: 68 minutes to <83 minutes
- 6 units: 83 minutes to <98 minutes (ASHA, n.d.-i)

Further information and examples of timed code use and documentation of these codes is found in other chapters in this book. As these coding rules apply specifically to Medicare B, Chapter 14 provides more detail.

Edits, Modifiers, and Other Rules for Current Procedural Terminology Codes

Correct Coding Initiative Edits and Medically Unlikely Edits

In addition to the guidelines about the use of diagnostic and procedure codes already mentioned, there are other coding rules that must be followed to facilitate reimbursement. These rules are found in two different kinds of edit tables: Correct Coding Initiative (CCI) edits and Medically Unlikely Edits.

The National CCI is an automated edit system to control specific CPT code pairs that can be reported on the same day. It is used for all Medicare Part B and all Medicaid claims. The goal of CCI is to eliminate two codes that would

Table 4-3

Example of Correct Coding Initiative Edits

Current Procedural Terminology Procedure 1	Paired With (One)	Can Be Performed on the Same Date?	If So, Use What Modifier?
92521 (fluency evaluation)	96105, 96125	Yes	-59 (Attach to code in column 2)
92612 (fiberoptic evaluation of swallowing)	31575, 92511, 92520, 92614	No	N/A

Adapted from American Speech-Language-Hearing Association. (n.d.). National Correct Coding Initiative (CCI) and Outpatient Code Editor (OCE) edit tables. Retrieved from http://www.asha.org/Practice/reimbursement/coding/CCI-Edit-Tables-SLP/

not normally make sense to be billed on the same date to the same client. Some codes can never be billed on the same day, whereas others can if a modifier is added. The modifier -59 can be added to indicate that although the two codes are not usually billed together, they were separate and distinct services on the date in question.

As seen in Table 4-3, 92521, fluency evaluation, and 96105, assessment of aphasia, can be performed and billed on the same date of service if the modifier -59 is applied. However, 92612, fiberoptic evaluation of swallowing, cannot be billed on the same day as 92520, laryngeal function studies, even if a modifier were applied (ASHA, n.d.-k).

Another set of edits are called Medically Unlikely Edits. These edits are a subset of the Outpatient Code Editor and indicate how many of a timed code can be billed on the same date of service. An upper limit of three is placed on assessment of aphasia (96105) and two on standardized cognitive performance testing (96125). If more than that number of codes is submitted, it would not be reimbursed (ASHA, n.d.-g).

Therapy Modifiers and Sometimes and Always Therapy Codes

When a procedure is performed by a rehabilitation professional, a therapy modifier must be attached to indicate who performed the procedure:

- GP = physical therapy
- GO = occupational therapy
- GN = speech-language pathology

There is no known explanation for why speech-language pathology uses GN and not a more logical GS.

CMS defines some codes as *always therapy* codes, regardless of who performs them; the therapy modifier must be applied. Other codes are *sometimes therapy* codes, and, if performed by a therapist, the modifier must be attached. If a procedure has the therapy modifier, all the documentation rules for therapy must be followed (e.g., plan of care, therapy cap). It might seem odd that someone who is not a speech-language pathologist would perform a procedure typically performed by the speech-language pathologist, but in physicians' offices, these procedures are sometimes performed by a nurse or nurse practitioner. An example of an always therapy code is 92507, individual therapy. An example of a sometimes therapy code is 92610, clinical swallow evaluation (ASHA, n.d.-m).

Modifiers Regarding Length of Service

Two other modifiers are used to indicate whether the service provided was more or less extensive than that described in the CPT code. Modifier -22 indicates that the service was more extensive (but don't expect to be reimbursed a higher rate). Modifier -52 indicates the service was less extensive and that not everything described in the code was completed. The payer may or may not decide to reimburse at a lower rate (Swanson, 2014).

Code for Habilitative

Beginning in 2017, states may require use of the SZ modifier to indicate that services were habilitative. This applies to patients with Affordable Care Act (ACA)-compliant health plans, Medicaid Managed Care, or those newly enrolled in Medicaid. At the time of this writing, specific guidelines had not been established. To locate ACA plans operating in your state, find the health insurance marketplace for your state online. When a patient presents requiring habilitation services and is enrolled in one of the ACA health plans, call the member services representative number on the card to ask whether the plan is an individual or small-group health plan. This is important because ACA-compliant plans only pertain to individual and small-group health insurance products. Having the patient's member ID will help the member representative locate that information. ACA-compliant plans can choose how to operationalize the separate visit limits for habilitation services and may not require use of the SZ modifier. Providers should not assume that they will because a claim could be returned unpaid if the plan is not set up to handle this modifier (Grooms, 2016).

Functional Outcomes Reporting: G-Codes

A requirement that began in 2012 as part of a law called the Middle Class Tax Relief and Job Creation Act is that therapists document the functional status of clients in the

Table 4-4

Severity Modifiers to Functional Outcomes Reporting

Functional Severity Modifier	Description in Functional Outcomes Reporting for G-Codes	Equivalent National Outcomes Measurement System Functional Communication Measure Level
CH	0% impaired, limited, or restricted	7
CI	At least 1% but less than 20% impaired, limited, or restricted	6
CJ	At least 20% but less than 40% impaired, limited, or restricted	5
CK	At least 40% but less than 60% impaired, limited, or restricted	4
CL	At least 60% but less than 80% impaired, limited, or restricted	3
CM	At least 80% but less than 100% impaired, limited, or restricted	2
CN	100% impaired, limited, or restricted	1

Adapted from American Speech-Language-Hearing Association. (n.d.). G-codes and severity modifiers for claims-based outcomes reporting. Retrieved from http://www.asha.org/Practice/reimbursement/medicare/G-Codes-and-Severity-Modifiers-for-Outcomes-Reporting/

areas they are addressing (e.g., receptive, expressive, swallowing, memory, motor speech) and measure change in that status at specific points in the treatment and at discharge. This reporting of functional outcomes, commonly referred to as *G-codes*, is done on the bill that is sent to Medicare for clients in the form of G-codes and modifiers. There are G-codes for seven functional areas and one *Other* to cover any other functional areas. Only one functional area can be reported at any one time, although it is likely that the speech-language pathologist is working on more than one area at once. For example, a client with aphasia might present with receptive and expressive language deficits along with some motor speech impairment. All three would be addressed simultaneously, but the clinician would have to select only one to report. That area is rated on a severity scale at specific points in therapy. The arbitrary scale has been mapped to the functional levels in the ASHA National Outcomes Measurement System (NOMS) (Table 4-4). At some point when the emphasis in therapy changes to one of the other areas, the clinician could close the initially reported G-code area with a discharge modifier and open another by reporting initial and projected status (ASHA, n.d.-b). Detailed information about G-codes can be found in Chapter 14.

Medicare Guidelines for Reimbursing Services

CMS establishes regulations that impose certain standards on providers. Many of these are explained in Chapter 15 of the Medicare Benefit Policy Manual (CMS, 2017a).

Although there are some national guidelines, some regulations are written by regional insurance companies contracted by CMS to administer the Medicare program. These contractors are called MACs and typically cover a multistate area (CMS, n.d.-a).

These guidelines are found in documents called LCDs. Most MACs write an LCD for speech-language services and a separate one for dysphagia services. The LCDs contain information about the type of service that is reimbursable, definitions of services, and typically a list of diagnostic and procedure codes covered by Medicare.

Some definitions found in the national Medicare Benefit Policy Manual are important concepts related to funding and reimbursement. Although these are Medicare regulations, most other payers impose similar guidelines. Speech-language pathologists need to check with the payer source and their facility and state regulations to determine which of these guidelines apply for clients whose services are not being reimbursed by Medicare B.

- *Under the care of a physician*: In order for Medicare to pay for the therapy service, the client must be under the care of a physician.
- *Medically necessary*: Services are medically necessary if the documentation indicates that they meet the requirements for medical necessity, including that they are skilled rehabilitative services provided by clinicians with the approval of a physician/non–physician provider, safe, and effective (i.e., progress indicates that the care is effective in rehabilitation of function).
- *Reasonable and necessary*: It should be expected that the individual's rehabilitation potential is significant in relation to the extent and duration of therapy services. If it is not, the services are not considered reasonable and necessary.
- *Skilled service*: Skilled services are those that require the services of a certified, licensed speech-language pathologist and could not be safely and effectively furnished by someone less skilled. For example, practicing an effortful swallow to clear residue throughout a meal would not be considered skilled. However, that same activity, when first introduced to the patient with the speech-language pathologist providing cues, changing the difficulty of the task based on the analysis of the client's performance, and providing reinforcement, indicates a level of skill that could not be provided by a caregiver or family member (CMS, 2017a). More information about documenting skilled service can be found in Chapter 8.
- *Expectation of improvement*: Historically, Medicare reimbursed for services only if the client was expected to make improvements, even with a chronic, progressive, degenerative, or terminal illness. If no improvement was expected, a maintenance program could be established, but therapy was not likely to be covered. In 2013, in the case of *Jimmo v. Sebelius*, the court determined that Medicare may not deny speech-language pathology services simply because the beneficiary shows no functional progress, such as those individuals with degenerative and progressive diseases (e.g., multiple sclerosis, Parkinson's disease, and amyotrophic lateral sclerosis). Rather, Medicare must cover skilled services that prevent deterioration and maintain functional levels, not just those that result in functional progress (CMS, n.d.-b). Chapters 11 and 12 contain information about the impact of this ruling when treating patients in palliative and hospice care.

Reimbursement for Speech-Language Pathologist Services

Regardless of the setting in which services are provided, someone has to pay for the services. Most often this is some type of insurance, called *third-party reimbursement*. The first party is the patient and the second is the provider. The three major third-party payers are Medicare, Medicaid, and private insurance companies. On rare occasions, the patient pays privately for services (i.e., private pay). Third-party payers have rules and regulations that must be followed in order for them to reimburse for speech-language pathology services. Medicare has the most stringent guidelines, and these are often adopted by other payers. Speech-language pathologists need to understand how funding for services works and must follow the regulations established by each payer.

Government-Sponsored Reimbursement Programs

A brief overview of the entities involved in establishing, implementing, and managing these programs is provided to facilitate understanding how speech-language pathology services are funded.

Congress enacted the laws that established the Medicare and Medicaid programs, and although these laws can be lengthy documents, they usually do not have all the details needed to implement the law. This level of detail is delegated to a regulatory agency. In regard to reimbursement, for example, Congress passed the laws establishing both Medicare and Medicaid but then delegated to CMS the task of writing all the regulations needed to interpret and implement the law. For Medicare, CMS then contracts with insurance companies to further define, interpret, and implement these regulations. These agencies are called MACs, and one MAC covers a region of the country. As Medicaid is a joint program of the federal and state governments, both CMS and the states have regulatory control of Medicaid.

Medicare

Medicare is insurance for individuals aged 65 years and older and also for younger people who are disabled and eligible for Social Security. Medicare was established in 1965 and was the first legislation to provide national health coverage. This original Medicare included only Parts A and B (Anderson, 2016).

Now there are four types of Medicare, and each covers a different type of care needed by the individual. They are as follows:

1. Medicare Part A: This covers what are considered inpatient services, including stays in acute care hospitals, skilled nursing facilities, inpatient rehabilitation facilities, and home health services. The facility is paid for all the services provided through a prospective payment arrangement, meaning that the amount of payment has been predetermined and is not dependent on how many services the client receives (CMS, n.d.-c).
2. Medicare Part B: This part of Medicare covers what are considered outpatient services. Not every person who has Part A Medicare also has Part B, because the beneficiary has to pay monthly premiums to have Part B. Medicare Part B services are currently reimbursed on a fee-for-service basis, and those fees are adjusted yearly and published in the MPFS (ASHA, n.d.-l).
3. Medicare Part C: Medicare Parts A and B are considered original or regular Medicare. Medicare Part C is a managed-care form of Medicare. It operates much like insurance that working-age adults have (e.g., a health maintenance organization). Medicare Part C was first established in the mid-1980s with two goals: Offering Medicare beneficiaries a choice of plans and transferring to Medicare some of the cost-saving strategies that had been achieved by managed care in the private sector (McGuire, Newhouse. & Sinaiko, 2011). Medicare Part C must offer the same coverage offered by Parts A and B but may also offer additional coverage.
4. Medicare Part D: This coverage, added in 2003, is for the cost of drugs (Oliver, Lee, & Lipton, 2004). Most beneficiaries pay a monthly premium, a yearly deductible, and a copayment for each prescription. However, some low-income Medicare beneficiaries can get help with Part D costs if they qualify for a low-income subsidy, called *Extra Help*, to help pay costs associated with Part D plans (Center for Medicare Advocacy, n.d.).

Many individuals who have Medicare Parts A and B choose to purchase a private insurance plan to act as a secondary insurance. These are called *Medicare supplemental policies* or *Medigap policies.* These supplemental policies pay for things that Medicare does not. For example, a Medigap policy often covers the copays and deductibles. Beneficiaries who use Medicare Part C (Medicare Advantage) cannot purchase a supplemental Medigap plan (CMS, 2014).

Medicaid

Medicaid is a federal-state partnership, created to provide health coverage for low-income families and children, pregnant women, elderly people, and people with disabilities. Eligibility is determined by household income. Working adults may qualify based on their income when they cannot afford private insurance. As part of the ACA (2010), some states expanded coverage, covering more working adults. Medicaid functions much like private insurance, and many states now have managed Medicaid plans, with requirements for preauthorizations, a limit on the number of therapy visits, and some copays. Although states are required to cover certain services, they may differ on what type of services are covered and how much Medicaid reimburses for those services (Medicaid.gov, 2018).

Private Insurance

Many individuals under the age of 65 have private insurance. This may be a benefit offered by the company at which they work, or they might purchase the insurance on their own to cover them and their families. Each insurance company can establish its own rules for what it covers, how much it will reimburse, and how it will reimburse. Companies may offer different kinds of plans for an individual to select. Most private insurance plans now are HMOs, preferred provider organizations, and high-deductible plans, which are all forms of managed care.

As each insurance plan is different, no specific details can be provided here about which companies cover speech-language services in outpatient settings. However, there are certain terms that apply to private insurance coverage for outpatient services. A deductible is the amount of money the insured individual has to pay him- or herself before insurance starts to cover. Once the deductible is met, the insurance company pays a percentage and the insured pays a percentage. For example, insurance might cover 80% and the insured 20%. The insured might also be responsible for a copay for each office visit or outpatient procedure. These copays are set at a specific dollar amount. For example, the insured might pay $25.00 for each office visit. These copays count toward the deductible the insured has to reach. Each policy period (usually a calendar year), there is an out-of-pocket limit. This is the most the individual will have to pay during that period. Once that limit is reached, the insurance company pays 100% (Figure 4-5).

Retrospective and Prospective Payment Systems

The payers described previously may utilize different methods, or systems, to reimburse for services. There are two basic ways that a service will be reimbursed by these third-party payers. The payer agrees to pay for each of the services that were delivered (retrospective), or can set reimbursement amounts before the services are rendered

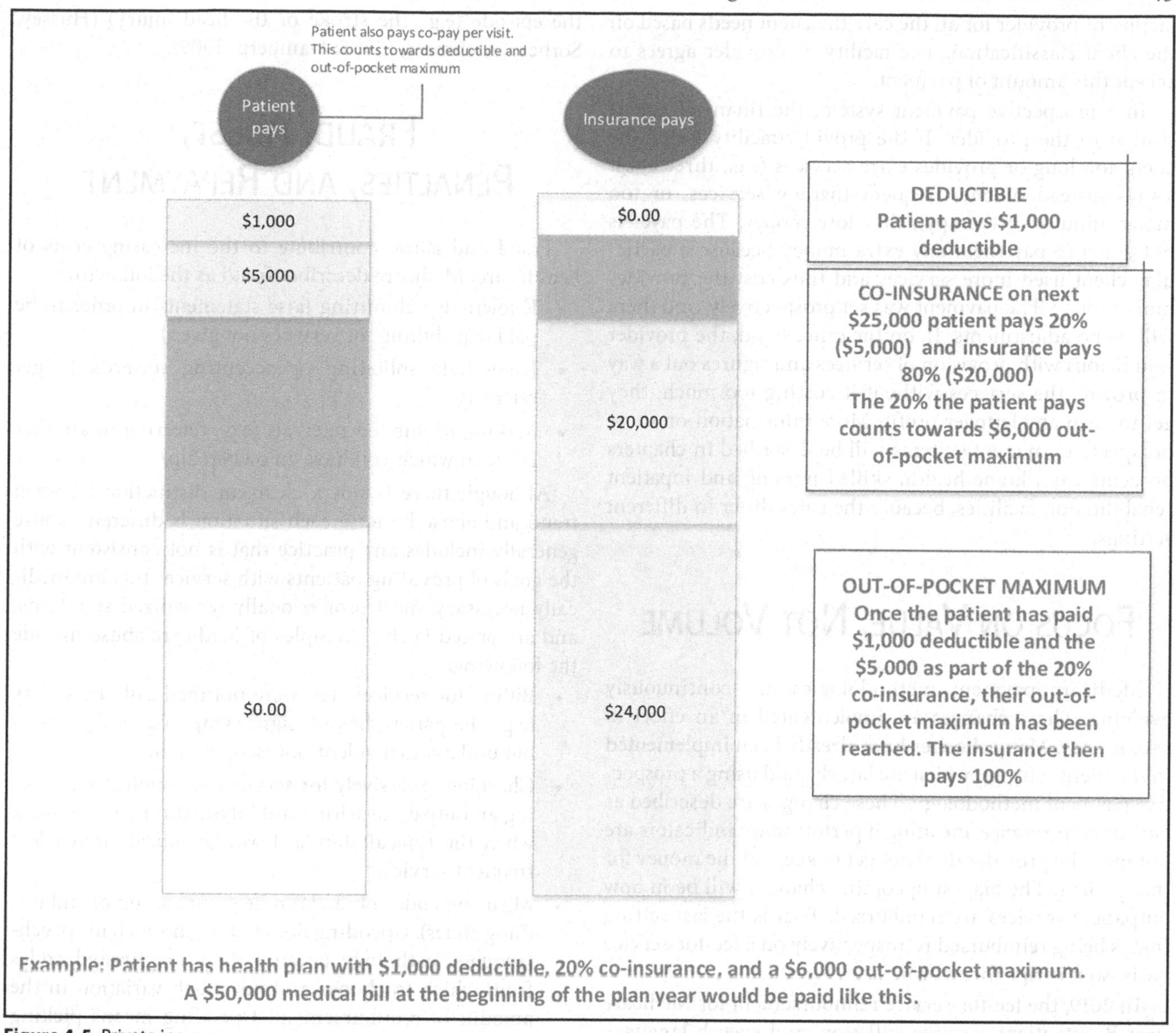

Figure 4-5. Private insurance.

(prospective). In a prospective payment system, the payment is still sent to the provider after the services are given.

Retrospective Payment

Simply put, a retrospective payment system means that the provider (e.g., the speech-language pathologist in private practice, rehabilitation agency, outpatient clinic) provides the services, and afterwards, perhaps at the end of each month, sends the bill to the third-party payer, who then reimburses the provider. In a retrospective payment system, there is no pressure on the provider to control costs. The provider is under no financial risk. Instead the focus is on volume. That is, the more services provided, the higher the bill and the more the facility or individual will be reimbursed. All financial risk is on the third-party payer because they have agreed to pay for the services provided after the fact (retrospectively). In retrospective payment systems, the payer may have attempted to control costs by establishing the amount (fee) they would pay for each service. They may also have also set a limit on the number of visits. When that happens, it is an example of a managed retrospective payment system.

Prospective Payment

As retrospective payment systems caused health care costs to spiral out of control, Medicare, Medicaid, and private insurance companies have largely switched to prospective payment systems in most inpatient settings. This means that in advance of a client ever needing a service, the insurer has determined what the payment should be. They pay per day, per stay, or per a predefined episode of care (e.g., 60 days). The payment is still sent to the provider after the stay, but the amount has been established prospectively. In each setting, there are different client classification systems that are used to help determine different rates. They prospectively set the amount they are willing to pay the facility or provider for all the care the client needs based on the client classification. The facility or provider agrees to accept this amount of payment.

In a prospective payment system, the financial risk is shifted to the provider. If the provider/facility keeps the client too long or provides extra services (e.g., three chest x-rays instead of one, frequent therapy services, or too many minutes of therapy), they lose money. The payer is not going to pay them any extra money because a particular client used more services and thus cost the provider more money. The payment was set prospectively, and there will be no adjustments. If, on the other hand, the provider is judicious with provision of services and figures out a way to provide the services without it costing too much, they get to keep any leftover profit. More information on these prospective payment systems will be described in chapters on acute care, home health, skilled nursing and inpatient rehabilitation facilities, because the rules differ in different settings.

Focus on Value, Not Volume

Medicare payment methodologies are continuously evolving. These changes are implemented in an effort to save money. Many changes have already been implemented in inpatient settings, which are largely paid using a prospective payment methodology. These changes are described as *pay for performance*, meaning if performance indicators are not met, the provider does not get to keep all the money for that patient. The biggest upcoming changes will be in how outpatient services are reimbursed. That is the last setting that is being reimbursed retrospectively on a fee-for-service basis, so it is ripe for reform.

In 2019, the fee-for-service reimbursement for Medicare Part B outpatient services will stop, and speech-language pathologists in health care settings will have to participate in one of two systems under Medicare's new Quality Payment Program. The provider can choose to participate in the Alternative Payment Models of the Merit-Based Incentive Payment System (Warren & Grooms, 2017).

Other changes may occur, such as reimbursement per an episode of care payment schema. In such a method, Medicare might provide a prospective payment to a group of facilities (e.g., acute care hospital, rehabilitation facility, home health agency, outpatient therapy provider) that will have to cover all the services provided to the patient at each of those settings across the continuum of care for the episode (e.g., the stroke or the head injury) (Hussey, Sorbero, Mehrotra, Liu, & Damberg, 2009).

Fraud, Abuse, Penalties, and Repayment

Fraud and abuse contribute to the increasing costs of health care. Medicare describes fraud as the following:

- Knowingly submitting false statements in order to be paid (e.g., billing for services not given)
- Knowingly soliciting or accepting rewards to get referrals
- Making prohibited referrals (e.g., referring to another clinic in which you have an ownership)

Although there is not a clear-cut distinction between fraud and abuse because each situation is different, abuse generally includes any practice that is not consistent with the goals of providing patients with services that are medically necessary, meet professionally recognized standards, and are priced fairly. Examples of Medicare abuse include the following:

- Billing for services that were not medically necessary (e.g., the patient has no signs/symptoms of dysphagia but undergoes a videofluoroscopic exam)
- Charging excessively for services or supplies (e.g., seeing an outpatient with a mild dysarthria 5 times/week when the typical standard would indicate much less frequent service)
- Misusing codes on a claim, (e.g., upcoding or unbundling codes). Upcoding does not occur much in speech-language pathology because there are limited codes from which to choose and not much variation in the amount of reimbursement. Upcoding means picking the code that will be reimbursed at a higher rate (CMS, 2017b).

CMS wants to ensure that the services they paid for were provided to the right clients at the right time, with the right intensity and for the proper length of time. They actively work to find fraud and abuse. Just because Medicare has paid a provider does not mean the provider necessarily gets to keep that money. CMS has contracted with agencies called Recovery Audit Contractors (RACs). The RACs' job is to audit claims sent to Medicare and uncover any questionable charges, which the facility then has to repay. RACs are paid a percentage of what they recover (CMS, 2016b).

The Speech-Language Pathologist's Responsibility in Compliance

Following Medicare reimbursement guidelines and carefully documenting service provided are the best way for a clinician and the facility to avoid being audited and having to repay funds.

Some places that employ speech-language pathologists do not involve the clinician in the coding and billing process. Someone else may be applying the diagnostic and procedure codes. They may even dictate the number of visits or how long the treatment should continue. However, these decisions are rightfully made by the treating speech-language pathologist, and it is the speech-language pathologist's license and certification that are in jeopardy if the rules of coding, documentation, and reimbursement are not followed. The speech-language pathologist should never agree to provide services that are not medically necessary, apply a code that is not accurate just to get reimbursed, continue services past the point of the client making measurable gains, or apply a diagnosis that is not accurate to maximize reimbursement.

Fraud and Abuse Applies With All Payers

ASHA's Issues in Ethics Statement: Representation of Services for Insurance Reimbursement, Funding, or Private Payment delineates the following specific situations related to reimbursement that would be unethical:

- Misrepresenting information to obtain reimbursement or funding, regardless of the motivation of the provider.
  - Do not select a CPT code for the sole purpose of getting reimbursed. The speech-language pathologist must select the code that most accurately describes the service provided.
  - Do not select an ICD-10 code because that diagnosis is covered by a payer when it is not the most accurate code to describe the communication or swallowing disorder.
- Providing service when there is no reasonable expectation of significant communication or swallowing benefit for the person served.
  - An example would be evaluating every resident in a skilled nursing facility.
- Scheduling services more frequently or for longer than is reasonably necessary.
- Scheduling more frequent visits/week than is necessary to achieve the goals.
- Requiring staff to provide more hours of care (e.g., the "3-hour rule") than can be justified in a Prospective Payment environment such as acute rehabilitation, long-term care, or home care.
- Supervision of students or other service providers in a fee-for-service environment.
- Providing professional courtesies or complementary care for referrals or otherwise
- Discounting care not based on documented need (ASHA, 2010).

References

All Things Medical Billing. (n.d.). The history of medical coding. Retrieved from http://www.all-things-medical-billing.com/history-of-medical-coding.html

American Medical Association. (2016a). About CPT coding. Retrieved from https://www.ama-assn.org/practice-management/cpt-current-procedural-terminology

American Medical Association. (2016b). CPT(R) process: How a code becomes a code. Retrieved from http://www.ama-assn.org/ama/pub/physician-resources/solutions-managing-your-practice/coding-billing-insurance/cpt/cpt-process-faq/code-becomes-cpt.page

American Speech-Language-Hearing Association. (n.d.-a). About ICD-10-CM for audiology and speech-language pathology. Retrieved from http://www.asha.org/Practice/reimbursement/coding/About-ICD-10-CM-for-Audiology-and-Speech-Language-Pathology/

American Speech-Language-Hearing Association. (n.d.-b). Claims-based outcomes reporting for Medicare Part B therapy services. Retrieved from http://www.asha.org/Practice/reimbursement/medicare/Claims-Based-Outcomes-Reporting-for-Medicare-Part-B/

American Speech-Language-Hearing Association. (n.d.-c). Coding for reimbursement. Retrieved from http://www.asha.org/practice/reimbursement/coding/

American Speech-Language-Hearing Association. (n.d.-d). Coding normal results frequently asked questions. Retrieved from http://www.asha.org/practice/reimbursement/coding/normalresults/

American Speech-Language-Hearing Association. (n.d.-e). Current Procedural Terminology (CPT) codes. Retrieved from http://www.asha.org/practice/reimbursement/coding/SLPCPT.htm

American Speech-Language-Hearing Association. (n.d.-f). Health Care Common Procedure Coding System (HCPCS) level II codes. Retrieved from http://www.asha.org/Practice/reimbursement/coding/hcpcs_slp/

American Speech-Language-Hearing Association. (n.d.-g). Medically unlikely edits for speech-language pathology services. Retrieved from http://www.asha.org/Practice/reimbursement/coding/Medically-Unlikely-Edits-SLP/

American Speech-Language-Hearing Association. (n.d.-h). Medicare coverage policy on speech-generating devices. Retrieved from http://www.asha.org/practice/reimbursement/medicare/sgd_policy/

American Speech-Language-Hearing Association. (n.d.-i). Medicare CPT coding rules for speech-language pathology services. Retrieved from http://www.asha.org/practice/reimbursement/medicare/SLP_coding_rules/

American Speech-Language-Hearing Association. (n.d.-j). Model speech-language pathology superbill. Retrieved from http://www.asha.org/uploadedFiles/Model-Superbill-SLP.docx

American Speech-Language-Hearing Association. (n.d.-k). National Correct Coding Initiative: Speech-language pathology edits. Retrieved from http://www.asha.org/Practice/reimbursement/coding/CCI_edits_SLP/

American Speech-Language-Hearing Association. (n.d.-l). The outpatient Medicare physician fee schedule. Retrieved from http://www.asha.org/practice/reimbursement/medicare/feeschedule/

American Speech-Language-Hearing Association. (n.d.-m). Overview of the Medicare physician fee schedule. Retrieved from http://www.asha.org/Practice/reimbursement/medicare/Overview-of-the-Medicare-Physician-Fee-Schedule/

American Speech-Language-Hearing Association. (2010). Issues in ethics: Representation of services for insurance reimbursement, funding, or private payment. Retrieved from http://www.asha.org/Practice/ethics/Representation-of-Services/

American Speech-Language-Hearing Association (2018). ICD-10-CM Diagnosis Codes for Audiology and Speech-Language Pathology. Retrieved from: https://www.asha.org/Practice/reimbursement/coding/ICD-10/

Anderson, S. (2016). A brief history of Medicare in America. Retrieved from https://www.medicareresources.org/basic-medicare-information/brief-history-of-medicare/

Centers for Disease Control and Prevention. (2017). ICD-10-CM official guidelines for coding and reporting FY 2017 (October 1, 2016 - September 30, 2017). Retrieved from https://www.cdc.gov/nchs/data/icd/10cmguidelines_2017_final.pdf

Center for Medicare Advocacy. (n.d.). Part D/Prescription Drug Benefits. Retrieved from http://www.medicareadvocacy.org/medicare-info/medicare-part-d/

Centers for Medicare & Medicaid Services. (n.d.-a). Contacts for Part B-Medicare Administrative Contractor (MAC-Part B) alphabetical index. Retrieved from https://www.cms.gov/medicare-coverage-database/indexes/contacts-part-b-medicare-administrative-contractor-index.aspx?bc=AgAAAAAAAAAA&

Centers for Medicare & Medicaid Services. (n.d.-b). *Jimmo v. Sebelius* settlement agreement fact sheet. Retrieved from https://www.cms.gov/medicare/medicare-fee-for-service-payment/SNFPPS/downloads/jimmo-factsheet.pdf.

Centers for Medicare & Medicaid Services. (n.d.-c). Long-term care hospitals. Retrieved from https://www.medicare.gov/coverage/long-term-care-hospitals.html

Centers for Medicare & Medicaid Services. (2014). Choosing a Medigap policy: A guide to health insurance for people with Medicare. Retrieved from https://www.medicare.gov/pubs/pdf/02110.pdf

Centers for Medicare & Medicaid Services. (2016a). Medicare coding: ICD-10. Retrieved from https://www.cms.gov/Medicare/Coding/ICD10/2016-ICD-10-CM-and-GEMs.html

Centers for Medicare & Medicaid Services. (2016b). Recovery Audit Contractors. Retrieved from https://www.cms.gov/research-statistics-data-and-systems/monitoring-programs/medicare-ffs-compliance-programs/recovery-audit-program/

Centers for Medicare & Medicaid Services. (2017a). Medicare Benefit Policy Manual: Chapter 15—Covered medical and other health services. Retrieved from https://www.cms.gov/Regulations-and-Guidance/Guidance/Manuals/downloads/bp102c15.pdf

Centers for Medicare & Medicaid Services. (2017b). Medicare fraud & abuse: Prevention, detection, and reporting. Retrieved from https://www.cms.gov/Outreach-and-Education/Medicare-Learning-Network-MLN/MLNProducts/downloads/Fraud_and_Abuse.pdf

Grooms, D. (2016). Get ready for new coding requirements for habilitation services. *ASHA Leader, 21*, 30–31. doi:10.1044/leader.BML.21102016.30

Hussey, P., Sorbero, M., Mehrotra, A., Liu, H., & Damberg, C. (2009). Using episodes of care as a basis for performance measurement and payment: Moving from concept to practice. *Health Affairs (Project Hope), 28*(5), 1406–1417. doi:10.1377/hlthaff.28.5.1406

Medicaid.gov. (2018). Keeping America Healthy. Retrieved from https://www.medicaid.gov/about-us/index.htmll

McGuire, T. G., Newhouse, J. P., & Sinaiko, A. D. (2011). An economic history of Medicare Part C. *Milbank Quarterly, 89*(2), 289–332.

Oliver, T. R., Lee, P. R., & Lipton, H. R. (2004). A political history of Medicare and prescription drug coverage. *Milbank Quarterly, 82*(2), 283–354.

Swanson, N. (2014). Bottom line: Cracking the new evaluation codes. *ASHA Leader, 19*, 30–31. doi:10.1044/leader.BML.19032014.30

University of Texas Department of Otorhinolaryngology. (n.d.). Current Procedural Technology: History, structure, process & controversies. Retrieved from https://med.uth.edu/orl/newsletter/current-procedural-technology-history-structure-process-controversies/

Warren, S., & Grooms, D. (2017). Change ahead for Medicare outpatient quality reporting and payment. *ASHA Leader, 22*, 26–28.

Review Questions

1. Describe the two major coding systems, who manages each, and the purposes of each.
2. Which code should be listed as primary on the speech-language pathologist's bill?
3. What is the relationship between CPT codes and HCPCS codes?
4. Describe the two government-sponsored third-party payers.
5. Discuss the difference between retrospective and prospective payment systems.
6. What is the difference between fraud and abuse?

Activity A

Download Medicare CPT Coding Rules for Speech-Language Pathology Services from ASHA's website (http://www.asha.org/practice/reimbursement/medicare/SLP_coding_rules.htm) and use it to answer the following questions:

1. Which code would you use if you were evaluating a patient with a tracheostomy for use of a speaking valve?
2. Which code can be used for an evaluation spanning more than 1 day?
3. How many individuals can be billed in the same group with the group therapy code?
4. Which code would be most appropriate to evaluate a client who had apraxia but no language involvement?
5. Which two codes can be used to describe different parts of a voice evaluation?
6. What document would you need to check to see if you could bill 97533, sensory integrative techniques, for a patient with Medicare Part B?
7. What codes are used for instrumental assessment of swallowing?
8. What are physical medicine codes, and can they be used by speech-language pathologists?
9. Which codes are timed?
10. What is the 8-minute rule?

Activity B

International Classification of Diseases, Tenth Revision, Clinical Modification *and Current Procedural Terminology Coding*

Download a copy of the ASHA Model Superbill (http://www.asha.org/uploadedFiles/Model-Superbill-SLP.docx). Hint: The code for pure tone hearing screening (92551) does not appear on the bill, so you may need to write this in. Note that if you are billing Medicare, Medicare does not pay for screening.

Also download the ICD-10 codes document (http://www.asha.org/uploadedFiles/ICD-10-Codes-SLP.pdf#search=%22for%22).

Using these two documents, fill out a bill for each of the following clients.

Preschooler Evaluation: Private Insurance

Four-year-old boy with multiple articulation errors and receptive and expressive language disorder is assessed. Has had multiple ear infections and surgery for placement of ventilation tubes. No other medical history. Hearing screening is also performed.

Dysphagia: Medicare

Seventy-four-year-old female with Parkinson's disease. Swallowing is getting worse. You assess the swallow clinically, and because she is showing signs of pharyngeal dysphagia, you are able to get her into radiology the same day for a videofluoroscopic swallowing study.

School-Aged Cleft Palate: Medicaid

Six-year-old female status post-repaired cleft of lip and palate. Fails hearing screening. You also assess articulation, resonance, and language skills. You note she is very hoarse, so you also complete a voice evaluation.

Preschoolers With Language and Phonological Awareness Deficits: Private Insurance

Three children, aged 3, 3.5, and 3.8 years, are seen together once/week for an hour-long session targeting their receptive language skills and phonological awareness. One child has a history of otitis media, one was born 2 months prematurely, and the other has no significant history. How is one of those sessions billed for each child?

Mild Cognitive Impairment Following Concussion: Medicare

Sixty-seven-year-old male suffered fall with no loss of consciousness, but diagnosed with concussion. Now has difficulty attending (particularly with distractions), comprehending complex reading material, and accessing short-term memory. You are with him 1 hour and 45 minutes during the evaluation and then spend another 40 minutes analyzing and writing the report. Hearing screening was completed.

5

Focus on Function and Outcomes

Nancy B. Swigert, MA, CCC-SLP, BCS-S

Focus on Function and Outcomes

It's all about the client: The services speech-language pathologists provide and how those services are documented. When clinicians keep that in mind, everything else falls into place. This chapter has purposely been placed at the end of Section I, "Basics of Documentation" and before the chapters that provide the details of documenting, coding, and billing different types of services in different settings. Keeping the focus on function informs decisions about which testing instruments to use, how goals are established, how progress is monitored, and how decisions about discharge are made.

Measuring and reporting outcomes also keeps the focus on function because outcomes are described in terms of what the client can do and what limitations the client may still have. Understanding outcome measurement tools and reporting systems will help the speech-language pathologist focus on an end goal important to the client. The stated outcome of intervention should not be an improvement in a few percentage points on a standardized test or a higher score on a scale, but on changes the client achieves that make a difference in his or her day-to-day life.

Models of Classification: The *International Classification of Diseases and Related Health Problems,* and the *International Classification of Functioning, Disability and Health*

Chapter 4 described the *International Classification of Diseases, Tenth Revision, Clinical Modification* (ICD-10-CM), which is the international system for coding diseases. The system focuses on what is wrong with the client that has resulted in him or her seeking health care services. It serves an important purpose in capturing data, but if that is the only classification system used by the clinician, the focus is on what is wrong and not at all on what the client's functional skills are and what other factors have an impact on her functioning (World Health Organization [WHO], 2016).

On the other hand, the *International Classification of Functioning, Disability and Health* (ICF) is a framework for classifying the consequences of disease, which then focuses

Swigert, N. B.
Documentation and Reimbursement for Speech-Language Pathologists: Principles and Practice (pp. 51-65).

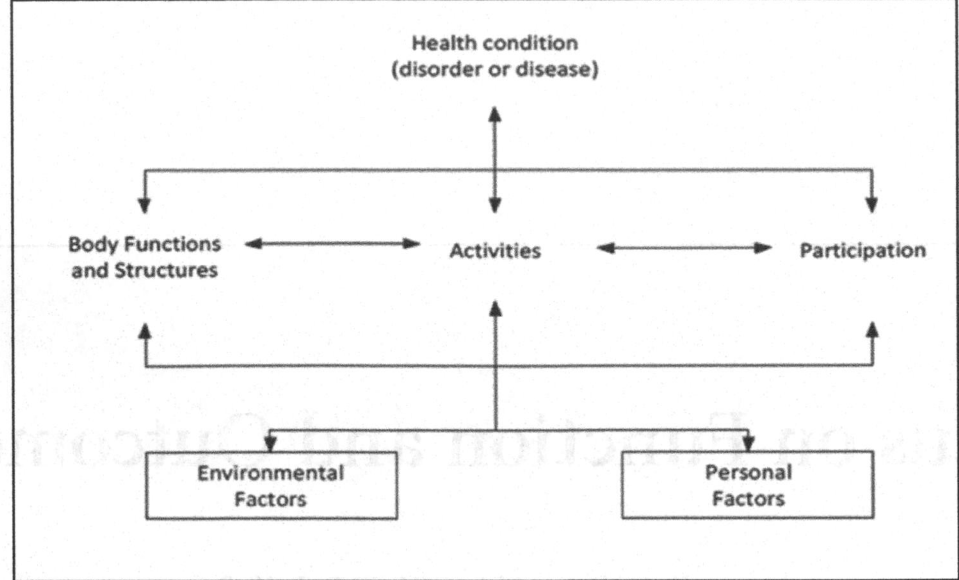

Figure 5-1. ICF model. (Reprinted with permission from World Health Organization. (2013). How to use the ICF: A practical manual for using the International Classification of Functioning Disability. Retrieved from http://www.who.int/classifications/drafticfpracticalmanual .pdf)

on function; that is, how the disease is impacting the client. The ICF complements the ICD-10-CM, and together they constitute the central classifications in the WHO's Family of International Classifications (Centers for Disease Control and Prevention, 2012).

International Classification of Functioning, Disability and Health Conceptual Model

In 2001, the WHO approved the *International Classification of Functioning, Disability and Health* and its abbreviation, ICF. The WHO was focused on the consequences of disease long before 2001; an earlier version of this classification system was first created in 1980. It was called the International Classification of *Impairments, Disabilities, and Handicaps* (ICIDH). The new ICF, however, reflected a major change in how the system was structured (Figure 5-1) (American Speech-Language-Hearing Association [ASHA], n.d.-a; WHO, 2013).

The ICF is structured around two comprehensive components:

1. Health conditions
   a. Body functions and structure (functioning at the level of the body; in the earlier model called *impairment*). These describe the anatomy and physiology/psychology of the human body.
   b. Activities (functioning at the level of the individual) and the activity limitations clients experience
   c. Participation in all areas of life (functioning of a person at the level of society) and the restrictions clients experience
4. Contextual factors
   a. Environmental factors that affect these experiences and whether these factors act as barriers or facilitators. These factors are not within the person's control, such as family, work, government agencies, laws, and cultural beliefs.
   b. Personal factors that influence how the disability is experienced, including things like age, race, gender, food preferences, habits, lifestyle, social background, and coping styles. Personal factors are not coded in the ICF because of the wide variability among cultures. They are represented in the framework, however, because they may have an influence on how a person functions. Personal factors can have a positive or negative impact on a person's function (Üstün, n.d.).

To help users further understand these factors, the WHO has developed definitions explaining how these terms are used in the context of health (Figure 5-2).

The system does not ignore the health condition and focus only on its impact, but relates the health condition to functioning and disability. Functioning and disability are considered part of a complex interaction between the health condition of the individual and the contextual factors of the environment and personal factors. It was designed to be relevant across cultures as well as age groups and genders, making it useful across heterogeneous populations (Centers for Disease Control and Prevention, 2012).

In the context of health:

Functioning is an umbrella term for body functions, body structures, activities and participation. It denotes the positive aspects of the interaction between an individual (with a health condition) and that individual's contextual factors (environmental and personal factors).

Disability is an umbrella term for impairments, activity limitations and participation restrictions. It denotes the negative aspects of the interaction between an individual (with a health condition) and that individual's contextual factors (environmental and personal factors).

Body functions - The physiological functions of body systems (including psychological functions).

Body structures - Anatomical parts of the body such as organs, limbs and their components.

Impairments - Problems in body function and structure such as significant deviation or loss.

Activity - The execution of a task or action by an individual.

Participation - Involvement in a life situation.

Activity limitations - Difficulties an individual may have in executing activities.

Participation restrictions - Problems an individual may experience in involvement in life situations.

Environmental factors - The physical, social and attitudinal environment in which people live and conduct their lives. These are either barriers to or facilitators of the person's functioning.

Figure 5-2. World Health Organization definitions for the International Classification of Functioning, Disability and Health. (Reprinted with permission from World Health Organization. (2013). How to use the ICF: A practical manual for using the International Classification of Functioning Disability. Retrieved from http://www.who.int/classifications/drafticfpracticalmanual .pdf)

Applying the International Classification of Functioning, Disability and Health *as a Conceptual Model in Daily Practice*

If clinicians fail to use the ICF framework, they may tend to focus on the impairment. Consider this impairment-based description provided by one speech-language pathologist to another, who will be working for the weekend.

> Mr. S is a 62-year-old who suffers from Parkinson's disease and has a moderate-severe dysphagia with reduced laryngeal elevation and hyolaryngeal excursion with resultant aspiration during the swallow and risk of aspiration after the swallow from residue in hypopharynx. He is on a pureed diet with small sips of thins.

Although this description may indeed tell the weekend speech-language pathologist what the impairment is and what needs to be worked on in therapy, does it really tell about Mr. S as a person? Using the ICF model, the hand-off might sound like this (with the ICF factors noted in bold):

> Mr. S is a 72-year-old who suffers from Parkinson's disease and has a moderate-severe dysphagia with reduced laryngeal elevation and hyolaryngeal excursion with resultant aspiration during the swallow and risk of aspiration after the swallow from residue in hypopharynx **(body functions and structure)**. He is on a pureed diet with small sips of thins and can eat this safely with minimal cues **(activity)**. He doesn't like to go to the dining room and sit with other residents because he has to eat so slowly **(participation)**. His wife will likely be here for all meals over the weekend, and she knows how to cue her husband though he is the patriarch of the family and doesn't really like taking suggestions from her **(environmental)**. However, he exhibits a good sense of humor and handles it well when she kids around with him **(personal)**.

If you were Mr. S, which description would you prefer the weekend speech-language pathologist have about you? Which comes closer to describing not just what is wrong with Mr. S, but also about how this disability has affected his functioning?

Purposes of the International Classification of Functioning, Disability and Health

Just as the ICD-10-CM has multiple purposes, so does the ICF. In a paper introducing the ICF, the WHO listed the aims of the ICF as follows:

- Providing a systematic coding system for health information
- Providing a basis for studying health and health-related states, outcomes, determinants, and changes in health status and functioning
- Establishing a common language for describing these health and health-related states, thus improving communication between different users (e.g., health care workers, researchers, policy makers)
- Permitting comparison of data across countries (Üstün, n.d.)

Using the International Classification of Functioning, Disability and Health *to Code Functioning Information*

Most speech-language pathologists use the ICF only as a conceptual model, but it also includes a coding system. It uses a system of numbers and letters, called *qualifiers*, to indicate things like severity and location. For example, structure of the pharynx is coded as s330, and structure of the oral pharynx is s3301 (Threats, 2007). There are similar codes for function, activities and participation, and environmental factors. The severity qualifiers range from 0 (no problem or within normal limits) to 4 (complete or profound problem). It is beyond the scope of this chapter to explain the ICF coding system, but speech-language pathologists should familiarize themselves with all aspects of the system (WHO, 2013). ASHA National Outcomes Measurement System (NOMS) users will be exposed to the ICF because clinicians will be requested to code body function/structure, activities/participation, and even environmental factors at admission and discharge. The goal is to stimulate use of the ICF with the intended impact of increasing clinicians' consideration of the patient perspective in planning treatment and evaluating its impact (Yorkston, 2015).

The ICF and ASHA Scope of Practice

The ASHA Scope of Practice includes a description of the WHO ICF framework and references how it interrelates with the following eight service delivery domains:

1. Collaboration
2. Counseling
3. Prevention and wellness
4. Screening
5. Assessment
6. Treatment
7. Modalities, technology, and instrumentation
8. Population and systems

The document states: "The ICF framework is useful in describing the breadth of the role of the SLP [speech-language pathologist] in the prevention, assessment, and habilitation/rehabilitation of communication and swallowing disorders and the enhancement and scientific investigation of those functions" (ASHA, 2016). The document also provides concrete examples of the components of the framework as applied to communication and swallowing disorders. These examples include the following:

- Body functions and structures: Craniofacial anomaly, vocal fold paralysis, cerebral palsy, stuttering, and language impairment
- Activity: Difficulties with swallowing safely for independent feeding, reading sentence-level material, and speaking intelligibly
- Participation: Eating with other residents in the dining room, participating actively in class, understanding a medical prescription, and accessing the general education curriculum
- Environmental factors: The role of the communication partner in augmentative and alternative communication, the influence of classroom acoustics on communication, and the impact of institutional dining environments on individuals' ability to safely maintain nutrition and hydration
- Personal factors: An individual's background or culture, if one or both influence his or her reaction to communication or swallowing

The document also reminds us that body structure and functions, activity, and participation exist on a continuum. For example, in body structure and functions, the range might be from normal variation to total impairment (ASHA, 2016).

Other ASHA Resources on the ICF

The ASHA website has numerous documents on person-centered treatment that guide a clinician through analyzing assessment data, using clinical reasoning, and goal setting. The handouts help the clinician see that assessment data should not just be those factors in body structures and function, but that information should also be gathered on activities and participation as well as on environmental and personal factors. The documents also lead the clinician through clinical reasoning in each of three areas: Body structure and function, activities and participation, and environmental and personal factors. They also show how to use this information for setting long-term and short-term goals (see Appendices 5-A and 5-B for examples) (ASHA, n.d.-a).

Outcomes: Results of Care and How These Are Reported

The focus on function aligns with seeking an outcome that is meaningful to the client. Many different types of results are often measured and reported in health care. Most speech-language pathology departments in health care organizations participate in the facility's performance improvement, or quality improvement, program. This typically involves identifying a process that is not working as effectively or efficiently as it should, identifying ways to improve the process, and then measuring the change in that process over time. Four different kinds of measures may be used in these performance improvement activities: Process measures, outcomes measures, patient satisfaction/patient experience measures, and patient reported outcome (PRO) measures.

Process Measures

Process measures capture things like meeting productivity standards or adhering to certain guidelines. For example, productivity standards at a facility might be set at having the speech-language pathologist spend 75% of his or her time with clients in billable activities. The performance of each clinician in the department might be measured and reported compared with that standard. Perhaps the department or practice has a guideline that all evaluation reports be written and in the chart within a certain number of days of the evaluation or that all calls from clients be returned within a certain number of hours. These are process measures.

Outcomes Measures

Outcomes measures are measures of the end result (i.e., the outcome) of what happens to clients as a result of their encounter(s) with the health care system (Rodenhauser, 2000). The same could be said for educational settings. These outcomes cannot be attributed to what happened during the encounter, just that after the encounter this is how the client is functioning. For example, imagine a client has a moderate phonological disorder and receives 6 months of speech-language therapy. At the end of that encounter, the client presents with phonological skills within functional limits. That information can be collected on an outcomes tool, but without experimental controls, it cannot be proved that the treatment the client received is what caused the improvement.

Outcomes data collected during the course of typical clinical practice are usually not accompanied by data from controls, as a typical research study would. A research study could be constructed to actually show that the intervention provided was responsible for the change in the client's phonological skills. Outcomes data become more powerful when collected for a large number of clients. The larger the data base, the more granular the conclusions. One can still not claim that the intervention is what resulted in the change. Generalized statements from outcomes data are typically made, such as the following:

- Clients who are 4 years old and present with moderate impairment in language progress to a mild impairment after at least X number of individual sessions.
- Males who are over 70 years old and have a stroke that results in severe apraxia typically improve to moderate apraxia in outpatient settings after X hours of individual treatment.
- X% of patients admitted to skilled nursing facilities with Parkinson's disease who are on a pureed diet and thickened liquids progress to a mechanical soft diet with thin liquids after X hours of treatment.

ASHA's NOMS is a voluntary data collection system developed to illustrate the value of speech-language pathology services provided to adults and children with communication and swallowing disorders. Speech-language pathologists or audiologists working in health care or school settings can register their organization in the NOMS program and become a participating data collection site. Speech-language pathology health care, currently in revision at the time of this printing, will have sections for adults, pre-Kindergarten, and K-12. Eventually there are plans to add an early intervention section as well. These planned revisions may also include PROs, economic modeling, and a taxonomy of treatment goals, targets, and ingredients to better understand the comparative effectiveness of different treatment approaches (Yorkston, 2015).

NOMS utilizes seven-point scales called Functional Communication Measures (FCMs). FCMs are disorder-specific rating scales designed to describe the change in an individual's functional communication and/or swallowing ability over time. Level 1 is the most impaired, Level 5 indicates a level of independence, and Level 7 is considered functional. Based on an individual's treatment plan/Individualized Education Program, FCMs are chosen and scored by a certified speech-language pathologist on admission and again at discharge from speech-language pathology services to depict the level at which the client is functioning in communication and/or swallowing abilities at each of those points in time. These data are submitted to ASHA's national registry. In addition to scoring the FCMs, speech-language pathologists also provide basic information on patient/client demographics and intervention characteristics (e.g., speech-language pathology diagnosis, frequency/intensity of treatment).

Speech-language pathologists and their participating facility(s) and/or school(s) have access to their data benchmarked by treatment setting and diagnosis against the national data and system data if applicable. Facilities can also generate customized analyses of their data, as well as national data, using the web-based reporting system (ASHA, n.d.-b).

The speech-language pathologist will also encounter other measurement tools in certain settings. For example, in skilled nursing facilities, the speech-language pathologist (and physical and occupational therapists) will be asked to help score patients on the Minimum Data Set, at inpatient rehabilitation settings on the Inpatient Rehabilitation Facility-Patient Assessment Instrument (IRF-PAI)/Functional Independence Measure (FIM) and in home health settings on the Outcomes Assessment Information Set (OASIS). These patient assessments were not designed to be used as outcomes tools, but the data derived from them have sometimes been used in that way. Other tools are in development. The Consultation and Relational Empathy (CARE) tool is being tested as a standardized patient assessment instrument to measure severity in hospitals and in post–acute care settings (Gage, 2014).

Medicare collects the information from those tools and, in outpatient settings, requires the clinician to collect information on the patient's functional limitations at the start of therapy, periodically throughout, and at the conclusion of therapy. This collection of functional limitations was designed to help the Centers for Medicare & Medicaid Services better understand beneficiaries' conditions, outcomes, and expenditures. This system is commonly referred to as *G-codes*, which are seven-point scales used to capture the beneficiary's limitations in communication and swallowing. Physical and occupational therapy also use G-codes specific to functional limitations in their areas (Centers for Medicare & Medicaid Services, 2014).

Patient Satisfaction/Patient Experience Measures

Patient satisfaction or patient experience often centers on the quality of services rendered. Think about the last time you completed a survey for a hotel or airline. Questions usually include topics like timeliness, friendliness of staff, and quality of food. On satisfaction instruments, consumers don't rate a service solely on the outcome, but on their perceptions of the entire process of service delivery. For example, the communication disorder for which they sought treatment is improved through therapy, but the office staff was rude and there was frequently a long wait time before each appointment. The outcome was good, but parts of the process were not. In addition, it is only the patient who can determine the criteria that matter when measuring satisfaction (Shelton, 2000). Shelton summarizes areas of patient satisfaction typically measured. Most of these are easily applicable to an outpatient setting in which speech-language pathology services are rendered. In addition to the patient's perception of the quality of the service received, these include the following:

- Access
  - How easy is it to schedule appointments by phone?
  - How easy is it to schedule the next appointment at the front desk?
  - Is there a long time between when the patient wants to be seen and when the appointment is set for?
- Convenience
  - Is the office located in an easy-to-reach area?
  - Are the hours of operation convenient?
  - Is parking available and easy to access?
- Communication
  - What is the patient's first impression of the provider?
  - How well does the provider explain the problem?
  - Does the provider listen?
  - Does the provider give necessary information for management of the problem?
- Personal caring
  - Were all staff in the office friendly?
  - Was the provider friendly?
  - Was the patient shown respect by all individuals?
- Facilities and equipment
  - What is the overall appearance of the office?
  - Is signage effective and easy to read?
  - Is the office clean?

Patient-Reported Outcomes

PRO measures differ from patient satisfaction/patient experience measures. PRO measures seek input from the client on the outcome of the service rendered. Whereas a clinician might determine the outcome of treatment was successful, the client's view might be entirely different. Suppose a client had a profound expressive language disorder following a stroke and was basically non-verbal. At the end of treatment, the client is able to use some single words and short phrases and supplements communication attempts with an augmentative system. The speech-language pathologist considers this a very successful outcome, but is that the view of the client and her family? Or consider a non-verbal 3-year-old with severe apraxia of speech who, at the conclusion of the preschool year, is using 50 words and signing short phrases. The clinician's view and the parent's view of the outcome of the intervention might differ significantly.

Funding agencies are interested in making sure that attention is being given to the patient's perspective when developing the treatment plan and in evaluating the outcomes. Because of this, PRO measures are gaining in popularity. Funding for research into PRO tools is increasing by federal health and research agencies. There is even an open-access journal on PROs, called *Patient Related Outcome Measures* (http://www.dovepress.com/patient-related-outcome-measures-journal).

PROs have been defined by the National Quality Forum as "any report of the status of a patient's health condition that comes directly from the patient, without interpretation of the patient's response by a clinician or anyone else" (National Quality Forum, n.d.). ASHA's National Center for Evidence-Based Practice in Communication Disorders uses a different operational definition because in some circumstances these data can be meaningful when completed by a caregiver, parent, or other proxy as long as it is transparent who is actually providing the data (Yorkston, 2015).

PRO tools measure what patients are able to do and how they feel by asking questions. These tools enable assessment of patient-reported health status for physical, mental, and social wellbeing. The National Quality Forum reports that a variety of patient-level instruments to measure PROs have been used for clinical research purposes and that many have been evaluated and catalogued within the National Institutes of Health's Patient-Reported Outcomes Measurement Information System.

PROs may include questions on the client's view of how well he or she is communicating or swallowing. These tools also often contain questions about the quality of life (QOL) the client is experiencing related to the communication or swallowing disorder. This mirrors the ICF model because the questions are not just about body structure and function. The QOL questions seek information about activities and participation. A primary principle of the ICF is that achieving the highest possible life functioning is the right of all human beings. The achievement of outcomes that are relevant to the person is more important than those outcomes chosen by the professional (Threats, 2012).

There are multiple examples of PROs that address communication and swallowing. Several examples of PROs in dysphagia are the SWAL-QOL, SWAL-CARE, MD Anderson Dysphagia Inventory (MDADI), and Eating Assessment Tool (EAT-10). Initially, the SWAL-QOL was a 93-item QOL and quality-of-care outcomes tool for dysphagia researchers and clinicians. Because its length made it impractical for clinical use, the researchers used psychometric techniques to reduce the 93-item instrument into two patient-centered outcomes tools: (1) the SWAL-QOL, a 44-item tool that assesses 10 QOL concepts; and (2) the SWAL-CARE, a 15-item tool that assesses quality of care and patient satisfaction. The scales have been shown to have good internal consistency, reliability, and short-term reproducibility. The scales differentiate normal swallowers from patients with oropharyngeal dysphagia and are sensitive to differences in the severity of dysphagia as clinically defined (McHorney et al., 2002).

The MDADI was the first validated and reliable self-administered questionnaire designed specifically for evaluating the impact of dysphagia on the QOL of patients with head and neck cancer. The MDADI is a 20-item, 5-point Likert questionnaire that assesses dysphagia in three domains (functional, emotional, and physical) (Chen et al., 2001). A Likert scale has a neutral point and then varying degrees of agree or disagree so that an individual can express how much he or she agrees or disagrees with a statement.

The EAT-10 is a self-administered, symptom-specific outcome instrument for dysphagia. The researchers concluded that the EAT-10 has good internal consistency, test-retest reproducibility, and criterion-based validity. The normative data suggest that an EAT-10 score of 3 or higher is indicative of dysphagia. The instrument may be utilized to document the initial dysphagia severity and monitor progress in treatment (Belafsky et al., 2008).

There are many other tools measuring QOL aspects related to communication and swallowing disorders. ASHA's Quality of Communication Life Scale was designed to be used with adults who have a range of communication disorders (Paul et al., 2004). A particular challenge is to gather PRO data from individuals with significant communication challenges. Irwin (2012) reported that different approaches to rehabilitation of aphasia have recognized that impairment-based and functional communication measures alone may not adequately catch some of the difficult-to-measure subjective benefits of aphasia treatment. Proponents of the social approach to aphasia advocate focusing on the social and personal consequences of aphasia, rather than focusing on the impairment itself (Irwin, 2012). This approach also supports the ICF model. Examples of such measures are the Burden of Stroke Scale (Doyle et al., 2003) and the Stroke and Aphasia Quality of Life Scale-39 (Hilari, Byng, Lamping, & Smith, 2003), both designed to be communicatively accessible to persons with aphasia.

The Washington Quality of Life (UWQOL) (Rinkel et al., 2009) for patients with head and neck cancer contains questions about speech and swallowing. The Voice Handicap Index (Jacobson et al., 1997) and Voice Related Quality of Life (V-RQOL) (Hogikyan & Sethuraman, 1999) are two instruments used with clients with voice disorders. The Voice Handicap Index is a 30-item self-administered questionnaire that asks an individual to describe his or her voice and the effects of his or her voice on his or her life. Three subscales cover the areas of functional, emotional, and physical aspects of voice disorders. Structured in this way, it captures information about body structure and function, and also about activities and participation. The emotional subscale also taps into what the ICF would designate as personal factors. The V-RQOL has questions about the functional impact of the voice disorder and questions about how the disorder is affecting the person's activity and participation.

In 2014, ASHA formed an ad hoc committee to make recommendations for evaluating, selecting, and implementing PRO measures. A search of the literature revealed over 100 instruments. The committee next devised guidelines for evaluating these measures. The long-term goal of this effort is to systematically identify and evaluate existing PRO measures related to communication and swallowing and to integrate these measures in the NOMS beginning in 2018 (Yorkston, 2015).

Unintended Consequences When Requiring Collection of Outcomes Data

As payers place more emphasis on outcomes related to reimbursement, it raises the risk of bias. Clinician-reported outcomes come into question because of the potential bias introduced by the increasing linkages between successful outcomes and successful reimbursement. That is one of the reasons for the increasing emphasis on PROs: That source of bias is greatly reduced. With PROs, payers often want the data to come directly to them, so that clinicians can't influence the data, and respondents feel they can respond truthfully. When the PRO data bypass the clinician, it can take away from the really valuable role that PROs can play in facilitating dialogue between the clinician and patient as to the latter's perspective (Yorkston, 2015).

References

American Speech-Language-Hearing Association. (n.d.-a). International Classification of Functioning, Disability and Health (ICF). Retrieved from http://www.asha.org/slp/icf/

American Speech-Language-Hearing Association. (n.d.-b). National Outcomes Measurement System (NOMS). Retrieved from http://www.asha.org/NOMS/

American Speech-Language-Hearing Association. (2016). Scope of practice in speech-language pathology. Retrieved from https://www.asha.org/policy/SP2016-00343/

Belafsky, P. C., Mouadeb, D. A., Rees, C. J., Pryor, J. C., Postma, G. N., Allen, J., & Leonard, R. J. (2008). Validity and reliability of the Eating Assessment Tool (EAT-10). *Annals of Otology, Rhinology, and Laryngology, 117*(12), 919–924.

Centers for Disease Control and Prevention. (2012). International Classification of Functioning, Disability and Health (ICF). Retrieved from http://www.cdc.gov/nchs/icd/icf.htm

Centers for Medicare & Medicaid Services. (2014). Functional reporting. Retrieved from https://www.cms.gov/Medicare/Billing/TherapyServices/Functional-Reporting.html

Chen, A. Y., Frankowski, R., Bishop-Leone, J., Hebert, T., Leyk, S., Lewin, J., & Goepfert, H. (2001). The development and validation of a dysphagia-specific quality-of-life questionnaire for patients with head and neck cancer: The MD Anderson dysphagia inventory. *Archives of Otolarynology—Head & Neck Surgery, 127*(7), 870–876.

Doyle, P. J., McNeil, M. R., Mikolic, J. M., Prieto, L., Hula, W. D., Lustig, A. P., . . . Elman, R. J. (2003). The Burden of Stroke Scale (BOSS) provides valid and reliable score estimates of functioning and well-being in stroke survivors with and without communication disorders. *Journal of Clinical Epidemiology, 57*(10), 997–1007. doi:10.1016/j.jclinepi.2003.11.016

Gage, B. (2014). Implementing standardized assessment for bundled payment and other integrated service approaches. Retrieved from http://www.paccr.org/wp-content/uploads/2014/11/Implementing-Standardized-Assessment-for-Bundled-Payment-and-Other-Integrated-Service-Approaches_GSA_November-7-2014.pdf

Hilari, K., Byng, S., Lamping, D. L., & Smith, S. C. (2003). Stroke and Aphasia Quality of Life Scale-39 (SAQOL-39): Evaluation of acceptability, reliability, and validity. *Stroke, 34*(8), 1944–1950. doi:10.1161/01.str.0000081987.46660.ed

Hogikyan, N. D., & Sethuraman G. (1999). Validation of an instrument to measure voice-related quality of life (V-RQOL). *Journal of Voice, 13*(4), 557–569.

Irwin, B. (2012). Patient-reported outcome measures in aphasia. *SIG 2 Perspectives on Neurophysiology and Neurogenic Speech and Language Disorders, 22*(4), 160–166. doi:10.1044/nnsld22.4.160

Jacobson, B. H., Johnson, A., Grywalski, C., Silbergleit, A., Jacobson, G., Benninger, M.S., & Newman, C. (1997). The Voice Handicap Index (VHI). *American Journal of Speech-Language Pathology, 6*, 66–70.

McHorney, C. A., Robbins, J., Lomax, K., Rosenbek, J. C., Chignell, K., Kramer, A. E., & Bricker, D. E. (2002). The SWAL-QOL and SWAL-CARE outcomes tool for oropharyngeal dysphagia in adults: III. Documentation of reliability and validity. *Dysphagia, 17*(2), 97–114.

National Quality Forum. (n.d.). Patient-reported outcomes. Retrieved from http://www.qualityforum.org/Projects/n-r/Patient-Reported_Outcomes/Patient-Reported_Outcomes.aspx

Paul, D. R., Frattali, C. M., Holland, A. L., Thompson, C. K., Caperton, C. J., & Slater, S. C. (2004). *The American speech-language-hearing association quality of communication life scale (QCL): Manual.* Rockville, MD: American Speech-Language-Hearing Association.

Rodenhauser, P. (2000). *Mental health care administration: A guide for practitioners.* Ann Arbor, MI: University of Michigan Press.

Shelton, P. J. (2000). *Measuring and improving patient satisfaction.* Burlington, MA: Jones & Bartlett Learning.

Threats, T. T. (2007). Use of the ICF in dysphagia management. *Seminars in Speech and Language, 28*(4), 323-333.

Threats, T. T. (2012). Use of the ICF for guiding patient-reported outcome measures. *SIG 2 Perspectives on Neurophysiology and Neurogenic Speech and Language Disorders, 22*(4), 128–135. doi:10.1044/nnsld22.4.128

Rinkel, R. N., Verdonck-de Leeuw, I. M., Langendijk, J. A., van Reij, E. J., Aaronson, N. K., & Leemans, C. R. (2009). The psychometric and clinical validity of the SWAL-QOL questionnaire in evaluating swallowing problems experienced by patients with oral and oropharyngeal cancer. *Oral Oncology, 45*(8), e67-e71.

Üstün, T. B. (n.d.). The ICF: An overview. Centers for Disease Control and Prevention. Retrieved from https://www.cdc.gov/nchs/data/icd/icfoverview_finalforwho10sept.pdf

World Health Organization. (2013). How to use the ICF: A practical manual for using the International Classification of Functioning Disability. Retrieved from http://www.who.int/classifications/drafticfpracticalmanual.pdf

World Health Organization. (2016). History of ICD. Retrieved from http://www.who.int/classifications/icd/en/

Yorkston, K. (2015). Selecting patient-reported outcomes measures: A committee update. American Speech-Language-Hearing Association. Retrieved from http://www.asha.org/Academic/questions/Selecting-Patient-Reported-Outcomes-Measures/

Suggested Readings

Ma, E. P. M., Threats, T. T., & Worrall, L. E. (2008). An introduction to the International Classification of Functioning, Disability and Health (ICF) for speech-language pathology: Its past, present and future. *International Journal of Speech-Language Pathology, 10*(1-2), 2-8.

Threats, T. T. (2008). Use of the ICF for clinical practice in speech-language pathology. *International Journal of Speech-Language Pathology, 10*(1-2), 50-60.

Review Questions

1. What are the stated purposes of the ICF?
2. Name the components of the ICF and describe why it is important for the speech-language pathologist to consider environmental and personal factors when assessing a client.
3. What are the four types of things measured to report the results of care (and used in performance improvement)?
4. Describe the difference between outcomes measures and PRO measures.
5. What is an FCM?

Activity A

For each of the following statements, indicate to which component of the ICF model it relates:
Body structure (BS)
Body function (BF)
Activity limitation (AL)
Participation limitation (PL)
Environmental factors (E)
Personal factors (P)

Component	Statement
	Hoarse voice
	Cleft lip and palate
	78 years old
	Moderate receptive language impairment
	Motivated to improve
	Lingual paresis
	Reduced jaw movement
	Cerebral palsy
	Male
	Gastroesophageal reflux disease
	Supportive spouse
	Difficulty in science class because of trouble understanding complex instructions
	Limited health benefits
	Vocal nodules
	Cannot chew solid foods
	Vegan
	Cannot recall words
	Cannot read multisyllabic words
	Access to augmentative communication device
	Closed head injury

Component	Statement
	Job requires telephone work
	Cannot play bridge with friends because of inability to recall words
	Easily frustrated
	Responds well to reinforcement
	Cannot follow three-step commands
	Will not eat in restaurants because friends are eating solid foods and client cannot
	Classroom acoustics
	Cannot understand a recipe
	No aids in the dining room to remind patient to take small sips
	Does not want to host family dinner requiring cooking from recipes
	Poor reading skills

Activity B

For each of the environmental and personal factors listed, indicate whether you think it would have a positive, negative, or no impact on the client's progress in therapy.

Personal and Environmental Factors	Likely Positive, Negative or No Impact
4-year-old with language impairment who has attention deficit hyperactivity disorder	
Former model now with dysphagia due to partial mandibulectomy	
78-year-old with aphasia	
No funds for augmentative communication device	
Motivated to improve	
Female who stutters	
Preschooler with language delay in home with no books and few toys	
Lives alone	
Male with Parkinson's disease and dysarthria	
Completes home practice activities	
Supportive spouse	
Toddler with visual impairment with feeding disorder	
Limited health benefits	
Basketball coach with voice disorder	
7-year-old who stutters whose father keeps correcting him	
Vegan	
Misses many treatment sessions due to transportation difficulties	
Child with feeding disorder willing to try new foods	
Access to augmentative communication device	
Client lives 50 miles from outpatient clinic	
Job requires telephone work	

Personal and Environmental Factors	Likely Positive, Negative or No Impact
Patient takes medication that makes her lethargic	
Easily frustrated	
Male who stutters	
Responds well to reinforcement	
Preschooler with severe verbal apraxia whose parents are supportive of using manual signs	
Client lives in rural area and has neighbor willing to drive him to therapy	
Classroom acoustics are good and client is teacher with voice disorder	
Mother of preschool child responds to child pointing rather than requiring verbalization	
No nursing aids in the dining room to remind patient to take small sips	
Patient with laryngectomy provided electrolarynx before leaving hospital	

Activity C

Go to the ASHA website and find information on NOMS (look in the Acute Care Hospital Data Report).

1. **List the 15 areas in the Adult Speech-Language Pathology Component for which there are functional communication measures.**
2. **List the six areas for which there are functional communication measures on the Pre-K component (look in the Pre-Kindergarten Data Report).**

Appendix 5-A

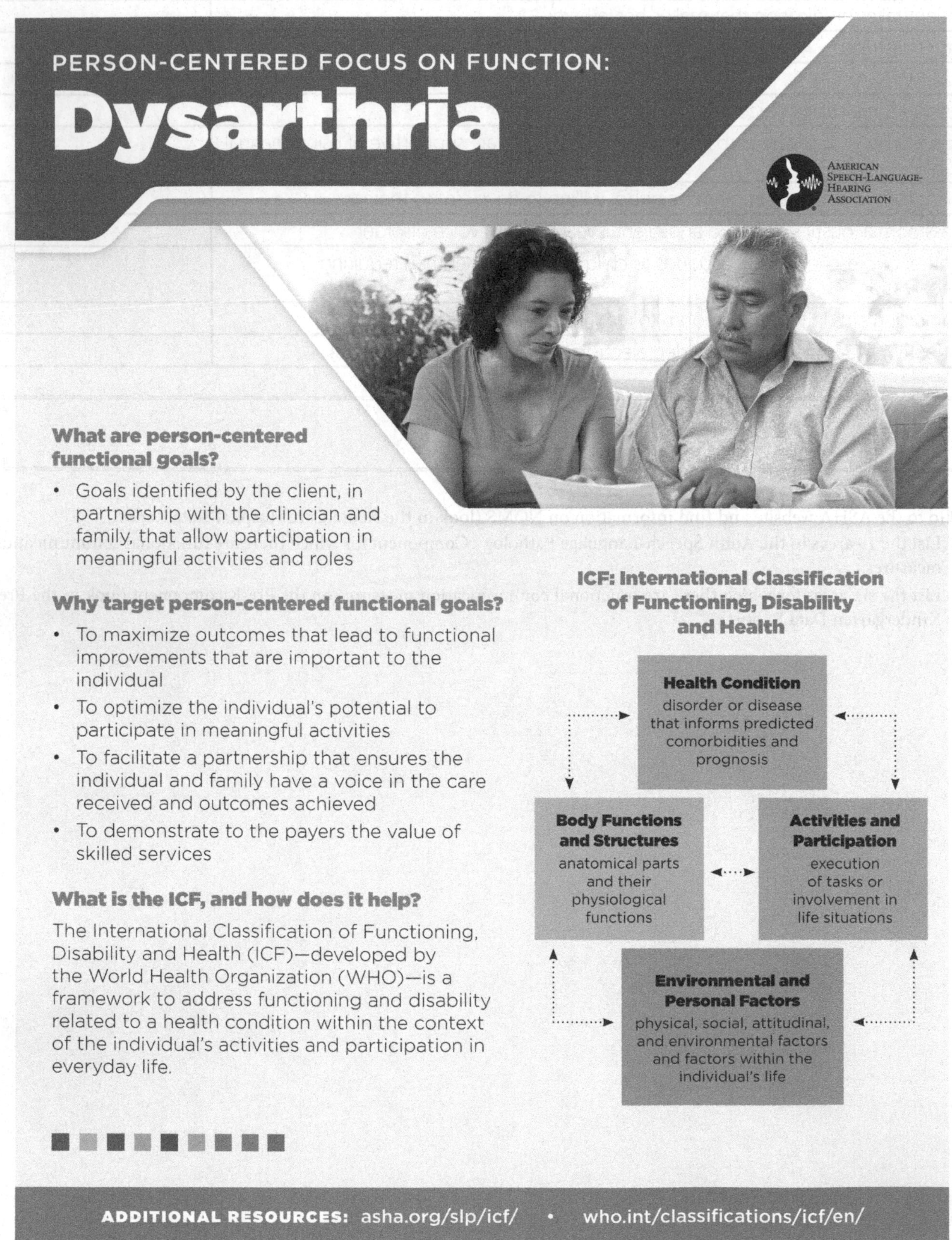

Reprinted with permission from American Speech-Language-Hearing Association. (n.d.) Person-centered focus on function: Dysarthria. Retrieved from https://www.asha.org/uploadedFiles/ICF-Dysarthria.pdf

Person-Centered Focus on Function: Dysarthria

Case study

Health Condition: Parkinson's disease with hypokinetic dysarthria

Assessment Data

Body Functions and Structures

- Rigidity of articulators
- Lingual tremors
- Reduced range of motion of articulators
- Poor respiratory support
- Monopitch
- Monoloudness
- Strained, breathy vocal quality
- Imprecise articulation
- Fluctuating rate of speech
- Difficulty initiating verbal productions
- Speech intelligibility[a]: 65%
- Functional hearing, vision, cognition, mobility

Activities and Participation

- Wife reports increased social isolation from frequent breakdown in communication resulting from reduced speech intelligibility.
- Patient reports[b] greater difficulty conversing over the telephone than in face-to-face conversations.
- Patient reports quickly fatiguing in verbal communicative contexts.

Environmental and Personal Factors

- Age: 57
- Motivated to communicate effectively with his children who live in different cities
- Hesitant to use technology to augment communication
- Reduced motivation for social communication due to stigma associated with speech intelligibility
- Had benefitted from SLP services previously but is currently discouraged given progression of disease
- Unable to communicate well in the presence of background noise

Clinical Reasoning

What impairments most affect function, based on clinician assessment & the individual's self-report?

What activities are most important to the individual in the current or discharge setting?

What environmental/personal factors are faciilitators or barriers to participation in the current or discharge setting?

Goal Setting

Person-Centered Functional Goals

Long-Term Goal:

Without external cues, Mr. J will use functional communication skills for social interactions with both familiar and unfamiliar partners.

Short-Term Goals:

- With moderate verbal cues from communication partners, Mr. J will increase respiratory support to produce intelligible phrase-level utterances.
- Mr. J will use a low-tech system with occasional cues to augment speech production in challenging environments (e.g., in the presence of background noise).
- Without cues, Mr. J will consistently initiate requests for appropriate environmental modifications (e.g., reduce background noise, use videoconferencing for phone calls) to improve communicative effectiveness.

[a] *Measured by sentence intelligibility subtest of the Assessment of Intelligibility of Dysarthric Speech (Yorkston & Beukelman, 1981)*
[b] *Reported on Communication Effectiveness Index-Modified (CETI-M; Yorkston., Beukelman, Strand, & Bell, 1999)*

10869

For clinical and documentation questions, contact **healthservices@asha.org**.
The interpretation of ICF and examples above are consensus based and provided as a resource for members of the American Speech-Language-Hearing Association.

Appendix 5-B

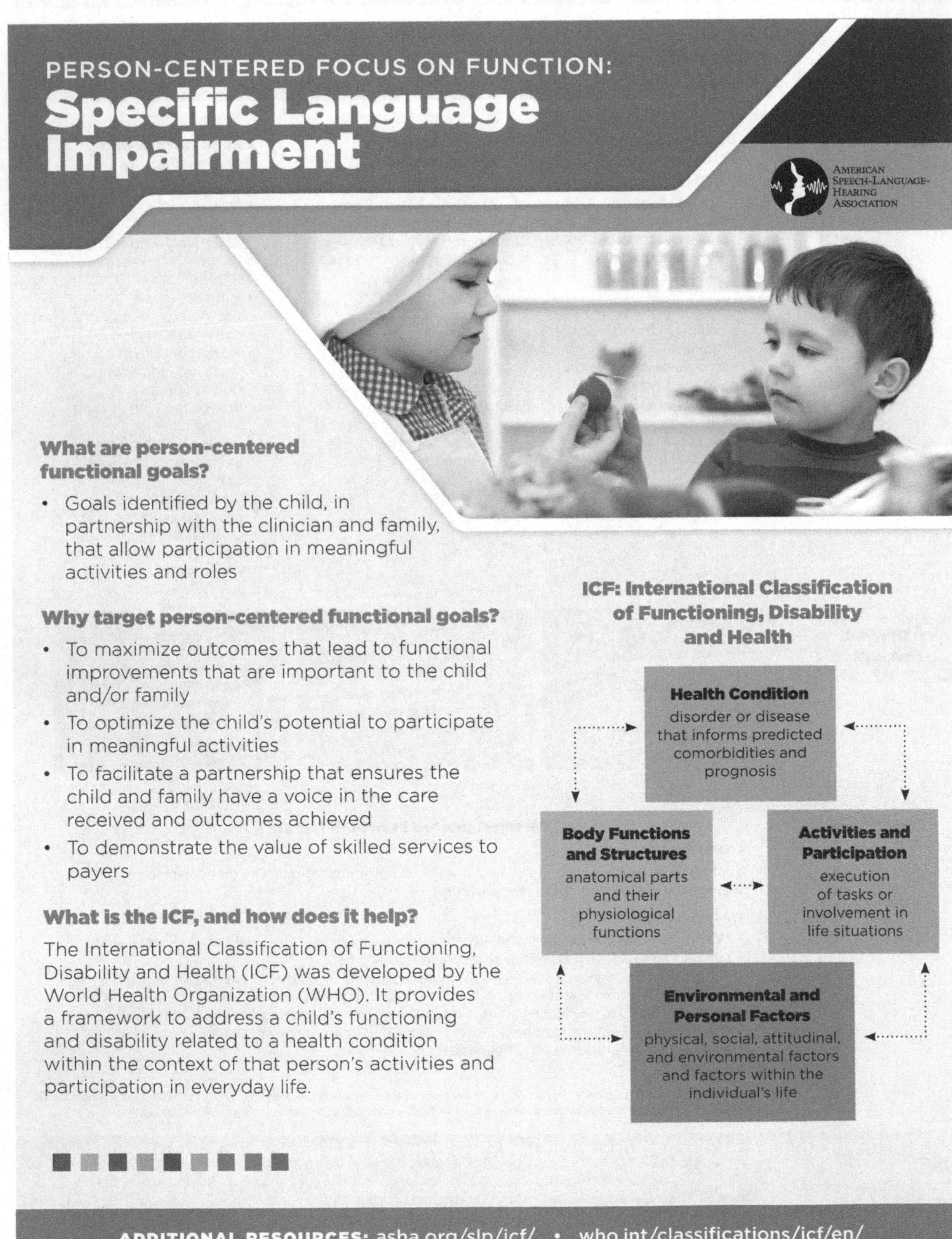

PERSON-CENTERED FOCUS ON FUNCTION:
Specific Language Impairment
American Speech-Language-Hearing Association
What are person-centered functional goals?
• Goals identified by the child, in partnership with the clinician and family, that allow participation in meaningful activities and roles
Why target person-centered functional goals?
• To maximize outcomes that lead to functional improvements that are important to the child and/or family
• To optimize the child's potential to participate in meaningful activities
• To facilitate a partnership that ensures the child and family have a voice in the care received and outcomes achieved
• To demonstrate the value of skilled services to payers
What is the ICF, and how does it help?
The International Classification of Functioning, Disability and Health (ICF) was developed by the World Health Organization (WHO). It provides a framework to address a child's functioning and disability related to a health condition within the context of that person's activities and participation in everyday life.
ICF: International Classification of Functioning, Disability and Health
Health Condition
disorder or disease that informs predicted comorbidities and prognosis
Body Functions and Structures
anatomical parts and their physiological functions
Activities and Participation
execution of tasks or involvement in life situations
Environmental and Personal Factors
physical, social, attitudinal, and environmental factors and factors within the individual's life
ADDITIONAL RESOURCES: asha.org/slp/icf/ • who.int/classifications/icf/en/

Person-Centered Focus on Function: Specific Language Impairment

Case study: Johnny

Health Condition: Specific Language Impairment

Assessment Data

Body Functions and Structures

(Formal/Informal Assessments)
Cognitive functioning

- Normal (KBIT2[a]); poor working memory (AWMA[b])

Language (CELF-P2[c])
Language (CELF-P2[c])

- Normal single-word receptive vocabulary (PPVT-4[d])
- Severe morphosyntax (CELF-P2) and narrative deficits (language sample)

Speech

- Mild speech sound disorder

Oromusculature, swallowing

- Normal structure + function

Voice/Resonance, Hearing

- Normal

Early literacy

- Poor print concepts (PALS[e])

Activities and Participation

(FOCUS[f], Child and Caregiver Interviews)

- Johnny has difficulty making friends and being included in other children's games.
- Johnny has difficulty telling adults about past events
- Johnny has difficulty joining in conversation with his peers.
- Johnny has difficulty communicating independently with unfamiliar adults.
- Johnny enjoys having family members read to him.

Environmental and Personal Factors

- 4 years old and attends Head Start preschool
- Lives with his mother, who has a learning disability, and his grandmother, who has a hearing impairment
- Is the younger of two children and is shy
- Is healthy, with an easygoing temperament
- Enjoys attending preschool, where he is more comfortable with teachers than with peers
- Lives in a low socioeconomic neighborhood
- He was born in the U.S., and only English is spoken at home

Clinical Reasoning

What impairments most affect function in this setting, based on clinician assessment and individual/family report?

What activities are most important to the individual in the current setting?

What environmental/ personal characteristics help or hinder participation in activities or situations in the current setting?

Goal Setting

Person-Centered Functional Goals

Long-Term Goal

Johnny will use age-appropriate grammar, pre-literacy, and social skills in everyday activities with family, peers, and unfamiliar adults 80% of the time in home and preschool settings by the end of the preschool year after receiving a block of language therapy and teacher-trained supports.

Short-Term Goals

- By the end of the preschool term, Johnny will use past tense correctly 90% of the time when he is telling news during group time with his classmates.
- By the end of the preschool term, Johnny will correctly identify rhyming words during book-reading activities with his mother, grandmother, and teacher 90% of the time.
- Johnny will take turns, make requests, and initiate conversations with his peers during snack time during a 10-minute period over 5 days.

[a]KBIT-2 = Kaufman Brief Intelligence Test-2 (Kaufman & Kaufman, 2004). [b]AWMA = Automated Working Memory Assessment (Alloway, 2007). [c]CELF-P2 = Clinical Evaluation of Language Fundamentals-Preschool (2nd ed.; Wiig, Secord, & Semel, 2004). [d]PPVT-4 = Peabody Picture Vocabulary Test-Fourth Edition (Dunn & Dunn, 2007). [e]PALS = Phonological Awareness Literacy Screening (Invernizzi, Juel, Swank, & Meier, 2004). [f]FOCUS = Focus on the Outcomes of Children Under Six (Thomas-Stonell, Robertson, Walker, Oddson, Washington, & Rosenbaum, 2012).

For clinical and documentation questions, contact **healthservices@asha.org**.

The interpretation of ICF and examples above are consensus based and provided as a resource for members of the American Speech-Language-Hearing Association.

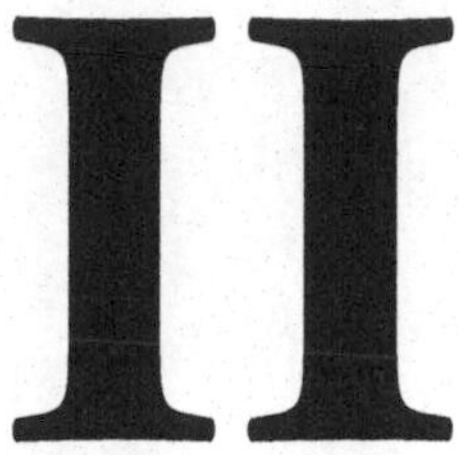

II

Documenting Different Types of Services

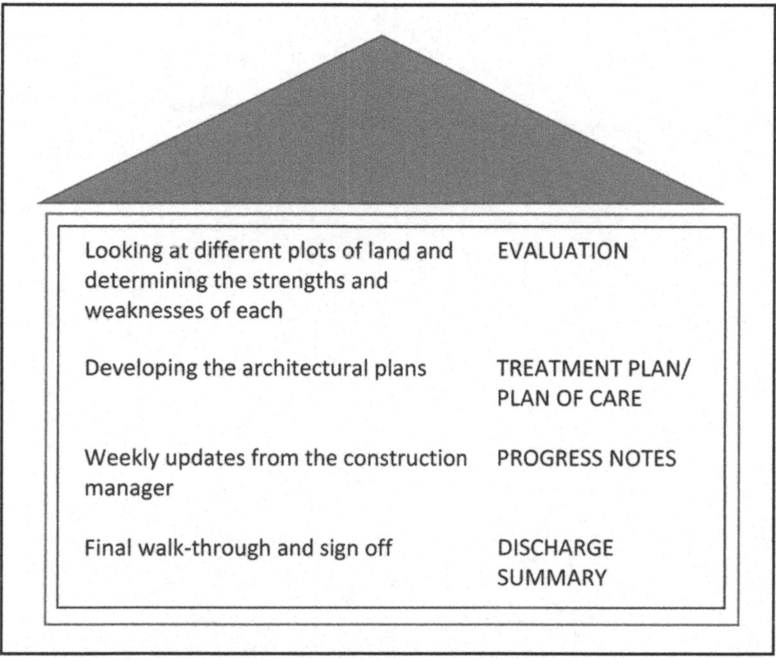

Figure II-1. Framework for client management and documentation.

In this section, we discuss the different types of services that the speech-language pathologist documents from initial evaluation through summarizing treatment in the discharge summary.

The evaluation report organizes and summarizes the information about the client's current state and gives a prognosis about achieving the goal state. The treatment plan is the framework that organizes the plan for intervention to work toward the goal state. Progress notes are the stepping stones demonstrating progress toward the goals. These three components of documentation, along with the discharge summary, form the framework for the management of the client.

Consider an analogy between building a new home and managing the care of a client (Figure II-1). The evaluation in this process involves visiting various developments and assessing the advantages and disadvantages of each building site. The plan is then developed by the architect. The client and architect collaborate until each agrees the plan is SMART: Specific, measurable, attainable, realistic, and has a time it will be completed (see Chapter 7). The construction manager sends weekly updates on progress. When the home is completed, the client and builder do a walk-through and double-check that the finished product matches the plan (i.e., the goals were met). If so, the project is complete, or discharge is achieved.

6

Evaluation Reports

Nancy B. Swigert, MA, CCC-SLP, BCS-S

Evaluation as Part of Overall Management of the Client

The evaluation is not only the beginning of contact with the client, but it is also inarguably the most important part of the management of the client. If the evaluation is not thorough and if the analysis of the findings is not accurate, the right goals will not be selected and appropriate treatment techniques will not be applied. In our construction analogy, if the right plot of land is not selected, it will be difficult for the architect to render plans to match the house imagined. For example, if a hilly plot of land is selected as a result of the evaluation of different plots, the architect can develop plans for a multistory house when what the client really intended was a one-story ranch.

Gathering Background Information Before the Evaluation

It is never appropriate to enter an evaluation session without at least some background information about the client. In outpatient settings, an intake form has probably been completed (see Chapters 14 and 17 for examples). In school settings, a specific referral process will have been followed (see Chapter 16). For inpatient medical settings, the physician or physician extender will have written an order for the evaluation and should provide some information about why the evaluation is needed. However, this is usually quite cursory, such as "Evaluate swallowing" or "Evaluate for speech after stroke." If the reason for referral is somewhat vague, the speech-language pathologist must seek more specific information before beginning the evaluation.

Medical Charts

Typically, the easiest place to find a good summary of the patient's current state is in the history and physical (H&P) written by the physician. The H&P gives the current medical complaint(s), background medical information, procedures/surgeries, and medications. The speech-language pathologist can then look to other specific areas in the chart to gain information more specifically related to the reason for referral. The nurse's notes contain specific information that is often essential. Examples of information that can be found in nursing documentation include level of independence prior to admission, level of alertness, ability to follow commands, any sensory deficits (e.g., visual, hearing), current diet, and supplemental oxygen. Consult reports from

Swigert, N. B.
Documentation and Reimbursement for Speech-Language Pathologists: Principles and Practice (pp. 69-83).

specialty physicians (e.g., neurology) can also contain vital information.

Case History Forms

In outpatient settings, it is customary to have the client/caregiver complete a case history form before the client arrives for his or her evaluation. A case history form collects demographic information as well as information about the presenting problem. The form can be basic and generic, and used for any type of client (see Appendix 6-A for an example).

Case history forms designed for specific disorders, however, can have more detailed information. The more information that can be obtained before the evaluation begins, the more efficient the speech-language pathologist can be during the evaluation session. The case history form can then also serve as the format for the clinician to interview the client to fill in any gaps in the information provided. Examples of disorder-specific case history forms are provided in the Appendices for Chapters 14 and 17.

Regardless of the form or format used to gather the information, the speech-language pathologist should be certain to learn the client's or caregiver's perspective on why the evaluation is needed. His or her perspective may be very different from that of the person who made the referral.

Client/Caregiver Interview

The written case history form can serve as the basis for interviewing the client or caregiver for more detailed information. The speech-language pathologist should look through the case history form before the evaluation and note any areas that might be unclear. The clinician can take notes in the margins of the case history form or use another questionnaire form to gather information. If a generic case history form has been used, the interview is a good time to delve into the specifics of the presenting problem.

Sometimes a detailed interview form can be used to guide the clinician through that part of the evaluation. Such interview forms are especially helpful to clinicians with less experience, or to a clinician beginning to see a new type of client. As the clinician gains experience and expertise with a particular patient population, the flow of the interview and types of questions to ask become second nature. The case history form should be worded with full sentences and questions for the client to read, whereas the interview form can include just terms or words to trigger the speech-language pathologist about what to ask.

Resources on the American Speech-Language-Hearing Association's Practice Portal

The American Speech-Language-Hearing Association's (ASHA's) webpage has a section called the *Practice Portal*. The portal contains reference documents on a variety of topics that have been developed by national office staff and subject matter experts. Many disorders for both adult and pediatric clients are addressed. There are templates to gather case history information (ASHA, n.d.-a) and detailed case history and assessment templates (ASHA, n.d.-b).

Necessary Components in an Evaluation Report

The format of evaluation reports varies depending on the setting in which the client is seen and whether the facility is using a paper format or an electronic health record (EHR), also called an *electronic medical record* (EMR). Regardless of the format in which the information is entered, the result should be a report that contains all necessary components. In an outpatient setting in which a paper report is generated, each section, usually with a clear header, is included. In an EHR, there should also be clear headers and grouping of information. Appendix 6-B provides an example of a template for an outpatient report using headers and categories to make it easy for the reader to find the information. Certain payer types or settings may have other templates you are required to use. Many other templates may be found in different settings. In an EHR, different category headings and sequence of information may be included.

Identifying Information

The top of the report should include all the information necessary to easily identify who the report is about and when the evaluation was completed. Typical information in this header includes the following:

- Client name
- Date of birth
- Age/adjusted age
- Gender
- Parent(s) names (if child)
- Address
- Telephone number

Table 6-1

Summary Statements: Client Participation in Evaluation

Observation Worded Objectively	Observation Worded Subjectively
Client was able to attend to tasks during the first part of the session, but attention waned as the evaluation continued.	Client was lazy and stopped working partway through the session.
Client exhibited signs of fatigue as the evaluation progressed.	Client obviously didn't get enough sleep because he kept nodding off.
Client was cooperative throughout the early part of the session, but level of cooperation decreased when harder tasks were presented.	Client gave the examiner a hard time whenever something challenging was presented.
Client only sometimes maintained eye contact during conversation.	Client exhibited rude behavior, failing to look the examiner in the eye.
Client did not appear to put forth full effort on tasks involving writing, giving only short responses.	Client didn't even try on writing tasks in the evaluation.

- Other facility required identifier (e.g., encounter or medical record number)
- Name of referral source
- Physician name (if different from referral source)
- Date of evaluation
- Time in/out, or just start time of evaluation (required in some settings for some payers)

Background Information/Reason for Referral

Based on the information gathered, whether from a medical chart, discussion with other members of the health care or education team, case history form, or interview with the client and/or caregivers, the speech-language pathologist has information about the reason for referral. This may be explicitly stated if a physician order has been given for the evaluation.

Background information is more detailed than simply stating a reason for referral. The background information includes pertinent related information. For example, perhaps the reason for referral on a preschool child is "unintelligible speech." The background information might include when specific developmental milestones were achieved, who is able to understand the child and in what situations, whether any siblings or anyone else in the family has a history of speech problems, and the child's response when not understood. It is helpful to include in the background and related information the client's and caregiver's views of what the problem is.

The related background information should include information such as the following:

- Onset of problem
- History of same problem in the past
- Any previous therapy and results
- Prior level of function
- Related medical conditions
- Any hospitalizations (related to the presenting problem)
- Any related medications
- Other services being received (e.g., physical or occupational therapy, special education)

If the client is a child, the following additional things should be included:

- Current educational performance
- Birth and developmental history

Behavioral Observations

In an outpatient report, the first paragraph often includes the examiner's behavioral observations of the client's participation in the evaluation. The speech-language pathologist may describe the client's level of effort, attentiveness, cooperation, and any effects of fatigue, for example. The statements should be factual and describe behaviors, and they should not include statements that might appear biased (Table 6-1). These summary statements by the speech-language pathologist help the reader of the report get a better picture of how the evaluation session went. A statement such "Client's behavior and responses during the assessment session today was typical/not typical of that seen in more familiar circumstances" tells the reader whether the results of the evaluation should be viewed as a reliable picture of the client's abilities. If the response was not typical, the speech-language pathologist should give examples.

This paragraph can also state who was present during the evaluation. This information is important for any evaluation done on a child because the parents' presence

The Kentucky Test of Motor Speech was designed to assess the degree and type of dysarthria. A variety of speech tasks are given to the client and performance is compared to speakers with no dysarthria and to a sample of speakers with a variety of types of dysarthria. Standard scores and percentiles are given for speakers with flaccid, spastic, ataxic, hypokinetic, hyperkinetic, and mixed dysarthria. The client's performance on each subtest is reported here:

Subtest	Client's Raw Score	Standard Score	Percentile Rank
Imitation of words			
Reading words			
Short phrase responses			
Connected speech			
Total score			

The client appears to exhibit a mild/moderate/severe/profound dysarthria most accurately described as flaccid/spastic/ataxic/hypokinetic/hyperkinetic/mixed.

Figure 6-1. Standard paragraph for fictional dysarthria test.

may have an impact on the child's performance. However, it can also be important to know about significant others who participated in or observed the evaluation of an adult.

Tests Given/Sources Used

To make the report easy to read, list the sources used that will be reported in the Test Results section and used to generate the impressions. This includes names of each standardized or criterion-referenced test administered, behavioral checklists, observations, and interviews.

Clinical Findings

The report should include the results and analysis of each of the tests given/sources used. This might mean including a paragraph for each of the testing instruments and tools within the body of the report. In a paper system, one way to save time is to utilize what might be called *standard paragraphs*. That is, the description of a particular test does not change from client to client; therefore, the clinician can construct a standard description of the test and then simply insert the findings from each client and put that information in the report. Figure 6-1 provides an example of a standard paragraph on a fictional test of dysarthria. The information to construct such standard paragraphs is found in the test manual. It is worth the time and effort to construct a bank of such standard paragraphs because the clinician will save time in the long run compared with typing or writing the same thing over and over with each new client.

To make reports shorter and more user friendly, instead of inserting a paragraph for each test given into the body of the report, this section of the report can provide an overall summary statement of the client's performance and state "See appendix for test descriptions and client scores." Then, these standard paragraphs can be placed together in an appendix. Many individuals who read the speech-language pathologist's report want to get to the bottom line quickly: How did the client perform, what is the speech-language pathologist's interpretation and summary, and what are the recommendations? When using the format of attaching the individual test results as appendices, the report can often be trimmed to one page of essential information. If more in-depth information is desired, the reader can study the attached appendices.

Hearing Screening

According to ASHA's Preferred Practice Patterns, the speech-language pathologist is limited to performing pure tone air conduction screening and screening tympanometry (ASHA, 2004b). Therefore, the speech-language pathologist's report should include only pass-fail information about hearing screening. Note that Medicare Part B does not pay for screening. Private insurance and Medicaid may reimburse for screening.

Diagnostic Code(s)

To make it easy for coders and third-party payers to find the information needed to process a claim, list the diagnoses and corresponding *International Classification of Diseases, Tenth Revision* (ICD-10) codes for the cognitive, communicative, and swallowing disorders for which the client was evaluated. See Chapter 4 for detailed information on coding.

Impressions

This is the most important part of the report. The speech-language pathologist analyzes all information obtained from multiple sources to form an impression: Patient characteristics, features, background/history, reason for referral, and of course results of the tests. Considering all of these factors, the speech-language pathologist applies clinical judgment to come to a conclusion. Referral sources are not interested in raw scores and percentiles. They want to know how you used that information to make an informed decision about the client's abilities and what you recommend. Think of the impressions section as your elevator speech about the evaluation. An *elevator speech* is something you can summarize and tell in the time it takes to get from one floor to the next in an elevator. Be clear and concise and share the most important information.

Prognosis

The report should include a prognostic statement, and this statement should not just be something like "excellent" or "fair." The prognostic statement should indicate a prognosis for what; that is, is the prognosis related to the client returning to baseline skills, communicating like same-age peers, eating a regular diet, eating a modified diet, or using communication skills in an occupation? Being specific with prognostic statements helps the client, referral source, and third-party payers know what the expectation is. The prognostic statement is your prediction of how likely it is that the client will achieve the long-term goal(s). The speech-language pathologist should also avoid terms that are not measurable when making a prognosis. Statements like the following are not measurable:

- The prognosis is good for client to eat an optimal diet. *(What is optimal?)*
- Prognosis is fair for client to communicate to the best of his ability. *(How would we know if that is the best of his ability?)*
- Prognosis is excellent for improved intelligibility. *(Improved compared with what? In what situations?)*

Instead, use statements that are measurable, such as the following:

- The prognosis is good for client to consume mechanical soft diet and thin liquids with minimal cues within 2 months. *(At the 2-month mark, this would be easy to determine.)*
- Prognosis is fair for client to communicate in short phrases in structured, familiar situations with no cues and guarded for communication in more complex situations. *(Now the reader understands that the client is expected to be limited to successful communication in only certain situations.)*
- Prognosis is excellent for speech that is intelligible to familiar and unfamiliar listeners 100% of the time. *(Listening to conversational speech at the conclusion of treatment would allow the listener to determine whether this prognosis was accurate.)*

Recommendations

Recommendations should address the next steps. They might include the following:

- Any other evaluations the client needs such as medical consultations, evaluations by other therapists, and full audiological evaluations.
- Treatment for the communication or swallowing disorder. The most important decision that will be made based on analysis of the evaluation results is whether to recommend that the client receive intervention services for his or her communication and/or swallowing problem. The ASHA document *Admission/Discharge Criteria in Speech-Language Pathology* provides guidance. For example, services might be recommended if the individual:
  - Cannot communicate functionally or optimally across settings
  - Cannot swallow safely to maintain adequate nutrition and hydration
  - Has skills that are not comparable to others of same age, gender, ethnicity, or cultural or linguistic background
  - Has a skill deficit that negatively affects his or her performance and participation or health status
  - Wants to maintain optimal communication or swallowing skills
  - Wants to enhance communication skills (ASHA, 2004a)

If recommending treatment, the report should specify the following (Centers for Medicare & Medicaid Services, 2017):

- Amount: Number of times per day, which typically only applies in inpatient settings
- Frequency: Number of times per week
- Duration: Number of weeks or number of treatment sessions
- Length of session is sometimes also indicated

Recommending Treatment When No Improvement Is Expected

Medicare requirements had historically held that for services to be reimbursed, there had to be an expectation that improvement would be made, often referenced as the *improvement standard*. In 2013, in the case of *Jimmo v. Sebelius*, the court held that Medicare could not deny services because the client showed no functional progress in cases of degenerative or progressive disorders, such as amyotrophic lateral sclerosis, multiple sclerosis, or Parkinson's disease. They stated that Medicare had to cover services to maintain skills and prevent deterioration (ASHA, 2016; Centers for Medicare & Medicaid Services, n.d.).

Note that these still need to be skilled services. Medicare will not cover services that are designed to practice or drill because these are activities that can be completed by caregivers. In the case of degenerative and progressive disorders, however, it may be appropriate for the speech-language pathologist to periodically reassess, intervene, and modify maintenance programs to address the client's current level of functioning in communication and swallowing. The speech-language pathologist's recommendations should specify the intent of the intervention in these cases. Recommendation statements might indicate short-term intervention to do the following:

- Adjust dysphagia recommendations and teach new strategies to assure continued safe intake by mouth
- Modify alternative communication system to account for decline in motor skills and teach caregivers use of modified system
- Provide refresher lessons on vocal loudness to re-establish speech that is understandable
- Provide new strategies for the caregiver to use to facilitate basic conversation with the client

The *International Classification of Functioning, Disability and Health* Framework and Evaluation Reports

Chapter 5 detailed the importance of keeping the focus on function. This tenet is important during the evaluation process and should be reflected in the evaluation report. Although the speech-language pathologist may not use section headers in the report that correspond to the *International Classification of Functioning, Disability and Health* (ICF) model directly, the evaluation and report should address each of the components. Consider where each of the components of the ICF framework might be included in the sections of the report (Table 6-2). To make it even more clear that the clinician has considered all aspects of the ICF model, the template and headers for a report can be modified to identify the ICF components more clearly (see Appendix 6-C). ASHA's Preferred Practice Patterns also address the ICF framework as part of the Fundamental Components and Guiding Principles (ASHA, 2004b). Whether or not the information is delineated with headers and categories, it is clear that the report should address each of the ICF components.

What Is Part of the Permanent Record?

Each facility may have guidelines about what forms actually become a part of the permanent medical or educational record. If not, the following are some things to consider when deciding whether a piece of documentation needs to go in the chart or be shredded:

- If all of the information is included in another way in the chart, it may not need to be kept.
    - Scoring booklets and test forms: If all of the pertinent results are in the report and/or appendices of the report, the test forms may not need to be a part of the permanent record. As an aside, note that test forms are typically copyrighted and should not be duplicated.
    - Interview forms: The pertinent information has been summarized in the report, so it is likely that the form on which the clinician took notes during the interview does not need to be kept. Forms like this can even be indicated with a watermark that states "Not a permanent part of the record."
    - Case history forms: The pertinent information has been summarized in the report, but there may be statements on the case history made by the client or caregivers that were not included in the report but the clinician deems important enough to keep permanently. In that case, do not discard the completed form.

When in doubt, keep rather than discard documents related to the evaluation.

References

American Speech-Language-Hearing Association. (n.d.-a). Demographics and history form. Retrieved from http://www.asha.org/uploadedFiles/slp/healthcare/AATDemographicsandHistory.pdf

American Speech-Language-Hearing Association. (n.d.-b). Pediatric feeding history and clinical assessment form. Retrieved from http://www.asha.org/uploadedFiles/Pediatric-Feeding-History-and-Clinical-Assessment-Form.pdf

American Speech-Language-Hearing Association. (2004a). Admission/discharge criteria in speech-language pathology. Retrieved from http://www.asha.org/policy/GL2004-00046.htm

American Speech-Language-Hearing Association. (2004b). Preferred practice patterns for the profession of speech-language pathology. Retrieved from http://www.asha.org/policy/PP2004-00191/

American Speech-Language-Hearing Association. (2016). *Jimmo v. Sebelius* plaintiffs return to court to urge enforcement. Retrieved from http://www.asha.org/News/2016/Jimmo-v-Sebelius-Plaintiffs-Return-to-Court-to-Urge-Enforcement/

Centers for Medicare & Medicaid Services. (n.d.). *Jimmo v. Sebelius* settlement agreement fact sheet. Retrieved from https://www.cms.gov/medicare/medicare-fee-for-service-payment/SNFPPS/downloads/jimmo-factsheet.pdf

Centers for Medicare & Medicaid Services. (2017). Therapy services. Retrieved from https://www.cms.gov/Medicare/Billing/TherapyServices/index.html

Table 6-2

Integrating *International Classification of Functioning, Disability and Health* Components Into the Evaluation Report

International Classification of Functioning, Disability and Health Component	Section of Evaluation Report	Example
Health condition (disorder or disease)	Background/reason for referral	Disease that has resulted in communication/swallowing problem
	Prognosis	What impact the health condition has on the prognosis
Body functions/structures	Background	Impact the disease/disorder has had on communication/swallowing
	Findings	Oral motor exam Oropharyngeal structure and function related to swallowing
	Prognosis	What impact the impaired body function/structure has on prognosis
Activities	Background/reason for referral	What activities are impacted by the disorder
	Summary	What specific problems noted during the evaluation have an impact on the client's ability to complete certain activities
	Recommendations	What will be done in therapy to help the client improve ability to complete activities
Participation	Background/reason for referral	What limitations on participation are caused by the disorder
	Summary	What specific problems noted during the evaluation have an impact on the client's ability to participate in daily life
	Recommendations	What will be done in therapy to help the client improve ability to participate in desired activities
Environmental Factors	Background/related information	What environmental factors play a role in how the disorder impacts the client
	Prognosis	What environmental factors are influencing the prognosis
	Recommendations	What environmental factors will help or hinder progress toward goals
Personal Factors	Background/related information	What personal factors play a role in how the disorder impacts the client
	Prognosis	What personal factors are influencing the prognosis
	Recommendations	What personal factors will help or hinder progress toward goals

Review Questions

1. Describe the ways background information can be obtained before the evaluation is begun, and discuss the advantages and disadvantages of each method.
2. What should be included in identifying information at the beginning of an evaluation report?
3. Describe the differences between reason for referral and background and related information.
4. Describe the different sources of information that can be used and reported in the results section of the report. Give a concrete example of each type of source.
5. What is the most important part of an evaluation report and why?

Activity A

For each background paragraph, edit to eliminate unnecessary information. Summarize several statements into one when possible. Keep only the essential information. Use only factual statements.

Client #1

Reason for Referral: Jimmy January, age 4.1, was referred by his pediatrician for evaluation of unintelligible speech.

Background and Related Information: Jimmy was accompanied to the evaluation by his mother and three siblings. The siblings range in age from 8 to 5. Jimmy is the youngest child. Jane, the oldest, never had any speech problems. Janet, the second oldest, never had any communication problems. John, who is 1 year older than Jimmy, also met all speech milestones at expected ages and never had speech problems. Jimmy attends preschool four mornings per week, where he reportedly likes physical activities and art. His teacher told his mother that Jimmy follows directions well and gets along well with the other children except for when he is trying to make himself understood and the other children can't understand him. At times like that, Jimmy has been known to strike out at the other children in frustration. It is not surprising that a child like Jimmy might hit other children when he can't be understood. This behavior is to be expected. Jimmy met all motor milestones within normal limits. He was born at 39 weeks' gestation and weighed 6 pounds 5 ounces at birth. He had surgery to remove a small cyst on his wrist at 3 years of age.

Client #2

Reason for Referral: Felicia February, age 42, was referred by her otolaryngologist for evaluation of hoarseness.

Background and Related Information: Ms. February is an elementary school teacher who reports she loses her voice at least once per school year. This has happened the last 3 years. She indicates this usually happens around November before holiday break. Ms. February is a gregarious individual who was observed in the waiting room to be talking loudly to the receptionist. She was laughing, and at times it didn't even seem like anything funny had been said. Ms. February has one child, age 9, who waited in the waiting room during the evaluation. He was pretty loud himself. Ms. February indicates she has to use her voice constantly during the school day and that her classroom, though painted a soothing grey, has hard floors and walls. She has to raise her voice to be heard in the back of the room. Ms. February had pneumonia last year and bronchitis the year before that. Ms. February also uses her voice to sing in a choir and probably to yell at her son, given the behaviors he exhibited in the waiting room.

Client #3

Reason for Referral: Maddie March, age 16, was referred for evaluation of her cognitive and executive function skills following a concussion suffered during a soccer game.

Background and Related Information: Maddie was accompanied to the evaluation by her father, who supplied some of the background information. It was unclear why her mother hadn't made time to accompany Maddie. Maddie plays on her high school soccer team and suffered a concussion 3 weeks ago. She was running toward the ball and another player ran into her. When Maddie fell, she hit her head pretty hard on the turf. She did not lose consciousness but did come out of the game. Luckily, her coach knew she should be on the sidelines because some coaches don't. Maddie met all developmental milestones within normal limits. She is a sophomore and gets average grades, although she admits she is not very good at algebra. Maddie complains that she is continuing to have headaches, is having trouble concentrating, and really has a lot of trouble when there is background noise, like other kids talking or the radio or television playing. She states that by the end of the school day she is exhausted, which of course is not surprising in a situation like this.

Activity B

American Speech-Language-Hearing Association Practice Portal

Go to the ASHA Practice Portal.

List the documentation templates available for use with adult clients.

List the documentation templates available for use with pediatric clients.

These items were found on the Motor Speech Assessment Template for adults. Fill in the information in columns 2 and 3:

Information Requested	Why Is It Important for a Motor Speech Evaluation?	Would These Same Items Be Needed on Any Type of Evaluation for an Adult (e.g., Voice, Aphasia, Memory)? Why or Why Not?
Medications		
Allergies		
Pain		
Primary languages spoken		
Educational history		
Occupation		
Hearing status		
Vision status		
Tracheostomy		
Mechanical ventilation		

Compare the templates for Pediatric Clinical Assessment Template (liquids only) and Pediatric Clinical Assessment Template (liquids, semi-solids, and solid foods). List five items that are different on the two templates and explain why.

Activity C

Write a Standard Paragraph

Select any standardized test from the clinic. Write a standardized paragraph for that test that includes the following:

- Name of test
- Authors
- Year
- Purpose of test
- Ages appropriate to use with
- Who test was normed on

Then develop a table to report raw scores, standard scores, percentiles, etc.

Appendix 6-A
Adult Client Case History

Name: ______________________________ Birthdate: ______________

Address: ____

____

Home phone: ______________________ Work/cell phone: ______________

Emergency contact (name, relationship, and phone number): ______________

____

Place of employment: ____

Occupation: ____

Education completed: ____

Describe your speech, voice, or swallowing problem(s): ______________

____

____

____

____

Have you had speech therapy before? Y N

If so, where and when: ____

Do you have any problems with your hearing? Y N

If yes, please explain: ____

Do any members of your family have (or had in the past) speech, language, or hearing problems? ______________

____

____

Who referred you for this evaluation? ______________________________

Who is your physician? ____

Physician's address: ____

____

APPENDIX 6-B
Outpatient Evaluation Template

Speech-Language Pathology Outpatient Evaluation

Name: ______________________________

Gender: __________ Facility identification number: __________

Date of birth: __________ Referral source: __________

Age: ______ (Adjusted age: ____) Physician(s): __________

Parent(s): __________ Date of evaluation: __________

__________ Time in/out: __________

Address: ______________________________

____

____

Telephone: __________

Background information related to referral: ______________________________

____

____

Reason for referral: ______________________________

____

____

Behavioral observations: ______________________________

____

____

Tests given/sources/measures used (see scores and comments attached):

____ Behavioral checklist

____ Standardized tests

____ Parent/client/caregiver interview

____ Criterion-referenced instrument

____ Observation

Clinical findings: ______________________________

____

____

Hearing screening: ______________________________

____

____

Diagnosis/ICD-10 code(s): ______________________________

____

____

Impressions: ______________________________

____

____

Prognosis: ______________________________

____

____

Recommendations: ______________________________

____

____

Frequency/duration of treatment: ______________________________

____

____

Speech-language pathologist signature, title, degree(s), credentials:

CC: Referral source

Physician(s)

APPENDIX 6-C

Outpatient Evaluation Template With International Classification of Functioning, Disability and Health *Categories*

Speech-Language Pathology

Name: ____

Gender: ______________ Facility identification number: ______________

Date of birth: ______________ Referral source: ______________

Age: ________ (Adjusted age: ______) Physician(s): ______________

Parent(s): ______________ Date of evaluation: ______________

______________ Time in/out: ______________

Address: ____

____

____

Telephone: ______________

Background information related to referral (including health condition): ______________

____

____

Reason for referral: ____

____

____

Behavioral observations: ____

____

____

Tests given/sources/measures used (see scores and comments attached):

_____ Behavioral checklist

_____ Standardized tests

_____ Parent/client/caregiver interview

_____ Criterion-referenced instrument

_____ Observation

Clinical findings (including body structure and function): ______________

____

____

Impact on activities and participation: ______________

____

____

Hearing screening: ____

____

____

Diagnosis/ICD-10 code(s): ____

____

____

Impressions: ____

____

____

Prognosis: ____

____

____

Personal and environmental factors impacting prognosis: ____

____

____

Recommendations: ____

____

____

Frequency/duration of treatment: ____

Speech-language pathologist signature, title, degree(s), credentials:

CC: Referral source

Physician(s)

7

Treatment Plans/Certifications

Nancy B. Swigert, MA, CCC-SLP, BCS-S

From Evaluation to Treatment Plan

The evaluation process should flow seamlessly into the treatment-planning process. In our housing analogy from Chapter 6, the treatment plan mirrors the development of the architectural plans. Treatment planning is establishing the framework for the intervention. Part of the evaluation included establishing the client's current state of functioning in all areas of communication and swallowing that are applicable. In addition, all prognostic factors are considered when discussing with the client and caregivers realistic expectations for the outcome of treatment.

Setting Goals

When developing a treatment plan, the speech-language pathologist should consider three points on a continuum of function: Baseline or prior level of function, current state/level of function, and goal state (Figure 7-1).

For a client who has previously had communication and/or swallowing skills that were within functional, age-appropriate limits, the baseline is that previously normal state. For children who have presented with the communication or feeding/swallowing disorder since birth, there is not a period of time in which the prior level of functioning was a normal baseline. For comparative purposes, the skills of a typically developing, same-age peer can be viewed as what the expected baseline might be. The current state information obtained during the evaluation serves as the benchmark against which progress will be measured. The baseline functioning helps in determining prognosis and setting a goal state.

In some cases, the goal state might be to return the client to the baseline level of functioning (Figure 7-2) or to help a child achieve the same functioning as typically developing same-age peers (Figure 7-3). In other situations, the goal state will be to improve function but not necessarily to return to baseline in the case of adults (Figure 7-4) or to catch up to peers (Figure 7-5). One of the challenges with goal setting for young children is that the target of reaching the level of typically developing peers keeps changing as the peers develop new skills.

Setting Goals When No Improvement Is Expected

For some clients with chronic or progressive conditions, no improvement is expected. Medicare requirements had historically held that for services to be reimbursed, there had to be an expectation that improvement would be made,

Swigert, N. B.
Documentation and Reimbursement for Speech-Language Pathologists: Principles and Practice (pp. 85-97).

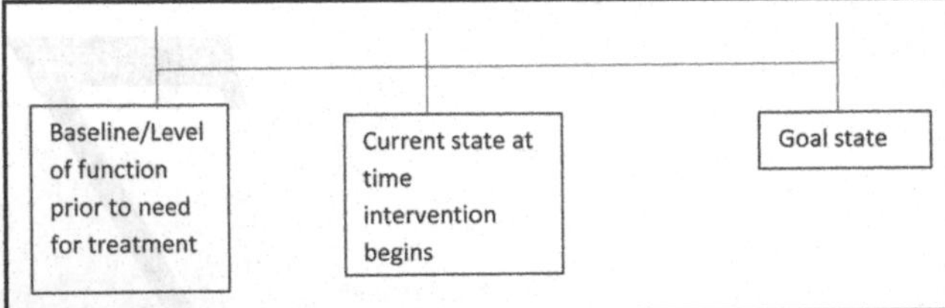

Figure 7-1. Timeline considerations when setting goals.

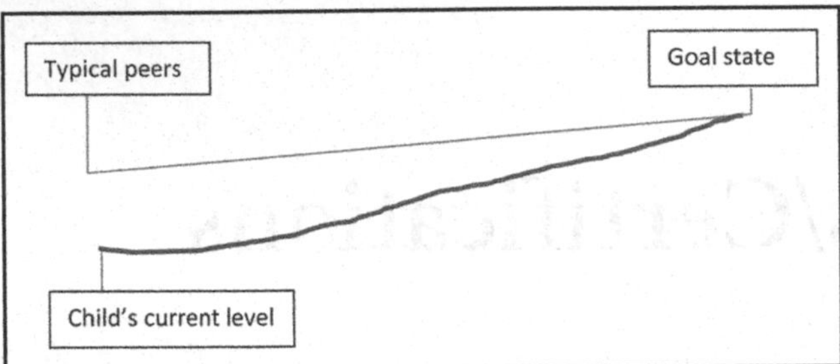

Figure 7-3. Child goal state is to reach level of typically developing peers.

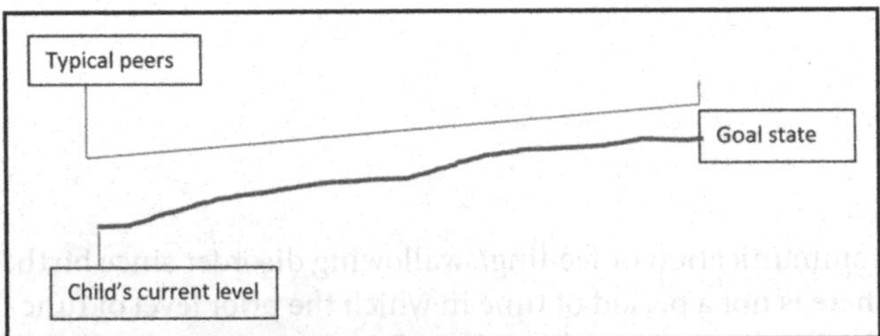

Figure 7-5. Child goal state is to improve, but not to reach level of typically developing peers.

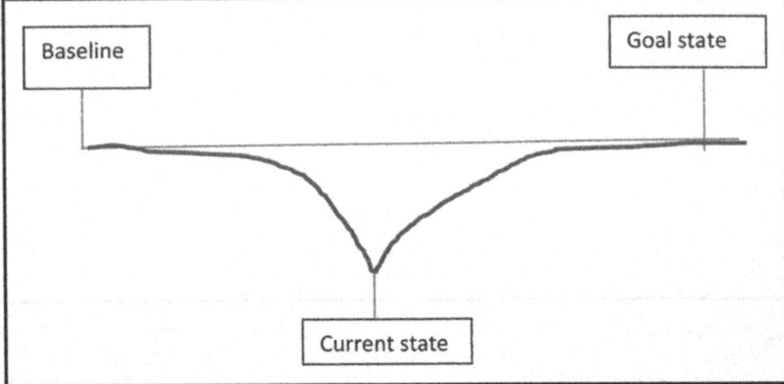

Figure 7-2. Adult goal state is to return to baseline/prior level of function.

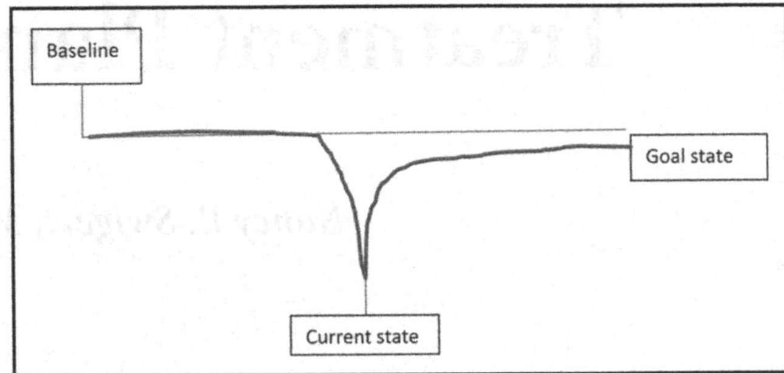

Figure 7-4. Adult goal state is to improve, but not to return to baseline/prior level of function.

often referenced as the *improvement standard.* In 2013, in the case of *Jimmo v. Sebelius*, the court held that Medicare could not deny services because the client showed no functional progress in cases of degenerative or progressive disorders, such as amyotrophic lateral sclerosis, multiple sclerosis, or Parkinson's disease. They stated that Medicare had to cover services to maintain skills and prevent deterioration (American Speech-Language-Hearing Association [ASHA], 2016; Centers for Medicare & Medicaid Services [CMS], n.d.).

Note that these still need to be skilled services. Medicare will not cover services that are designed to practice or drill because these are activities that can be completed by caregivers. In the case of degenerative and progressive disorders, however, it may be appropriate for the speech-language pathologist to periodically reassess, intervene, and modify maintenance programs to address the client's current level of functioning in communication and swallowing.

For the client with a chronic disorder who is not functioning at an optimal level, the focus of a short course of treatment might be on teaching compensatory strategies and helping the client and caregiver learn ways to maximize function. The same is true for a client with a progressive disorder for which intermittent courses of treatment are indicated at various stages of the disease.

When no improvement is expected, the goals are worded to reflect not an expected improvement in skill, but improved use of compensations and adaptations. Goals might also be written for a change in caregiver behaviors such as cueing. For example, instead of a goal stating, "*Client will improve ability to use single words to express needs,*" the goal might state, "*Client will compensate for reduced ability to use verbalization to communicate by pointing to pictures to indicate needs,*" or "*Caregiver will present client a choice of three pictures from which to choose to indicate basic needs.*"

Goal Setting With the Client

Clinicians often discuss treatment goals with the client and caregivers, but may not always get a commitment from them on what they are willing to work toward. Too often, the speech-language pathologist is setting goals he or she expects the patient to achieve in the therapy sessions with him or her, which may be a focus at the level of impairment in body structure and function. With the changing health care environment, speech-language pathologists should develop treatment plans with a focus on the patient working on the goals outside of the therapy session as much as possible.

Table 7-1

Principles of Patient Self-Management in Chronic Disease Compared With Applying Those Principles to Patient Participating More Actively in Management of the Communication or Swallowing Problem

Patient Self-Management of Chronic Disease	More Active Client Self-Management of Communication or Swallowing Disorder
• Management of chronic disease over time is essential. • Client must engage in different health care practices. • Client knows the most about consequences of chronic disease and must apply that knowledge to manage the disease over time. • The client and health care professional must share knowledge and authority for managing the disease.	• Client engagement and participation over the course of treatment is essential. • In order to generalize skills learned in treatment, the client must engage in carryover activities. • Client and caregivers know the most about communication and swallowing needs in day-to-day situations and must apply what they learn in treatment over time. • The client, caregivers, and speech-language pathologist must share knowledge and authority for reaching goals.

Adapted from Holman, H., & Lorig, K. (2004). Patient self-management: A key to effectiveness and efficiency in care of chronic disease. *Public Health Reports*, 119(3), 239.

Placing more responsibility on the patient for managing his or her disorders is called *patient self-management*. This has been applied mainly to helping patients manage a chronic disease (Holman & Lorig, 2004). Management of a chronic disease differs from the way an acute event is managed, which places most of the responsibility in the hands of the medical professionals. With a chronic disease, the patient must take a more active role. Although most clients seen by a speech-language pathologist do not have a chronic communication or swallowing problem, some of the principles of patient self-management can be applied to clients with communication and swallowing disorders and their caregivers. The speech-language pathologist must actively work to achieve buy-in from the client and caregivers to participate not only in therapy, but also outside the therapy session to achieve the agreed upon goals (Table 7-1).

In addition, goals must be measurable and meaningful to the patient, caregivers, and other health professionals, and especially to payers. Documentation should clearly reflect the focus on outcomes important to the patient and centered on function, not centered on impairment.

SMART Goals

One framework that is helpful in writing good goals is the SMART criteria, commonly attributed to Peter Drucker's management by objectives concept (Boudreaux, 2005; Bovend'Eerdt, Botell, & Wade, 2009). SMART is an acronym that stands for specific, measurable, attainable, realistic, timely (Figure 7-6). This acronym is often used in project management settings to help an individual identify

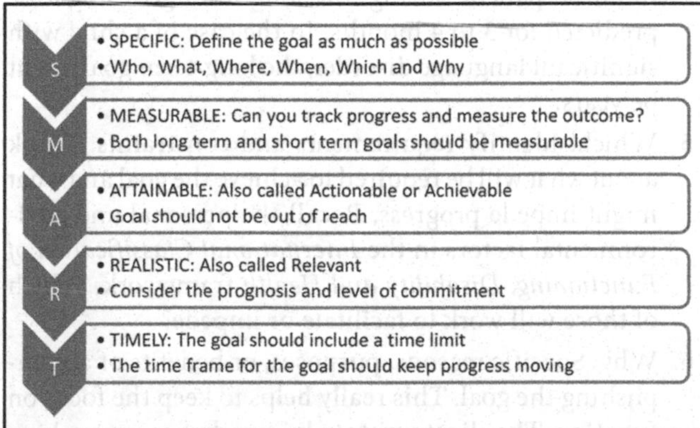

Figure 7-6. SMART goals.

goals and the necessary steps needed to accomplish a given task. Employees may be asked to establish SMART goals for their individual growth over the next year. Their progress toward achieving the goal is assessed as the annual performance appraisal.

SMART goals are being used increasingly in health care to help patients learn to manage their own health, especially related to chronic conditions. Perform an internet search for SMART goals for hypertension, weight loss, or diabetes management for examples of how this is applied to patient self-management. Facilities using SMART goals state that this format helps to engage patients in an interactive discussion about their health care and results in patients more committed to reaching these goals.

Let's look more closely at each of the steps in writing SMART goals.

Specific

A specific goal has a much greater chance of being accomplished than a general goal. To set a specific goal, you must answer the six "W" questions:

1. Who: Who is involved? Almost always this is the client. In certain cases, only the caregiver may be involved. For example, a patient with moderate dementia may not be able to actively participate in treatment but a goal may be written for the caregiver to implement. In many cases, the client and caregiver(s) are involved in the treatment.
2. What: What do I want to accomplish? Keeping the focus on function, this question should be, "What do the client and I agree we should work to accomplish?"
3. Where: Identify a location. Is this a goal to be achieved in the treatment setting? Transferred to settings outside the treatment room? Generalized to all settings?
4. When: Establish a time frame. Depending on the setting, short-term goals are written for a period of weeks or months. Long-term goals are usually set for the time frame the client will be at that level of care. For example, in an acute care hospital, the long term goal might be at time of discharge in 4 to 5 days, whereas in an outpatient setting, the long-term goal might be predicted for 3 to 4 months. In the case of a child with significant language disorder, the long-term goal might be years.
5. Which: Identify requirements and constraints. Think about what will be required to achieve the goal and what might impede progress. Recall the personal and environmental factors in the *International Classification of Functioning, Disability and Health* framework. Which of those will work to facilitate or impede?
6. Why: Specific reasons, purposes, or benefits of accomplishing the goal. This really helps to keep the focus on function. The client wants to know why we are working on a specific task.

As an example, a general goal would be, "Client's verbal skills will improve," but a specific goal would say, "Client's verbal skills will improve through increased ability to recall names of objects so that he can interact with family during mealtimes to request desired food and drink 90% of trials with no cues within 4 weeks."

1. Who? The client and the caregivers
2. What? Wants to interact at meals
3. Where? At family meals
4. When? Within a month
5. Which? Will need support of family members. May need picture cues in the environment.
6. Why? So that the client feels engaged in family mealtime activities.

Measurable

There must be tangible criteria for measuring progress toward the attainment of each goal you set. In addition, terms must be operationally defined. For example, if a goal uses words like *fluently, intelligibly, smoothly, accurately,* or *concisely,* these must be defined. If not, how would one know when the goal was achieved?

To determine whether a goal is measurable, ask questions such as the following:

- How much?
- How many?
- How will you know when it is accomplished?

Long-term goals sometimes pose the biggest challenge for making them measurable. Consider the following long-terms goals and decide whether you would know when the patient had achieved them. Some probing questions are listed after each goal.

- Patient will eat optimal diet. *(What is optimal?)*
- Patient will advance diet as far as possible. *(How far is it possible for the patient to go?)*
- Patient will eat foods like same-age peers. *(In children, there is a wide range of what is eaten. Consider a 2-year-old: Does the goal imply soft, mashed table foods? Finger foods? Peeled apple slices?)*
- Patient will safely consume thin liquids. *(How will you know if it is safe? No coughing? No pneumonia? No upper respiratory infection?)*

Short-term goals in particular are written with a percent accuracy or number of times a response needs to be accurate. The goals often need to indicate level and type of cueing required. If that information is omitted, it will make it difficult to measure success. Consider the following goal and scenario:

Goal: Child will follow two-step directions with 90% accuracy when given by parent during activities of daily living (ADL).

You are observing the father and the child in a home setting, and as the father gives a direction to the child (e.g., "Find your truck and put it in the toy box"), he points to the truck in the corner and then gestures to the toy box. When the child gets the truck, the father then gestures to the toy box and opens the lid. The child puts the truck in the toy box. Is that following a two-step direction? If the goal had been written as, *Child will follow two-step directions given* ***moderate gestural cues*** *with 90% accuracy when given by parent during ADL,* then this scenario represents one accurate completion of the task. If the goal was, *Child will follow two-step directions with* ***no cues*** *with 90% accuracy when given by parent during ADL,* then this is not an accurate completion of the task. If this information about cueing is not included, it makes measuring success inaccurate.

It is not sufficient to use terms like *minimal, mild, moderate,* or *maximum assist* without describing what kind of assist is being given. What would this goal mean? *Client will answer simple questions with maximum cues.* Is the client being given a printed word with the answer? Is the clinician gesturing to indicate the answer? Is the clinician showing a picture of the answer? It is much more meaningful to describe the type of cue the client requires.

Attainable

This goal is sometimes called *actionable* or *achievable.* A goal can be written that is specific and measurable, but if it is not attainable, it is not a good goal. Consider an elementary school–aged child with severe cerebral palsy who is fed by G-tube with concomitant severely impaired oral skills: No lip closure, no lingual lateralization, severe tongue thrust movement to propel boluses posteriorly with significant loss of most of the bolus. A long-term goal for the child to receive all nutrition and hydration by mouth is not an attainable goal. On the other hand, a long-term goal for the child to take small amounts of smooth foods by spoon with jaw and lip assist may be attainable. If the clinician has discussed prognosis with the caregiver, and the caregiver understands and accepts the prognosis, it is more likely that attainable goals will be set.

ASHA's National Outcomes Measurement System (NOMS) Adult Component has a new feature that gives clinicians access to real-time national benchmarking data to help the speech-language pathologist establish an attainable goal. When the patient's information is entered into the NOMS system and the Functional Communication Measure (FCM) rating is given, the speech-language pathologist can select "View National Goal Setting." These national data indicate what percentage of patients who have also started at this same FCM level and were treated in the same setting achieved each FCM level. The NOMS system also includes a reporting feature that allows clinicians to receive more detailed information, such as how many sessions or what length of time it took on average for patients with similar characteristics (e.g., medical diagnosis, severity level) receiving treatment in my facility to reach that level compared with patients receiving treatment nationally (ASHA, n.d.-b).

Realistic

A realistic goal is one that is attainable, and also one the patient agrees he or she is willing to work toward. Setting a realistic goal requires significant discussion with the client and caregivers. Not only must the prognosis be considered, but the level of commitment of the client and caregivers has an impact. Consider a fitness goal that an adult might set. She might set a goal to run an upcoming 10K race. She is fairly fit and walks 3 times/week. However, in order to run the 10K, she will need to start running a couple of miles a day. Realistic? Only if she is committed to doing so.

The same is true of setting communication and swallowing goals. Perhaps a client with a fluency disorder who successfully uses fluency-enhancing strategies in one-on-one conversations agrees to a goal of using fluency-enhancing techniques on phone calls, but continues to avoid phone call interactions. The goal is not realistic.

Clients cannot achieve goals if they only work on them with the speech-language pathologist during treatment sessions. If a child's caregivers agree they will stop providing negative reinforcement to the child's tantrums when child is presented with a food the child does not like, it may be realistic that the tantrums can be eliminated. However, if the caregivers' reinforcement of that response continues, what the speech-language pathologist does in the treatment session is not likely to change the behavior.

Timely

A goal should be grounded within a time frame. The time frame for short- and long-term goals is influenced by the setting in which the client is seen. In acute care, the patient may only be in the facility for several days. Most short-term goals, then, would be set for that period of time. In other inpatient settings where the patient might be seen for weeks or a month or more, the short-term goals might be written for shorter periods during that time and then updated as the patient makes progress. In outpatient settings, the short-term goals are likely updated and changed periodically as dictated by the payer. Medicare, for example, requires that the treatment plan (called a *certification* in Medicare terms) be updated and re-signed by the physician. Even at points not required by a third-party payer, the clinician may want to update the treatment plan. It might be determined that one of the goals was too challenging, one was achieved, or the clinician wants to add goals and treatment objectives. If a third-party payer required update is imminent, make those changes at that time. If there are no requirements for periodic updating of the treatment plan, the clinician can make those changes at any time (Figure 7-7).

Increasing Efficiency in Developing Treatment Plans

Because the same goals are typically used for clients with similar deficits, clinicians can develop *goal banks.* A goal bank is a list of long- and short-term goals specific to a disorder. They can be written with blanks for percent accuracy, type and amount of cueing, etc. The speech-language pathologist can select appropriate goals for the client and modify the wording as needed. Commercially available therapy resource books often contain goal banks for the disorder addressed (Swigert, 1997, 2000, 2003, 2005, 2010).

SPEECH-LANGUAGE PATHOLOGY
TREATMENT PLAN

Patient Name: James Randall
DOB: 10-9-62
Patient #:
Medical Diagnosis/ICD-9: Hoarseness R49.0
Problem areas to be addressed: Client's voice gives out by mid-day
Date treatment initiated: 6-4-17
Estimated amount, frequency and duration of treatment: 1x week; ½ hour to 1 hour; 4-6 weeks
Reasonable expectation to meet treatment goals: Excellent as hoarseness is new onset and client motivated
Date of report: 6-4-17; updated 7-2-17 **At discharge, total # treatment units:**

Long Term Goal Functional Goal(s):
Patient will be able to use voice for vocational and avocational activities.

Date established	Speech therapy/swallowing therapy for these short term goals in functional/measurable terms	Progress/ Date
6-4-17	1. Patient will eliminate vocally abusive behaviors: a. decrease coughing 2. Patient will institute vocal hygiene techniques: b. increase water intake to 64 ounces/day c. substitute swallow or silent cough for coughing 3. Patient will reduce hyperfunctional use of the vocal mechanism via: a. Improved use of diaphragmatic breathing in supine and standing with verbal cues b. Reducing tension in oro-pharyngeal area by applying digital manipulation without cues c. Improving tone focus for easy phonation through use of vocal function exercises	2.a Achieved 6-15-17
Added: 7-2-17	4. Patient will utilize amplification in the classroom for any class of over 10 students.	

Speech-language Pathologist Signature ______________________ Date ________

CC: O.T. Laryngol, M.D.
Date sent: 6-4-17

Figure 7-7. Adjusting goals during treatment.

Medical Necessity

The treatment being planned should meet the requirements of being medically necessary. Medicare indicates that to be medically necessary, the care must be the following:

- Reasonable: Provided with appropriate amount, frequency, duration, and accepted standards of practice
- Necessary: Appropriate treatment for the patient's medical and treatment diagnoses and prior level of function
- Specific: Targeted to a particular treatment goal
- Effective: Expectation for functional improvement within a reasonable time or maintenance of function in the case of degenerative conditions; patient's prior level of function serves as the baseline
- Skilled: Requires the knowledge, skills, and judgment of a speech-language pathologist. When establishing a treatment plan, the goals should be those that the client can only achieve through the provision of skilled service by the speech-language pathologist. Medicare (and other plans that adopt Medicare documentation guidelines) requires that services eligible for reimbursement must be at a level of complexity and sophistication that requires the specific expertise and clinical judgment of the qualified speech-language pathologist, thus meeting the definition of skilled services. Goals such as, *"Client will participate fully in the treatment session"* or *"Client will improve communication skills"* do not imply that any level of skill of the speech-language pathologist is required in order to meet the goal (ASHA, n.d.-a). More information on skilled services is provided in Chapter 8.

Focus on Function

When collaborating with the client and caregiver to select and write long- and short-term goals, the focus should remain on function. What is it that the client wants to be able to do, and in what situations? What is important to one client will not be important to another, and yet each might have similar skill deficits. Consider two individuals with a muscle tension dysphonia, rendering their voices quite hoarse and impairing their ability to speak and be heard over any background noise. At the level of impairment, their disorders are very similar. However, one client is a retired accountant who desires to be able to use his voice to carry on conversations over the phone with his grandchildren. The other is an amateur country singer who performs in clubs on the weekends and wants to be able to sing and not lose her voice over the course of the show. Not only are the long-term goals different for these two individuals, but the short-term goals may differ significantly as well. If the goals were written only to address the impairment, the clients' functional needs would not have been addressed.

Long- and Short-Term Goals and Treatment Objectives

Long-Term Goals

Typically, long-term goals are written that are long term based on the level of care. What level of skill and function do you and the client agree is realistic and attainable by the time the client moves to the next level of care? For children, the long-term goals might be established for the anticipated end date of services or for a more arbitrary midpoint such as the end of each school year.

Long-term goals should be established for each of the areas of swallowing and communication being addressed. If the client is working on receptive and expressive language and articulation, a long-term goal would be established for each. For example, a child might have these long-term goals:

- By the end of the school year, child's speech will be understandable to peers and adults in 100% of situations without cues.
- By April 1, child will follow directions as well as same-grade peers in classroom situations.
- By the end of the school year, child will use complex and compound sentences in spoken language as well as same-grade peers in classroom situations.

Long-term goals should meet all of the SMART criteria and focus on function.

Short-Term Goals

If the clinician is following the SMART criteria, short-term goals will be written in functional terms and tell what and why. A functional goal tells *why* you are working on something. It should be written in terms that a non-speech-language pathologist can understand. Not functional: "Client will accurately produce sibilants, affricates, and fricatives." Functional: "Patient will accurately produce sibilants, affricates, and fricatives in conversation so he can be understood by peers and adults."

Write short-term goals as the smaller steps needed to reach the long-term goal. There may be multiple short-terms goals for each long-term goal. Short-term goals should be measurable, and, in addition to answering *why*, should answer *what*. What does the patient have to be able to do in order to achieve the long-term goal? For example, for the long-term goal, *By the end of the school year, child's speech will be understandable to peers and adults in 100% of situations without cues*, you might have short-term goals such as the following:

- Short-term goal: Child will produce sibilants and affricates in all positions of words accurately.
  - Short-term goal SMART terms: Within 10 weeks, child will produce sibilants and affricates in all positions of words during structured activities in the treatment session with minimal visual cues on 90% of trials to contribute to increased intelligibility.
- Short-term goal: Child will produce sibilants and affricates at sentence level.
  - Short-term goal SMART terms: Within 16 weeks, child will produce sibilants and affricates when answering a question with a sentence in the treatment session with minimal visual cues on 85% of trials to contribute to increased intelligibility.
- Short-term goal: Child will produce sibilants and affricates in conversation.
  - Short-term goal SMART terms: By spring break, child will produce sibilants and affricates in conversational speech in the classroom with no cues on 85% of trials to contribute to increased intelligibility.

Treatment Objectives

You can break short-term goals into more measurable steps called *treatment objectives*, which are the steps to achieve the short-term goal and are often equivalent to therapeutic activities. The treatment objectives put the focus on the *how*. How are you going to help the patient reach that short-term goal? What activities will be used to achieve the goal? One short-term goal might have several treatment objectives.

For example, for the short-term goal, *Within 10 weeks, child will produce sibilants and affricates in all positions of words during structured activities in the treatment session with minimal visual cues on 90% of trials to contribute to increased intelligibility*, you might have the following (and more) measureable treatment objectives:

- Client will produce sibilants in initial position of words when naming pictures with minimal visual cues 90%.
- Client will produce sibilants in medial position of words in imitation with moderate tactile cues 95%.
- Client will produce sibilants in final position of words with no cues when answering questions with a single word 90%.

Combining Short-Term Goals and Treatment Objectives

If your charting system does not accommodate both short-term goals and treatment objectives, the short-term goal and treatment objective can be combined. For example: *Within 10 weeks, child will produce sibilants and affricates in all positions of words during structured activities* ***by naming pictures and completing open-ended sentences*** *in the treatment session with minimal visual cues on 90% of trials to contribute to increased intelligibility.*

Treatment Plans, Certifications, and Recertifications

The treatment plan can be documented in various ways depending on the setting in which the services are being provided. Each electronic health record differs in how the information is entered and what a printout might look like. Other inpatient settings not using an electronic health record may have specific forms that need to be used for the treatment plan/certification. A useful format in outpatient settings includes spaces for all the required information in a table format that can be used for the goals (see Appendices 7-A and 7-B for examples). This same form can then be used as updates (recertifications) and for the discharge summary.

Regardless of the format, the treatment plan should contain the following:

- Client identifying information
- Diagnoses
- Date the plan was established
- Period of time the plan will cover
- Type, amount, frequency, and duration of services
    - Type: Individual, group
    - Amount: Number of times per day
    - Frequency: How many times per day or week
    - Duration: For what period of time; number of weeks or months
- Long-term goal(s)
- Short-term goal(s)
- Treatment objectives (or short-term goals with the objectives embedded)
- Signature, date, and professional designation of the person who established the plan (CMS, 2012)

In settings in which the services are provided to clients with Medicare as the payment source, the treatment plan is called a *certification* and requires a physician's signature on the plan. The plan must be updated periodically, at different time frames depending on the setting, and signed again. This is referred to as *recertification.*

References

American Speech-Language-Hearing Association. (n.d.-a). Documentation in health care. Retrieved from http://www.asha.org/PRPSpecificTopic.aspx?folderid=8589935365§ion=Key_Issues

American Speech-Language-Hearing Association. (n.d.-b). National Outcomes Measurement System (NOMS). Retrieved from http://www.asha.org/NOMS/

American Speech-Language-Hearing Association. (2016). *Jimmo v. Sebelius* plaintiffs return to court to urge enforcement. Retrieved from http://www.asha.org/News/2016/Jimmo-v-Sebelius-Plaintiffs-Return-to-Court-to-Urge-Enforcement/

Boudreaux, G. (2005). Peter Drucker's continuing relevance for electric cooperatives. *Management Quarterly, 46*(4), 18.

Bovend'Eerdt, T. J., Botell, R. E., & Wade, D. T. (2009). Writing SMART rehabilitation goals and achieving goal attainment scaling: A practical guide. *Clinical Rehabilitation, 23*(4), 352–361.

Centers for Medicare & Medicaid Services. (n.d.). *Jimmo v. Sebelius* settlement agreement fact sheet. Retrieved from https://www.cms.gov/medicare/medicare-fee-for-service-payment/SNFPPS/downloads/jimmo-factsheet.pdf

Centers for Medicare & Medicaid Services. (2012). Physical, occupational, and speech therapy services. Retrieved from https://www.cms.gov/Research-Statistics-Data-and-Systems/Monitoring-Programs/Medical-Review/Downloads/TherapyCapSlidesv10_09052012.pdf

Holman, H., & Lorig, K. (2004). Patient self-management: A key to effectiveness and efficiency in care of chronic disease. *Public Health Reports, 119*(3), 239.

Swigert, N. B. (1997). *The source for dysarthria.* Austin, TX: LinguiSystems.

Swigert, N. B. (2000). *The source for dysphagia.* Austin, TX: LinguiSystems.

Swigert, N. B. (2003). *The source for reading fluency.* Austin, TX: LinguiSystems.

Swigert, N. B. (2005). *The source for children's voice disorders.* Austin, TX: LinguiSystems.

Swigert, N. B. (2010). *The source for pediatric dysphagia.* Austin, TX: LinguiSystems.

Review Questions

1. Why is it important to involve the client and caregivers when establishing a treatment plan?
2. What are some factors that determine the length of time set to achieve short- and long-term goals?
3. What questions should the speech-language pathologist ask him- or herself to make sure the goal being written is specific?
4. What is the difference in a goal being attainable and being realistic?
5. What are treatment objectives, and how are they related to short-term goals?
6. How does the concept of patient self-management relate to goal setting?
7. What components are required to meet the definition of medical necessity?

Activity A

Which of the following goals are measurable? If not clearly measurable, what needs to change to make them more measurable?

1. Patient will eat an optimal diet daily.
2. Client will speak clearly 75% of the time.
3. Client will answer simple questions with moderate cues 95% accurately.
4. Client will reduce the occurrence of backing to less than 20% at word level.
5. Client will not stutter on the phone.
6. Client will be able to participate in meetings at work.
7. Patient will answer simple questions with one-word answer when given phonemic cues on 90% of trials.
8. Client will answer complex questions about paragraph-level material he has read with no cues on 95% of trials.
9. Client will not try to talk in situations with excessive background noise.
10. Client will use reduce rate of speech to 50% of typical rate on sentence-level responses on 90% of situations.
11. Client will comprehend a short grade-level story she has read.
12. Client's caregiver will provide a gestural or visual cue 85% of the time when the client is having trouble retrieving a word during conversation.
13. Child will complete open-ended sentences with an appropriate word or phrase given minimal cues during treatment on 90% of trials.
14. Client will use multiple swallows with pureed texture.
15. When provided with an action picture, client will construct a sentence with correct verb and verb tense with no cues on 90% of trials.
16. When provided with a visual cue to look to the left of the paper, the client will be able to read a sentence aloud correctly.
17. Child will be able to determine whether two words are the same or different when presented the words aloud.
18. Client will match a printed word to one of three pictures without cueing on 95% of trials.
19. Client will utilize fluency-enhancing techniques when encountering challenging speaking situations.
20. Client will select correct picture on augmentative device to match the word spoken by the clinician when given moderate physical cues.

Activity B

Evaluating Goal Statements

Determine which of the following goals have all of the components of a SMART goal. For each goal that is incomplete or inaccurate, describe what it lacks.

1. By the time of discharge in 1 week, client will be able to answer yes/no questions about basic needs with no prompts.
   _____ This goal has all the SMART components.
   _____ This goal lacks ______________________________
2. Client will read fluently.
   _____ This goal has all the SMART components.
   _____ This goal lacks ______________________________
3. Speech-language pathologist will instruct family in cueing techniques.
   _____ This goal has all the SMART components.
   _____ This goal lacks ______________________________
4. By the end of the school year, the student will be able to read multi-paragraph passages from social studies text and write complete sentences to answer the questions with no cues.
   _____ This goal has all the SMART components.
   _____ This goal lacks ______________________________
5. In order to be able to eat safely, only pureed food will be presented to the client in the dining room at each meal.
   _____ This goal has all the SMART components.
   _____ This goal lacks ______________________________
6. Client will remember to use vocal hygiene strategies every day.
   _____ This goal has all the SMART components.
   _____ This goal lacks ______________________________
7. In order to increase intelligibility, within 4 weeks, client will produce phrases with /s/ blends accurately.
   _____ This goal has all the SMART components.
   _____ This goal lacks ______________________________
8. Within 45 days, client will be able to engage in short (3- to 4-minute) conversations with spouse while exhibiting fewer than five word retrieval deficits in the conversation.
   _____ This goal has all the SMART components.
   _____ This goal lacks ______________________________
9. Within 6 months, client will be able to use 15 single words when prompted with a gestural cue.
   _____ This goal has all the SMART components.
   _____ This goal lacks ______________________________
10. Client will demonstrate improved ability to answer questions.
   _____ This goal has all the SMART components.
   _____ This goal lacks ______________________________

Activity C

Writing SMART Long-Term Goals

Review the scenarios below and write a long-term goal that is specific, measurable, attainable, realistic, and timely. Each client might need more than one long-term goal (to address different deficit areas), but you only need to select one area to address.

1. Your client suffered a severe stroke with resultant profound receptive and expressive aphasia. His husband wants him to be able to come home after his stay in rehabilitation, but he will need to be able to stay alone at home for a period of several hours each day. He will likely be at the rehabilitation facility for 5 weeks.
2. Your client, a 4-year-old, has significantly impaired phonological awareness skills, a moderate articulation disorder, and a mild receptive language disorder. Next year he will start a kindergarten program, and his mother wants him to be able to learn to read along with his classmates.
3. Your client has Parkinson's disease, which has impaired the intelligibility of his speech. He is coming to your outpatient clinic for therapy because he is no longer able to play cards with his friends due to his speech.
4. Your client was just discharged from a rehabilitation facility to home, where you begin his home health treatment. He has a moderate pharyngeal dysphagia related to a head injury and is on a mechanical soft diet with nectar thick liquids. He wants to be able to enjoy Thanksgiving dinner with his family.
5. Your client suffered a concussion during a high school football game and is experiencing difficulty with concentration and memory that are interfering with his ability to participate in class. He has finals in 6 weeks.

Appendix 7-A

Example Treatment Plan: Motor Speech Outpatient

Speech-Language Pathology Treatment Plan

Patient name: Spring Sneeze **DOB:** 1/23/2003 **Patient #:** XXXX

Medical diagnosis/ICD-10: Oral dysphagia R13.11; Dysarthria R47.1; Secondary to status post-surgery for malocclusion M26.4; Late effect of complications from that surgery T89.9XXS

Problem areas to be addressed: Drooling, can't drink from cup, impaired oral phase, impaired articulation interfering with school performance

Date treatment initiated/plan established: 2/12/17 **Intervention time frame:** 2/12/17 through 5/1/17

Estimated amount, frequency, and duration of treatment: Individual 1-hour sessions; 2-3x week for 5 weeks; then 1-2x/week for 6 weeks

Reasonable expectation to meet treatment goals: Guarded given uncertain etiology and probable nerve damage

Date of report: 2/12/17

Long-term functional goal(s):

1. Spring will be able to eat and drink without difficulty.
2. Spring will be able to correctly articulate all sounds

Date Established	Short-Term Goal(s) and Treatment Objectives	Progress/ Date*
2/12/17	1. Spring will improve lip movement for speech and swallowing, including the ability to: a. Achieve and maintain lip closure for 2-3 minutes without visual cues b. Consistently close lips to produce bilabial phonemes /p,b,m/ in all positions of words at conversational level without visual cues c. Pucker lips and maintain that position for 30 seconds without visual cues d. Lateralize pursed lips side to side without visual cues on 10/10 trials e. Retract top lip to show teeth without visual cues on 10/10 trials 2. Spring will improve tongue movement for speech and swallowing, including the ability to: a. Protrude tongue and maintain for 10 seconds without visual cues b. Lateralize tongue tip to corner of lips bilaterally without visual cues 10/10 times c. Lateralize tongue tip into lateral buccal cavity without visual cues 10/10 times d. Elevate tongue tip to alveolar ridge and maintain for 10 seconds without visual cues e. Forcefully "pop" tongue against roof of mouth 10/10 trials f. Elevate back of tongue to produce /k/ with force at beginning and end of words 100%	

*Progress on goals: A = Achieved; I = Improved; N/C = No change

Speech-language pathologist signature: ____________

Date: ________

CC: G. Surgeon, MD; K. Adolespeds, MD

Date sent: 2/18/17

Appendix 7-B
Example Treatment Plan: Pediatric Feeding Outpatient

Speech-Language Pathology Treatment Plan

Patient name: Malika Fazal **Patient #:** XXXX
Medical diagnosis/ICD-10: R13.11 Oral dysphagia
Problem areas to be addressed: Noisy sucking with excess gas; refusing spoon feeding
Date treatment initiated: 08-24-17
Estimated amount, frequency, and duration of treatment: 1x/week; 6 weeks; then 1x/mos for 3 mos
Reasonable expectation to meet treatment goals:
Date of report: 08-18-17
At discharge, total # treatment units:

Long-term functional goal(s):
1. Child will eat and drink age-appropriate foods and liquids in typical amount of time.

Date Established	Speech Therapy/Swallowing Therapy for Short-Term Goals in Functional/ Measurable Terms	Progress/ Date*
08-18-17	1. Infant will increase efficiency with bottle feeding. a. Infant will be provided minimal jaw support while sucking. b. Infant will use bottle/nipple that reduces intake of air. 2. Infant will take runny pureed foods from spoon. a. Food will be placed mid-tongue. b. Lip closure will be encouraged with physical assist as needed.	

*Progress on goals: A = Achieved; I = Improved; N/C = No change.
Speech-language pathologist signature: ________________
Date: ____________
CC: Paul Pediatrician, MD
Date sent: 08-18-17

8

Progress Notes

Nancy B. Swigert, MA, CCC-SLP, BCS-S

Treatment Notes and Progress Notes as Part of the Overall Management of the Client

The evaluation has been completed, the treatment plan devised, and now treatment is beginning. In our analogy from Chapter 6 about building a house and managing a client's care, the progress note is the weekly update from the construction manager. As the person paying for the house that is being built, you are anxious to know that your money is being well spent. You want to know that the builder is following the plans you approved and that steady progress is being made. Third-party payers think the same thing about therapy. Is the clinician following the agreed upon plan of care, and is the client making steady progress toward goals? The treatment notes and progress notes are where this documentation takes place. A treatment note is one that is written for each session. A progress note is written less frequently (e.g., weekly or every tenth visit) and summarizes what has happened over the course of several treatment sessions.

SOAP Format

In health care settings, the standard format for documenting services provided is the SOAP note. SOAP stands for subjective data (S), objective data (O), assessment of the data (A), and plan for next steps (P). These notes provide accountability, support the clinical decisions that were made, and corroborate the delivery of appropriate services (Cameron & Turtle-Song, 2002). They are intended to enhance communication among health care professionals, and thus improve the continuity of care. These notes also help the clinician recall the specific details of the case (Kettenbach, 1990). Advantages of using a standard format like a SOAP note include the ability to follow a logical format each time, the speed at which the note can be completed, and the ability for others who read the note to quickly orient to where specific information can be found (Konin & Frederick, 2017).

SOAP notes can vary in length and style depending on the setting but should contain information in each of the four components. In some settings, the notes may be short phrases (Figure 8-1), but in most outpatient rehabilitation settings, the format contains full sentences (Figure 8-2). The note should be complete enough that someone who was not present for the session can tell what happened and why.

Swigert, N. B.
Documentation and Reimbursement for Speech-Language Pathologists: Principles and Practice (pp. 99-112).

SWIGERT & ASSOCIATES, INC.
PROGRESS NOTE
PARADOXICAL VOCAL FOLD MOTION

February 14, 2017

Winter Freeze

S: No bad attacks
Using techniques in sports
No use of inhalers

O: Taught diaphragmatic breathing—all positions
Best standing and supine
Answered questions about exhalation and practiced

A: Analyzed performance
Gave tactile cues
Doing well with all techniques

P: Appointment next week
Can cancel if doing well
Pick up the pace in running
Practice techniques in fast walking/stair climbing.

Nancy B. Swigert, MA, CCC-SLP

Figure 8-1. Abbreviated SOAP note.

SWIGERT & ASSOCIATES, INC.
PROGRESS NOTE
PARADOXICAL VOCAL FOLD MOTION

February 14, 2017

Winter Freeze

S: Winter reports that she has not had any bad "attacks". She has felt tightness and implemented the sniff inhalation techniques. Uses techniques in sports. Has slowed down, but not come out of the game. No attacks at school. No use of inhalers.

O: Taught diaphragmatic breathing in supine, standing, and sitting. She did well with all positions. Using diaphragmatic breathing well, though best in supine and standing.
Answered questions she had (e.g., how long should the exhalation be) and practiced as appropriate.

A: Analyzed Winter's technique with abdominal breathing and altered cues provided by giving tactile cues for inhalation and this improved performance. Winter seems to be applying the strategies well.

P: Set an appointment for next week, but she can call and cancel if she is doing this well. She is to start picking up the pace with her running, but using the technique throughout. If she has to come in next week, practice techniques in fast walking and stair climbing.

Nancy B. Swigert, MA, CCC-SLP

Figure 8-2. SOAP note more typical of rehabilitation settings.

It should be understandable not only to another speech-language pathologist, but to other health care professionals and non–health care professionals, such as third-party payers or regulatory agencies, as well. However, the clinician must balance the need for thoroughness with the demand for efficiency (Hsu & Sánchez, 2016). It should not take more than a few minutes to write, type, or enter a progress note, and ideally this should be done within the session.

S: Subjective

This section of the note contains information provided by the client or those accompanying the client. It is considered subjective because there is not a way to measure or verify what the client reports. Typically, these statements occur at the start of the session, but they might occur at any point during the session. They might include statements by the client about symptoms, experiences related to the communication or swallowing disorder since last seen by the speech-language pathologist, reports of applying strategies or techniques, or specific questions raised. Do not repeat inflammatory statements made about other health care professionals or the quality of services, because these can compromise the client's care by antagonizing other staff or be viewed as malicious or damaging to the reputation of the other party (Cameron & Turtle-Song, 2002). For example, don't include a statement such as, "Client's mother reported they are appalled at the way the pediatrician's staff treats them when client acts out in their waiting room." Instead, use a more general statement such as, "Client's mother reported concerns about the way some individuals respond to client's outbursts."

Not everything the client reports is pertinent. The clinician develops skill at extracting what is pertinent and recording it in a succinct and accurate fashion (Figure 8-3). It is not necessary to use quotation marks, and in fact they should be kept to a minimum. Overuse of quotation marks makes the record more difficult to review for patterns of information shared. In addition, when reviewed by outside readers like auditors or attorneys, the accuracy of the notes might be questioned. It is helpful to use words like *reports*, *states*, *says*, *describes*, *indicates*, *complains of*, and *indicated*. The clinician does not have to refer to him- or herself because it is implied that the clinician is the author of the note. For example, do not document things like, "Client reported to this clinician" or "Client's mother described to the speech-language pathologist…" (Cameron & Turtle-Song, 2002).

Recording everything the patient reports regarding her voice disorder

Client reported that her voice lasted through third period on Tuesday, Wednesday, and Thursday, but by Friday she became hoarse after second period. Her fellow teachers noticed this as well and mentioned it during lunch on Friday. She has talked to the principal twice about getting an amplification system and has more forms to fill out which she indicates she will do over the holiday weekend and get them turned in. She reported attending her daughter's soccer matches and admits to forgetting and yelling a few times. She said that her caffeine intake is down to 2 cups/day.

Editing the client reports to just what is pertinent for the S section

Reports voice lasting through partial days, less at end of week. Continues talks with principal about amplification. Has forms to complete. Still occasional yelling at sports. Caffeine intake down.

Figure 8-3. S section of SOAP note edited to what is pertinent.

O: Objective

This section of the note contains objective, measurable information about what occurred during the session. One of the ways to streamline documentation but also keep the focus on the goals specified on the treatment plan is to use the O section of the note to chart against each of the goals or treatment objectives that were addressed during that session. This is easy to do in an electronic health record (EHR) if it is built correctly. The clinician clicks on each goal/treatment objective and simply inserts the percentage of accuracy achieved for that treatment activity. If progress notes are being typed (i.e., not in an EHR), the goals/treatment objectives can be copied and pasted from the treatment plan into the O section of the note. Then, the speech-language pathologist simply inserts the correct percentage next to each (Figure 8-4). However, in order to document that a skilled service was provided, the clinician also has to document additional information that might be included in the O section of the note, such as commenting on cues, level of independence, or latency of response, which demonstrate that the speech-language pathologist was utilizing his knowledge and skills (American Speech-Language-Hearing Association [ASHA], n.d.). If the speech-language pathologist is working in a setting in which progress notes are handwritten rather than typed, a template can be produced with the O section of the note prepopulated with the treatment objectives, and copies of the template can be made. Then, each session, the speech-language pathologist can fill in the correct percentages and complete the S, A, and P sections of the note.

A: Assessment

This section of the note is where the speech-language pathologist demonstrates his or her knowledge and skills. Someone without the level of expertise of a speech-language pathologist could probably complete the S and O sections of the note, writing down what the client reports and tallying the number of correct responses. However, the assessment can only be done well by the speech-language pathologist. The clinician synthesizes information provided by the client and analyzes the client's performance throughout the session. This section can contain the speech-language pathologist's impressions. The report of the objective data needs to be supplemented with information that demonstrates the clinician's involvement in the session, recording the adjustments made throughout the treatment session that could only be done by a skilled speech-language pathologist. The synthesis, analysis, and adjustments (e.g., cues, changing level of difficulty) are reported in the A section of the note. More information on documenting skilled care follows.

The A section of the note can be used to provide summary statements of the client's performance. The speech-language pathologist should support such judgment statements with objective data. Using the phrase *as evidenced by* is a good way to accomplish this. For example, the speech-language pathologist might document, "Client's word retrieval skills are much improved *as evidenced by accuracy of 90% with no cues needed.*" The A section is also a good place to summarize the client's progress toward goals. The clinician can also use this section to justify continued treatment, especially if writing a periodic progress note. See Chapter 16 for more information on treatment notes vs progress notes.

If the clinician also needs to describe something about the client that is having an impact on performance in therapy, it is important to avoid value-laden language and opinionated statements. Avoid words that have a negative connotation such as *manipulative*, *obnoxious*, *spoiled*, *dysfunctional*, *obstinate*, *out of control*, or *rude*. Instead, record observations of behaviors that would lead the reader to a similar conclusion. For example, instead of recording, "Client was off the wall today, acting like a spoiled brat," the clinician could document, "Client refused to sit down, threw toys, and demanded to get a prize from the surprise box" (Cameron & Turtle-Song, 2002).

P: Plan

This part of the note specifies what is to happen next, both in terms of activities between sessions and at the next session. It is not acceptable to simply put "continue per plan" as the P section of the note. This part of the note

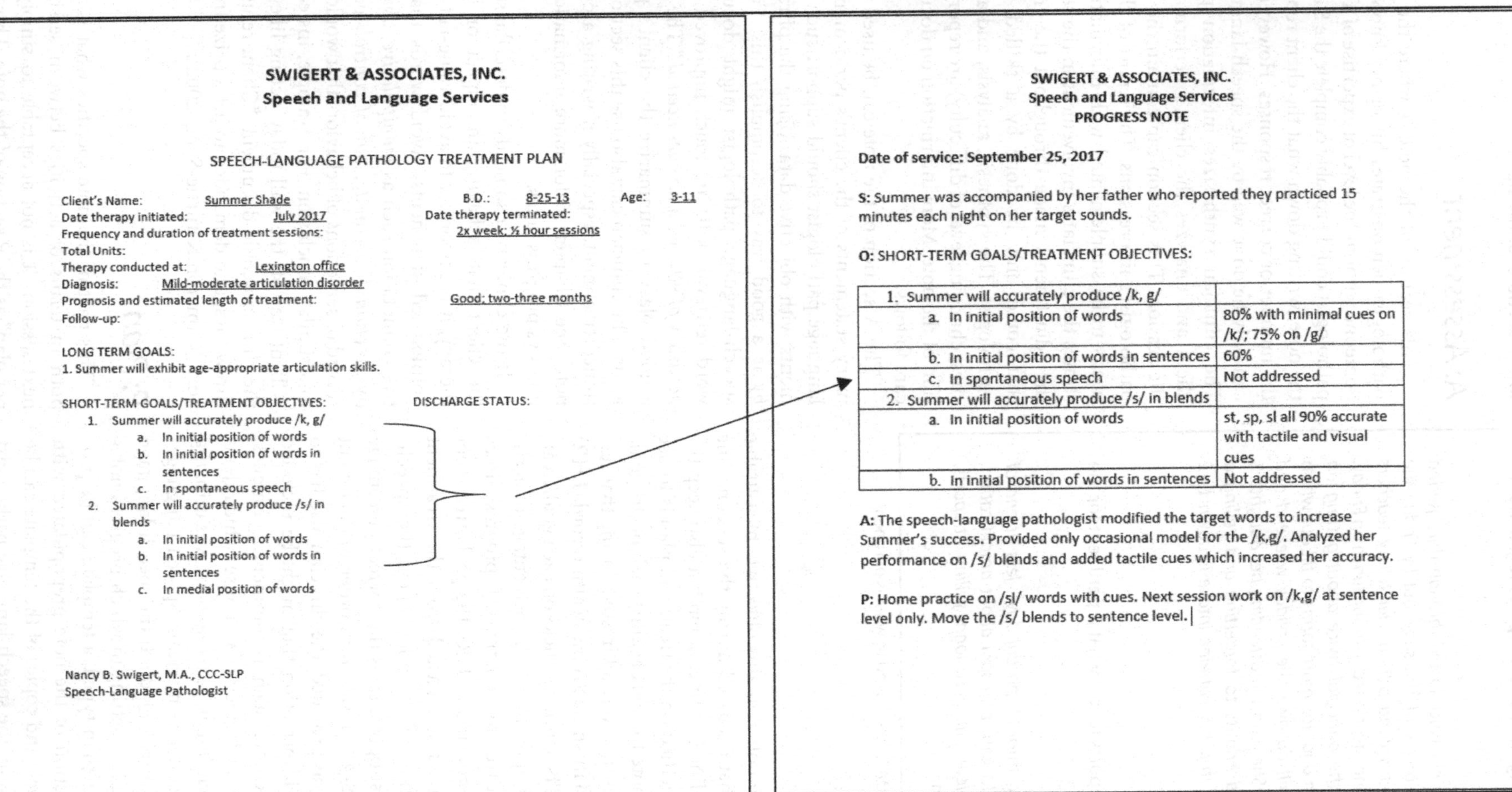

SWIGERT & ASSOCIATES, INC.
Speech and Language Services

SPEECH-LANGUAGE PATHOLOGY TREATMENT PLAN

Client's Name: Summer Shade B.D.: 8-25-13 Age: 3-11
Date therapy initiated: July 2017 Date therapy terminated:
Frequency and duration of treatment sessions: 2x week; ½ hour sessions
Total Units:
Therapy conducted at: Lexington office
Diagnosis: Mild-moderate articulation disorder
Prognosis and estimated length of treatment: Good; two-three months
Follow-up:

LONG TERM GOALS:
1. Summer will exhibit age-appropriate articulation skills.

SHORT-TERM GOALS/TREATMENT OBJECTIVES: DISCHARGE STATUS:

1. Summer will accurately produce /k, g/
   a. In initial position of words
   b. In initial position of words in sentences
   c. In spontaneous speech
2. Summer will accurately produce /s/ in blends
   a. In initial position of words
   b. In initial position of words in sentences
   c. In medial position of words

Nancy B. Swigert, M.A., CCC-SLP
Speech-Language Pathologist

SWIGERT & ASSOCIATES, INC.
Speech and Language Services
PROGRESS NOTE

Date of service: September 25, 2017

S: Summer was accompanied by her father who reported they practiced 15 minutes each night on her target sounds.

O: SHORT-TERM GOALS/TREATMENT OBJECTIVES:

1. Summer will accurately produce /k, g/	
a. In initial position of words	80% with minimal cues on /k/; 75% on /g/
b. In initial position of words in sentences	60%
c. In spontaneous speech	Not addressed
2. Summer will accurately produce /s/ in blends	
a. In initial position of words	st, sp, sl all 90% accurate with tactile and visual cues
b. In initial position of words in sentences	Not addressed

A: The speech-language pathologist modified the target words to increase Summer's success. Provided only occasional model for the /k,g/. Analyzed her performance on /s/ blends and added tactile cues which increased her accuracy.

P: Home practice on /sl/ words with cues. Next session work on /k,g/ at sentence level only. Move the /s/ blends to sentence level.

Figure 8-4. Treatment plan to O section of progress note.

Table 8-1

Tips for Point-of-Care Documentation

Try This	Think About This
Change your perception.	Charting is not something extra done after the session; it is an integral part of the session.
Arrange the treatment room so that you and the client are sitting next to each other.	This allows the client to see what you are documenting as you chart.
Tell the client what you are charting and why.	This keeps the client informed about progress.
Seek input from the client on what to chart.	Ask the client his or her impression of how he or she did on a particular activity.
Pre-load the treatment note.	Having the computer on and the progress note already open makes the session more efficient.
If narrative/annotation is needed, enter short phrases.	You can always take a minute later to expand into full sentences if needed.

should be so accurate and precise that another speech-language pathologist could step in and take over the care of the client without missing a beat. Typically, this section includes date of next appointment, any homework or home activities, any follow-up the client needs to complete (e.g., physician appointment), any referrals being made by the speech-language pathologist (e.g., referral to another health care or educational professional for assessment or intervention), and the direction for the next session. Also include mention of any changes in the treatment plan, such as a change in frequency or intensity of services. Prognostic statements might also be included as indicated to provide information about how the client is responding to the intervention.

Point-of-Care Documentation

Point-of-care documentation, or documenting while the provider is with the client, is a growing practice in health care. It is typically done when an EHR is used but can also be done in a paper charting system. There is an impact on the interaction between patient and provider when the provider is documenting on a computer during the session. It alters the visual, postural, and verbal connection between clinician and patient (Als, 1997). Als (1997) found that the physician took a time out from the conversation with the patient to document. Physicians and other health care professionals express concern that using a computer to document might depersonalize the care (Aydin, Anderson, Rosen, Felitti, & Weng, 1998). Despite reservations about point of care documentation, there are advantages to documenting at the time the service is rendered.

Charting is something the clinician does as a part of the service provided, not something extra that is done after the service is completed and the client has left or the speech-language pathologist has left the patient's room. If done correctly, point-of-care documentation can increase the collaboration between the clinician and the client. It is also a more accurate way to chart than trying to remember all that happened at the end of the session or, worse yet, after seeing three or four clients and then charting all the visits at once. The goal is to be able to log off or close the paper chart when the treatment session is over, or to need only a minute or 2 to flesh out narrative sections (Table 8-1).

The treatment session can be compared with a conversation in which the participants take turns and information is exchanged. Taking time to document throughout the session should not feel as if something is being taken away from the interaction, but instead that something is being added (Table 8-2).

Documenting during treatment takes practice and is easier with some client than others. The clinician should explain to the client and caregivers that notes will be taken throughout the session. It is likely the client has already experienced point-of-care documentation at his or her physician's office or even dentist's office. The speech-language pathologist can use a standard phrase to introduce the client to this type of documentation, such as the following:

- I'll be making notes throughout the session to be sure I capture everything we do.
- I'll stop here and there during the session to record information on how you are doing.
- It's important that I record how you are doing, so I'll be taking notes as we go.
- I'll be sure and let you know how things are going as I take some notes during the session.

It can be particularly challenging with a pediatric client if a parent is not in the session. If the child is older, he or she can be given a break to play with a toy for a minute here and

Table 8-2

Flow of Session With Point-of-Care Documentation

Part of Note	What Happens	What Client/Caregiver Says	What Is Charted	What the Speech-Language Pathologist Says While Charting
S	Speech-language pathologist asks how things have been going since the last session.	Father says, "Randy and I have practiced about 10 minutes each day, usually in the car on the way home from school. He has a little trouble with the /r/ when it is in the middle of the word. His teacher said she has heard him say some words with /r/."	Home practice completed with father. /r/ medial most difficult. Some carryover per teacher.	"That's great work. Let me jot down how you all have practiced and what the teacher said."
O	Child completes activity naming pictures with /r/ all positions of words, and /r/ initial in phrases while speech-language pathologist notes accuracy. Father practices the /r/ medial cards with Randy.		/r/ initial 90% /r/ initial phrases 75% /r/ medial 80% /r/ final 85%	"That's improved on all positions from last session. Let me note that while you go over the medial /r/ once more with Randy."
A	During the naming activity, the speech-language pathologist provides tactile cues on medial /r/. When Randy has particular difficulty with a word, the speech-language pathologist also has Randy look in the mirror, and this improves accuracy.		Analyzed client's responses and added tactile and visual cues as needed for medial /r/.	"I'm making a note that touching Randy under the chin helped him make the /r/ sound in the middle."
	Speech-language pathologist asks father how he thinks the session went	"I can see how that touch helps Randy."		
	The speech-language pathologist reminds the father to have Randy look in the mirror.	"The mirror helps too."	Provided feedback to provide more cues.	"So glad to see you use the mirror."
P	The speech-language pathologist provides homework sheet with /r/ initial phrases.		Homework /r/ initial phrases. Next session final /r/ phrases.	"So the plan is to work on /r/ in phrases. Use the touch cue when you need to. Next session we'll even try phrases with /r/ at the end."

there throughout the session while charting takes place. Ideally, the caregiver will be in the treatment session, and the speech-language pathologist can engage in dialogue with the caregiver while charting.

Treatment That Is Medically Necessary

Medicare requires (and most third-party payers adopt the same requirement) that to be reimbursed, treatment must be medically necessary. Services are medically necessary if they are the following:

- Skilled, rehabilitative services;
- Provided by clinicians (or qualified professionals when appropriate);
- With the approval of a physician/non–physician provider, safe; and
- Effective (i.e., progress indicates that the care is effective in rehabilitation of function) (Centers for Medicare & Medicaid Services [CMS], 2017).

Documentation in the progress notes is one place that a reviewer or auditor would look to support medical necessity.

Demonstrating Skilled Care

Treatment for any client with any disorder should only be given if the skilled services of a speech-language pathologist are required. Medicare indicates that skilled therapy services may be necessary to improve a patient's current condition, to maintain the patient's current condition, or to prevent or slow further deterioration of the condition.

Medicare regulations are the most stringent in this regard, but the best practice for any client with any payer is to ensure that the progress note demonstrates that skilled care was provided. Just because the service was provided by a speech-language pathologist does not make it skilled. If the service could be self-administered (e.g., client practices a swallowing exercise that she already knows how to perform), or safely and effectively provided by an unskilled person without the direct or general supervision of the speech-language pathologist (e.g., client's spouse reminds client to reduce rate of speech when reading), it is not considered skilled, even if it is the speech-language pathologist performing these tasks. Medicare also indicates that just because there is not a competent unskilled person to practice with the client, the service is not skilled if the speech-language pathologist instead practices with the client (CMS, 2017).

ASHA's website provides detailed information on how the speech-language pathologist can demonstrate skilled services in the progress notes, such as the following:

- The documentation of treatment activities should show that the activities:
  - Followed a hierarchy of complexity
  - Were focused on achieving the target skills for a functional goal
- Based on the speech-language pathologist's expert observation, modify activities during treatment sessions to maintain patient motivation and facilitate success.
  - Increase or decrease complexity of treatment task
  - Increase or decrease amount or type of cueing needed
  - Increase or decrease criteria for successful performance (e.g., accuracy, number of repetitions, response latency)
  - Introduce new tasks to evaluate patient's ability to generalize skill
- Help clients practice behaviors. Note that this practice should be combined with explaining the rationale and expected results and/or providing reinforcement.
- During the session, continually assess patient response in order to modify intervention as needed.
- Develop, program, and modify an augmentative and alternative communication system (low or high tech) (ASHA, n.d.).

See Table 8-3 for examples of documenting skill in different parts of the treatment note.

Skilled services that are not adequately documented may appear to be unskilled, such as the following:

- Reporting on performance during activities without describing modification, feedback, or caregiver training that was provided during the session
- Repeating the same activities as in previous sessions without noting modifications or observations that would alter future sessions, length of treatment, or point of care
- Reporting on activity without connecting the task to the long- or short-term functional goals
- Observing caregivers without providing education or feedback and/or without modifying the plan (ASHA, n.d.)

For more information and examples on documenting skilled services, visit the ASHA Portal Page on documentation for speech-language pathologists (www.asha.org/Practice-Portal/Professional-Issues/Documentation-in-Health-Care/).

Table 8-3

Ways to Show Skilled Care in Progress Notes

What the Speech-Language Pathologist Might Document to Support Skilled Care	Example	Section of SOAP Note Where This Might Appear
Terminology that demonstrates the clinician's level of skill	Demonstrated and explained super-supraglottic swallow and impact on timing as well as closure.	O
Explain how an activity relates to a goal	Client's performance of vocal function exercises was improved with ability to produce nasalized, front focus "eee" at 12 seconds. This will help client maintain front focus in speech.	O, A
Report Objective Data		
Report accuracy on a task[a]	Client at 80% on using manual sign to request "more" and "eat" and less than 50% on "drink."	O
Report speed of response[a]	Client demonstrated significantly reduced latency of response, with only 1- to 2-second delay before following 2-step direction.	O, A
Report number of responses[a]	Client read 8/10 sentences with easy onset.	O
Report number of cues	Cued client on 60% of responses.	O, A
Report type of cues	Provided tactile cues to indicate that client should extend production of sibilants and that increased accuracy to 90% on words.	O, A
Report level of independence	Client now independent with monitoring and eliminating throat clearing.	A
Report physiologic changes	Client's performance decreased when sibling was in the room due to increased distractibility.	A
Specify feedback given	Provided feedback to client on performance on contrasting word pairs, instructing client to use mirror for cues as needed.	A
Explain Why Modifications to Treatment Plan or Activities Were Made		
Resulted in functional change	When client is cued to take a breath before starting to talk, loudness is maintained for the whole utterance, making it easier for others to understand her.	A
New goals could be added	Because client achieved 95% accuracy on sibilants, have added goal to work on affricates.	A
Activities added or dropped	Client doing so well on naming items within a category (divergent) that task will be dropped and convergent task added instead.	A
Criteria changed	Client able to answer questions about story read to him in quiet environment, so will add background noise to same task.	A

(continued)

Table 8-3 (continued)

Ways to Show Skilled Care in Progress Notes		
What the Speech-Language Pathologist Might Document to Support Skilled Care	**Example**	**Section of SOAP Note Where This Might Appear**
Client/Caregiver Training		
Elaborate on training	Trained client's mother to model manual sign and use physical cues as needed and to stop responding to pointing at objects.	A
Evaluate response to training	After showing client's son how to cue client to reduce rate, the son was able to use the cues in a 5-minute conversation with his father.	A

[a]The speech-language pathologist should also report on modifications, feedback, and caregiver training and not simply on accuracy, speed, or number of responses.

Adapted from American Speech-Language-Hearing Association. (n.d.) Documentation of skilled versus unskilled care for Medicare beneficiaries. Retrieved from http://www.asha.org/Practice/reimbursement/medicare/Documentation-of-Skilled-Versus-Unskilled-Care-for-Medicare-Beneficiaries/

Documenting Teaching as Part of the Treatment Session

Sometimes clinicians mistakenly assume that teaching the client and caregivers is something that happens after treatment. However, this engagement of the client and caregivers is an essential part of treatment and should ideally occur throughout the session, not just at the end. In fact, documenting this client and caregiver engagement is another way to demonstrate skilled care. Documentation could address the following:

- Training and providing feedback to patient/caregiver in use of compensatory skills and strategies (e.g., feeding and swallowing strategies, cognitive strategies for memory and executive function)
- Training caregiver to facilitate carryover and generalization of skills
- Instructing patient and caregiver in use and care of communication system

Documenting Each Visit

The typical practice in most settings is for the speech-language pathologist to write a full progress note each time the client is seen. However, in some settings, mostly inpatient, the clinician simply documents that the service was provided. Then, the clinician writes a summary note once/week. (For more information on periodic progress reports required by Medicare, see Chapter 16.) Medicare does not require a note each visit. However, they do require the following information be documented for each visit:

- Date of service
- The procedure(s) performed (including the Current Procedural Terminology [CPT] code)
- The length of each procedure performed (which would be crucial only if a timed CPT code was used; otherwise, the length of the session generally is equal to the length of the one procedure code used during that session)
- The signature and professional identification of the provider of the procedure(s) (CMS, 2017)

If you are writing a progress note for each visit, that information should also be contained in the note, in addition to much more detailed information described here.

Documenting Non-Patient Contact

Sessions with the client are not the only ones that should be documented. Sometimes there is important information about the case that is discussed over the phone, in face-to-face conversations, or via email. This information should be included in the chart. Email correspondence can be stored electronically in an EHR and printed for a paper chart. Face-to-face discussions and phone conversations should be noted in the chart. If it is a quick exchange, for instance in the hall with another member of the treatment team in which no substantial information is discussed, it is not necessary to record it. For example, you might see the physical therapist, who reports to you that the client was using gestures appropriately in the physical therapy session. You might just include this in the S section the next time you see the client. If, on the other hand, the physical therapist shares significant information, a separate entry, which is dated/timed to reflect the time of the conversation, should be placed in the chart. Perhaps the physical therapist tells you that he heard from the client's mother that the seizure activity had significantly increased in the past few days and that the client's level of alertness has declined. This could be entered in a note in the chart. It is not necessary to use SOAP format for an entry like this. It should be dated and timed and have your full signature/authentication.

References

Als, A. B. (1997). The desk-top computer as a magic box: patterns of behaviour connected with the desk-top computer; GPs' and patients' perceptions. *Family Practice, 14*(1), 17–23.

American Speech-Language-Hearing Association. (n.d.) Documentation of skilled versus unskilled care for Medicare beneficiaries. Retrieved from http://www.asha.org/Practice/reimbursement/medicare/Documentation-of-Skilled-Versus-Unskilled-Care-for-Medicare-Beneficiaries/

Aydin, C. E., Anderson, J. G., Rosen, P. N., Felitti, V. J., & Weng, H. C. (1998). Computers in the consulting room: a case study of clinician and patient perspectives. *Health Care Management Science, 1*(1), 61–74.

Cameron, S., & Turtle-Song, I. (2002). Learning to write case notes using the SOAP format. *Journal of Counseling and Development, 80*(3), 286.

Centers for Medicare & Medicaid Services. (2017). Medicare Benefit Policy Manual: Chapter 15—Covered medical and other health services. Retrieved from https://www.cms.gov/Regulations-and-Guidance/Guidance/Manuals/downloads/bp102c15.pdf

Hsu, L., & Sánchez, F. (2016). SOAP notes. Retrieved from https://owl.english.purdue.edu/owl/resource/1003/01/

Kettenbach, G. (1990). *Writing SOAP notes*. Philadelphia, PA: FA Davis Company.

Konin, J. G., & Frederick, M. A. (2017). *Documentation for athletic training* (3rd ed.). Thorofare, NJ: SLACK Incorporated.

Review Questions

1. What is the difference between a treatment note and a progress note?
2. List two challenges and two advantages to using point-of-care documentation.
3. Why is a standard format like SOAP used for charting?
4. What does each part of the acronym SOAP stand for?
5. List four things speech-language pathologists should keep in mind when documenting so that the note demonstrates that skilled care was provided.

Activity A

Summarize and rewrite each S example so that it is no more than two to three short sentences. Extract what is pertinent to the disorder being treated. Include only pertinent, factual information and descriptions of behavior, not judgments.

Case #1: A Pediatric Expressive Language Accompanied by His Father

S: Emory's father reported that Emory gave a book report this week. He is interested in dinosaurs so the family got a couple of books from the local library. One was a little above his level, so Emory's dad actually read most of that one to him. His parents helped him write out what he wanted to say and reminded him to use complete sentences. His dad ran into his teacher at the store and she told him that Emory still rambled a little bit but did a much better job at giving the topic and using connecting phrases. His last oral book report 3 weeks ago was very unorganized per the teacher.

Case #2: A Young Adult Status Post-Concussion With Memory and Attention Deficits

S: Lien was 10 minutes late for her session, which is so typical of her. She seems flighty and I suspect this was the case before her concussion. She had not completed the memory activity assigned on the computer game and said she just didn't have time (or did she just not make it a priority?). Lien said she has had fewer headaches and was actually able to read the front page of the paper in one sitting. Had filled in her calendar on her smartphone for daily activities as requested.

Case #3: A 2-Year-Old With Receptive and Expressive Language Delays Seen in the Home of His Grandmother

S: Randy's grandmother answered the door in her bathrobe (it was 10:00 a.m.!). She said that Randy had not slept well the night before and she suspected he was coming down with something, perhaps the cold that his siblings have had. She reported he has used the signs for "up" and "eat" pretty consistently with her but said she doubts that Randy's mother makes him do this at all when he is with her. She said because he was tired, she expected him to be a real handful during the session.

Case #4: An 82-Year-Old With Mild Cognitive Impairment Accompanied by His Wife

S: Mrs. Kim reported that her husband got very upset a few days ago when he could not balance the checkbook. He wanted to get that done before their daughter came over because she usually checks on them and sees what they might need to go to the store to buy. Mr. Kim denied getting upset and said there was something wrong with the calculator and that was why he couldn't get the checkbook balanced. Mrs. Kim stood behind him and shook her head while he was saying this.

Case #5: A 45-Year-Old Physical Education Teacher With Muscle Tension Dysphonia

S: Ms. Martinez said that she used her amplification system in all but one of the periods she taught last week. The exception was one class she took outside for laps around the building. Stated it was such a nice day she hated to keep the children in the gym, and that day the third graders were particularly active and needed to run off some of that energy. She indicated she was at a family dinner and by the end of the evening her throat hurt to talk. She described her family as "full of loud talkers!"

Case #6: A 7-Year-Old With Dysfluency Dropped Off for Therapy (Parent Not Present)

S: Jabari told me his dad had dropped him off and couldn't come in. The weeks he is with his dad, this clinician rarely gets to see the father, which is disappointing to say the least because his father also has dysfluency and would really like to get him involved in supporting Jabari's treatment. Jabari's grandmother, on the other hand, is a bit overinvolved. She is always correcting Jabari. Jabari said he saw the school speech-language pathologist in group this week and worked on practicing his smooth speech during a board game. The other two students in the group have more severe dysfluency per the speech-language pathologist. Jabari reported that his soccer team had won their game last week (he had talked about it during therapy last week). He seemed very excited about that.

Case #7: A 68-Year-Old Male With Parkinson's Disease and Dysarthria

S: Mr. James and his husband both reported good success with the practice of loud speech at their weekly bridge game. They are avid bridge players and have been with the same group for over 20 years. Mr. James said that he had also had lunch with an old business colleague and admitted the friend did have to ask him to repeat himself several times during the meal. They were at Full Bloom, a particularly noisy restaurant in town, so not surprising he might have been hard to hear.

Case #8: A 78-Year-Old Status Post-Cerebrovascular Accident With Moderate Receptive and Expressive Aphasia

S: Mrs. Murray's husband (he is so dedicated to his wife!) had completed the home activities provided to them at the last session: Answering moderately complex yes/no questions, naming familiar objects described by attributes, and following two-step directions. He is one of the most accurate at recording responses that this speech-language pathologist has seen. Mrs. Murray tried her best to express that they had been to visit their daughter and family over the holidays. She sure puts forth great effort and maintains a positive attitude.

Case #9: A 13-Month-Old With a Feeding Disorder

S: Hagen's mother brought along some of the foods she has tried with him this past week: Fork-mashed tofu, pieces of banana, dissolvable snacks, and small pieces of cheese. She reports that Hagen was willing to try everything but spit out the pieces of cheese and made his typical "I'm about to gag" face (which is so adorable, but you can tell he's faking it because he doesn't really gag anymore). His mother reported that he took milk from sippy cup, and, as requested, she is holding liquids until the end of the meal.

Activity B

For each of the statement(s) listed, indicate in which section of the SOAP note it would go:

S	O	A	P	
				Patient states she had practiced overnight and thinks the voice is better. She is still whispering.
				Patient did very well today. She is able to modify her productions with less cueing.
				Reviewed exercises from yesterday and switched gears to more nasal productions in hopes of using resonant voice therapy techniques to reinforce less tension.
				She's to practice the homework 5 minutes of every hour.
				Client is to practice the patterns taught. He is also to begin a list of words that are hard for him to pronounce (e.g., spirit).
				Client states he is very eager to get started in treatment.
				Provided feedback to client's daughter regarding ways to cue client on word retrieval.
				Client and her husband attended the session. She reported they had reviewed the sentences she had been practicing.
				Initial trials with Mendelsohn maneuver with sips of water unsuccessful. Modified instruction and provided tactile cues and performance improved.
				Audio record some sentences for intonation work and bring to next session.
				Patient reports she is doing a little singing with her group at church. She saw her ear-nose-throat doctor today, and he indicated the proton pump inhibitor should start taking effect soon.
				She was able to perceive the difference in focus and how it changed the quality of her voice.
				She's to call in 1 week. I suspect she won't need to be seen. If she does need another appointment, work on projection and changing volume for singing.
				Accuracy on expressive language tasks: Completing open-ended sentences 75% with cues; providing 3 items in a category no cues 80%; describing simple objects with adjective and verb no cues 75%.
				Client states the problem has been going on for several years. Between May and September, the symptoms resolved (but not this spring.)
				A variety of facilitation techniques were attempted, and none were successful in consistently achieving phonation: Yawn-sigh, inhalation phonation, digital manipulation, glottal fry, resonant voice therapy.
				Patient to follow up with otolaryngologist before next visit.
				Analyzed client's performance on vocal function exercises and modified task to increase success.
				Articulation work on words with /p/ and /f/ and then sentences with both. 90% to 95% accuracy at word level and 75% at sentence level. She did great unless a word with an /m/ also occurred and then accuracy dropped to 60%.
				Observe eating at next visit to see if he applies compensatory strategies without cues.
				Client has not been seen in almost a month. States she has been continuing to drill with her exercises and articulation at sentence level.
				See tracking sheet for data. Continued to concentrate on lip closure activities, with most activities at 90% to 95% accuracy.
				Will call for appointment first of the year. That session, try initial /z/ and then on to "th" in phrases in common words like "this" and "these".
				Client reports he has practiced some. He shared several frequently used words that confuse listeners (e.g., polymer).
				Demonstrated to client's wife how to pause and give client time to respond before cueing. After demonstration, she was able to do this.

Activity C

Which of the following statements in the progress note support that skilled care was provided? For each that *does* support skilled care, explain why it documents skill. Tip: Use Table 8-3 to select the way the statement(s) support skilled care.

1. Based on client's performance, added cues and encouraged her to monitor "vibrations" with hand on larynx.
2. The client seemed to understand the principals and improved his production of stress with repetition.
3. Observed client's wife practice activity designed to improve word recall and provided instruction to her on how to provide cues only when needed.
4. Explained to client's grandmother that use of the repeat reading technique is designed to build toward automaticity, reading fluency, and improved comprehension.
5. Seems like she is doing better on the open-ended questions this session compared with last.
6. She was able to perceive the difference in correct vs incorrect productions.
7. Analyzed client's production of target sounds and modified the target words to help client achieve success.
8. Doing very well. Eating is better.
9. Client 95% accurate on receptive language tasks.
10. After client completed receptive language task of two-step directions, had his mother explain the purpose of the task using teach-back methodology.
11. Decreased complexity of articulation task by dropping to phrase level, and this increased client's accuracy.
12. Client doing better at spotting patterns and hearing his errors.
13. Client 90% accurate on receptive language tasks designed to increase independence in activities of daily living. Explained to client's wife how these practice tasks are similar to those directions given by nursing staff.
14. Client demonstrated 5-second latency in response to simple yes/no questions, but when picture cues added, latency decreased to 2 seconds.
15. With verbal cues only, client fluent on 60% of responses, but when a visual cue was added via biofeedback, accuracy increased to 78%.
16. Doing very well. In spontaneous speech, she is achieving lip closure and acoustic accuracy for bilabials about 95% of the time.
17. Explained purpose of the effortful swallow to clear residue and client practiced the technique.
18. Watched client's wife practice the activity of client reading sentences with reduced rate.
19. Client accuracy at 80% on production of clusters, up from 60%.
20. Client demonstrated ability to use reduced rate and increased loudness independently without cues, indicating carryover of strategies taught.

9

Discharge Summaries and Maintenance Programs

Nancy B. Swigert, MA, CCC-SLP, BCS-S

Discharge Plans as the Wrap-Up

The discharge plan is the speech-language pathologist's final documentation on the client for that period of intervention. It should tell the story of the intervention so that other health care professionals, or the client and caregivers, can easily tell what happened. In our housing analogy from Chapter 6, it is the final walk-through with the builder, during which the work that has been completed is summarized and any remaining things that need to be done are pointed out.

Knowing When to Discharge

In health care settings, the determination of when to discharge can be straightforward or quite challenging. For inpatient settings, the timing of discharge from speech-language pathology services is often the same as the discharge date from the facility. In outpatient settings, the timing of discharge might be dictated by the third-party payer. Perhaps a limited number of sessions were approved and the client does not want to continue services on a private pay basis. If the timing of discharge is not dictated by setting or reimbursement, the speech-language pathologist must determine when the client has reached maximum gain from the intervention. The American Speech-Language-Hearing Association (ASHA) document *Admission/Discharge Criteria in Speech-Language Pathology* suggests the following considerations for discharge:

- Skills are now within normal limits or at premorbid status
- Goals and objectives have been met
- Skills are commensurate with others of the same age, gender, ethnicity, or cultural or linguistic background
- Deficits no longer negatively impact client's activity, participation, or health
- Desired level of enhanced skills has been met (ASHA, 2004)

Of course, there are instances in which the intervention will be terminated before maximum or optimal gain has been reached. Sometimes these are client-related reasons, such as lack of transportation or lack of cooperation. When those issues present, the clinician should address them in an effort to help the client continue in treatment. When the issues cannot be solved, the treatment may need to be terminated.

Swigert, N. B.
Documentation and Reimbursement for Speech-Language Pathologists: Principles and Practice (pp. 113-127).

When to Start Planning Discharge

Regardless of the setting, the speech-language pathologist should be thinking about discharge from the day of the evaluation. Whether limited by setting or third-party payer regulations, duration of therapy is not infinite. The clinician should discuss with the client and caregivers at the time of the evaluation and establishment of the treatment plan what the estimated duration of therapy will be. The criteria for discharge should also be discussed at that time. In addition, the clinician should be teaching the client and caregiver throughout the course of the intervention on how to complete carryover activities.

When to Discharge When No Improvement Was Expected

Medicare requirements had historically held that for services to be reimbursed, there had to be an expectation that improvement would be made, often referenced as the *improvement standard*. In 2013, in the case of *Jimmo v. Sebelius*, a federal court held that Medicare could not deny services because the client showed no functional progress in cases of degenerative or progressive disorders, such as amyotrophic lateral sclerosis, multiple sclerosis, or Parkinson's disease. They stated that Medicare had to cover services to maintain skills and prevent deterioration (ASHA, 2016; Centers for Medicare & Medicaid Services [CMS], n.d.). When enrolling a client in short-term intervention to maintain skills and prevent deterioration, the discussion of how long the intervention will be should also occur at the time of the evaluation. The goals should be made clear regarding maintaining skills so that the client and caregiver are not under the mistaken impression that improvement is expected.

Formats for Discharge Summaries

If using an electronic health record, the format for the discharge summary will be predetermined but should include all essential elements. In paper charting systems, the discharge summary can be written in one of several formats. Utilizing the SOAP (subjective, objective, assessment, plan) format cues the clinician about all the information that should be included (Table 9-1). The discharge summary should provide a succinct but complete picture of what occurred during the course of intervention, including the following:

- Client's and caregiver's view of what was accomplished in treatment
- Objective data (e.g., testing or measures of success on goals)
- Treatment methodologies used
- Impact the intervention had on function
- Remaining problems/challenges
- Reason for discharge
- Plans for further intervention or evaluations/consults

The treatment plan is another format that can be used for the discharge summary. The table for goals and objectives in the treatment plan format cues the clinician to include specific objective data about the status on the goals but may not provide as much structure to remember to include other elements. That information can be added to reflect the S, A, and P sections. Appendices 9-A and 9-B provide examples.

Reporting Subjective Data

At the conclusion of intervention, the client's and caregiver's impression of what was accomplished during the intervention should be sought. If the treatment plan and intervention have focused on function, it should be relatively easy for the client and caregiver to report on changes they notice in day-to-day activities. You are not seeking their input on how they think the client did on specific treatment activities (e.g., using the effortful swallow, speaking more slowly), but instead on the impact these improvements have had in daily life (e.g., eating more types of foods, being understood by neighbors and friends). Try to relate these statements to what the client and caregiver described as the impact on function at the beginning of the intervention. Gather information on their view of the client's current status compared with when intervention started and perhaps as compared with baseline. In the case of children, compare with when intervention started and with peers.

In addition to gathering information informally from the client and caregiver, the speech-language pathologist might utilize a specific tool to gather this information. This might be a self-designed customer satisfaction tool to gather input. The speech-language pathologist might also use one of several patient-reported outcomes (PRO) tools. See Chapter 5 for more information on PRO tools.

Reporting Objective Progress in the Discharge Summary

If specific treatment methodologies were used, the clinician should briefly mention and describe them. This could be very helpful to another speech-language pathologist who will be seeing the client in a different setting. For example, if surface electromyography was used to provide biofeedback during swallowing treatment or if a phonological approach was used to address unintelligibility, the methodology should be listed.

Table 9-1

Discharge Summary Template Using SOAP Format

S	• Client/caregiver statements about client's current status, amount of improvement made. • Statements about client's change in functional status: How the communication and/or swallowing problem improvement has had an impact on daily activities, participation. • Relate the statements to the initial complaints about impact on function in daily activities and participation. • Other statements about client's final status.
O	• Document results of any standardized or criterion-referenced tests administered at end of treatment. • Document objective data on long-term goal(s). • Document objective data on short-term goal(s). This does not mean you have to have the client work on each short-term goal in the last session so percent accuracy can be tallied; you can report the percent from a recent session. • Summarize the treatment methodologies used during this episode of care in general terms. For example: Vocal function exercises and instruction in vocal hygiene techniques utilized throughout treatment; life participation approach used as framework for treatment; naturalistic approach using intrinsic reinforcement was utilized.

A	• State the reason for discharge, such as treatment terminated due to the following:
	  ◦ Lack of continued funding
	  ◦ Client relocating
	  ◦ Client will receive services at another facility
	  ◦ Client being discharged from care at this level
	  ◦ Client has achieved all long- and short-term goals
	  ◦ Client has achieved maximum gain from intervention
	  ◦ Client/caregiver has demonstrated ability to follow through on maintenance activities
	  ◦ Client wishes to stop treatment at this time
	  ◦ Client withdrawing from treatment against clinician's recommendation
	  ◦ Client attendance has been poor and efforts to address unsuccessful
	  ◦ Client unwilling to participate in treatment and efforts to address unsuccessful
	  ◦ Other personal reasons (e.g., lack of transportation)
	• Summarize the effects of the intervention on impairment (body function), activities, and participation.
	• Summarize any personal and/or environmental factors that had an influence on progress during intervention.
	• Summarize what the objective changes reported in the O section mean (e.g., what a score on a certain test means related to function; what achieving a certain percent accuracy on a short-term goal means related to function).
	• Describe the client's current state of communication/swallowing.
	• Describe any remaining problems or goals that have not been addressed and explain why they have not been addressed.
	(continued)

Table 9-1 (continued)	
Discharge Summary Template Using SOAP Format	
P	• Describe any home program/maintenance activities that have been established and who will work with the client on these. • If the client is going to receive further intervention (e.g., at another level of care), state and list what should be addressed in that setting. • List any other evaluations or interventions the client needs (e.g., see the otolaryngologist, enroll in preschool). • List any recommendations for re-evaluations (e.g., re-evaluate swallowing after chemoradiation treatment completed, re-evaluate articulation skills in 6 months to determine whether client is demonstrating age-appropriate skills).

Long-Term Goals

The long-term goals, in collaboration with the client, were written for this episode of care. These goals were where you thought the client would be in each functional area being addressed. Long-term goals, although written in measurable terms, often are not reflected in percentages. To gather objective data on each of the long-term goals, rely on client and caregiver reports and on observations you have made.

Short-Term Goals and Treatment Objectives

The short-term goals and treatment objectives, if written in SMART format (specific, measurable, attainable, realistic, time bound), make it easy to report measurable gains. It is not necessary to repeat activities for each of the treatment objectives during the last session. That is, the speech-language pathologist does not need to posttest each of the goals and objectives. Data would have been collected in each session reflecting level of accuracy for the objectives addressed during that session. The speech-language pathologist can refer to the progress notes to see when each objective was achieved. The treatment plan may have been updated during the course of treatment, with some goals discharged and others added. This information can also be used to determine current status on a particular goal or objective (Figure 9-1).

Re-Evaluation Versus Measurement of Progress on Goals

It is not necessary to administer standardized tests at the conclusion of treatment, but if that was done, the results of the testing should be included in the objective section of the discharge summary. It is more typical to report the current status on the goals. Medicare does not pay for re-evaluations unless there has been a significant change in the client's status. That is not typically the case when preparing a discharge summary because the change over the course of intervention has been gradual. Of course, standardized tests can be administered and the session coded as treatment. If not restricted by the payer, and if administering a standardized test would be the best way to capture the client's progress, share the results of the standardized test in the discharge summary.

Analyzing and Summarizing What Occurred During the Intervention

Just as in a treatment progress note, the A section is where the speech-language pathologist demonstrates skill and judgment in reporting what happened in intervention and states why the intervention is coming to an end. The following are the main categories of reasons that intervention is concluded:

- All goals and objectives have been met
- Although not all goals and objectives have been met, client has achieved maximal gain
- Reimbursement dictates discharge
- Client is leaving/being discharged from that particular setting
- Client decides to discontinue for a variety of personal reasons

Summarize any personal or environmental factors that had an impact on the client's performance in treatment and the impact the treatment has had on impairment, activity, and participation. Explain what the objective data reported means to the client, particularly in terms of functional gains. If there are remaining problems to be addressed and goals there were not met, discuss these and give a prognosis

SPEECH-LANGUAGE PATHOLOGY
TREATMENT PLAN

Patient Name: James Randall
DOB: 10-9-62
Patient #:
Medical Diagnosis/ICD-9: Hoarseness R49.0
Problem areas to be addressed: Client's voice gives out by mid-day
Date treatment initiated: 6-4-17
Estimated amount, frequency and duration of treatment: 1x week; ½ hour to 1 hour; 4-6 weeks
Reasonable expectation to meet treatment goals: Excellent as hoarseness is new onset and client motivated

Date of report: 6-4-17; updated 7-2-17 **At discharge, total # treatment units:**

Long Term Goal Functional Goal(s):
Patient will be able to use voice for vocational and avocational activities.

Date established	Speech therapy/swallowing therapy for these short term goals in functional/measurable terms	Progress/ Date
6-4-17	1. Patient will eliminate vocally abusive behaviors: a. decrease coughing 2. Patient will institute vocal hygiene techniques: b. increase water intake to 64 ounces/day c. substitute swallow or silent cough for coughing 3. Patient will reduce hyperfunctional use of the vocal mechanism via: a. Improved use of diaphragmatic breathing in supine and standing with verbal cues b. Reducing tension in oro-pharyngeal area by applying digital manipulation without cues c. Improving tone focus for easy phonation through use of vocal function exercises	2.a Achieved 6-15-17
Added: 7-2-17	4. Patient will utilize amplification in the classroom for any class of over 10 students.	

Speech-language Pathologist Signature ______________________ Date

CC: O.T. Laryngol, M.D.
Date sent: 6-4-17

Figure 9-1. Periodic updates to treatment plan help when preparing a discharge summary.

for continued improvement. Describe the client's current state related to the communication/swallowing disorder.

Describing Next Steps for the Client

As in the P section of the progress note, address next steps for the client. If the client will receive services in another setting or at another level of care, state that. It can be helpful to the speech-language pathologist who will see the client next if you also mention what might be appropriate goals at that level of care. If the client needs other evaluations or consultations, list them. If a re-evaluation is indicated (e.g., to see whether client is maintaining skills after a period of time or whether adjustments need to be made in the home program due to possible improvement or deterioration in function), report when that should be scheduled and specifically what should be assessed. Finally, if a home program has been developed for the client and caregiver, describe it here.

Sharing the Discharge Summary

The discharge summary is the last opportunity to communicate with other health care professionals about this client. The summary should be shared with any health care professional who received the evaluation and treatment plan and any updated reports (e.g., recertifications). This summary provides these professionals with a picture of the client's current state and informs them of the next steps for the client. Too often in a clinician's busy schedule, completion of discharge summaries is viewed as less important than other documentation such as evaluations and progress notes. This results in a backlog of clients for whom the discharge summaries have not been completed. Sending a discharge summary to a physician months after treatment was concluded does not make a good impression. In addition, the client may have been to see the physician in the interim, and the physician would have had no information about the client. Every piece of documentation the speech-language pathologist sends to other providers provides an insight into the quality of the speech-language pathologist's work. The discharge summary is equally as important as all other documentation.

Outcomes Data

Outcomes data and PROs were described in detail in Chapter 6. If outcomes data are collected on one or more of the tools described, including that data in the discharge summary can be meaningful. If the measure was used at admission and repeated at discharge, reporting each of the scores/results allows the reader to compare the client's level of functioning at these different points in time. If participating in ASHA National Outcomes Measurement System data collection, the Functional Communication Measures would be scored again at discharge (ASHA, n.d.).

Maintenance Programs

Many times at the conclusion of treatment, there are things the speech-language pathologist wants the client to continue to practice and address so that the skill will be maintained. Perhaps the client just needs to carry over the skill into more settings. The client might need to complete activities designed to help the client progress further or to keep the client's skills from deteriorating. For patients with Medicare Part B, the speech-language pathologist may establish what they call a *functional maintenance program* and provide instruction on how to carry out the program. After that instruction has taken place, the skilled services of the speech-language pathologist are no longer needed (CMS, 2017).

Of course, Medicare beneficiaries are not the only clients who can benefit from a maintenance program. These maintenance, or home, programs can take many forms depending on the needs of the client. For example, a client with a voice disorder might be given a CD of vocal exercises to continue to practice (Stemple, 2002). A child with an articulation disorder might be tasked with practicing the accurate production of sounds in particular settings. A client with mild cognitive impairment might have a home program requiring that he and his spouse use a daily planner to help with memory loss. Some clients might even be given a packet of homework sheets to continue to practice language activities. Regardless of the format or specifics of the home program, the fact that one was designed should be documented in the chart. The discharge summary is a good place to do this. If a detailed written maintenance program was given, a copy of that program should be placed in the chart. It is not necessary, however, to include copies of any homework pages in the chart. Appendices 9-C through 9-E are examples of home programs.

In some instances, the home program might refer the client to a website for video examples of exercises. The National Foundation on Swallowing Disorders, a consumer advocacy organization, has clips of various dysphagia exercises that the client can watch to help with practice (National Foundation of Swallowing Disorders, n.d.). For patients who have completed Lee Silverman Voice Treatments (LSVT), LSVT Global has a video series of homework exercises to help them maintain speech and voice gains (LSVT Global, n.d.).

References

American Speech-Language-Hearing Association. (n.d.). National Outcomes Measurement System (NOMS). Retrieved from http://www.asha.org/NOMS/

American Speech-Language-Hearing Association. (2004). Admission/discharge criteria in speech-language pathology. Retrieved from http://www.asha.org/policy/GL2004-00046.htm

American Speech-Language-Hearing Association. (2016). *Jimmo v. Sebelius* plaintiffs return to court to urge enforcement. Retrieved from http://www.asha.org/News/2016/Jimmo-v-Sebelius-Plaintiffs-Return-to-Court-to-Urge-Enforcement/

Centers for Medicare & Medicaid Services. (n.d.). *Jimmo v. Sebelius* settlement agreement fact sheet. Retrieved from https://www.cms.gov/medicare/medicare-fee-for-service-payment/SNFPPS/downloads/jimmo-factsheet.pdf

Centers for Medicare & Medicaid Services. (2017). Medicare Benefit Policy Manual: Chapter 15—Covered medical and other health services. Retrieved from https://www.cms.gov/Regulations-and-Guidance/Guidance/Manuals/downloads/bp102c15.pdf.

LSVT Global. (n.d.) LSVT homework helper exercise videos. Retrieved from https://www.lsvtglobal.com/homework-helper-videos

National Foundation of Swallowing Disorders. (n.d.). Swallowing exercises. Retrieved from http://swallowingdisorderfoundation.com/oral-exercises-to-strengthen-the-swallowing-function-entry-page/

Stemple, J. C. (2002). *Vocal function exercises.* San Diego, CA: Plural Publishing Inc.

Review Questions

1. Describe two formats that can be used to prepare a discharge summary, and discuss advantages and disadvantages of each.
2. Give an example of something subjective that might be reported in a discharge summary.
3. State two ways objective data can be obtained for the discharge summary.
4. Why is it important to include analysis statements in the discharge summary rather than just reporting objective change?
5. What are some reasons a maintenance program might be established for a client?

Activity A

For each of the cases below, sort the statements into the correct section of a SOAP format discharge summary; that is, indicate whether the statement belongs in subjective (S), objective (O), assessment (A), or plan (P).

Case #1

Haylee, a 5-year-old, has completed articulation therapy.

	Haylee still only inconsistently produces /r/ accurately.
	Haylee's score on the Goldman-Fristoe Test of Articulation is now within functional limits for her age.
	Treatment is being discontinued because Haylee's skills are considered within age-appropriate limits.
	Although Haylee's mom, Mrs. Amanda, had some challenges in bringing Haylee to treatment due to transportation, she was diligent in completing homework activities.
	Mrs. Amanda reports that the other children in her pre-kindergarten class can understand Haylee all the time.
	Haylee should be re-evaluated in 6 months to determine whether she has mastered the production of /r/.
	Mrs. Amanda has been given a variety of homework pages to practice with Haylee to help her continue to improve production of /r/.
	Compared with when treatment started, Mrs. Amanda stated that Haylee is more outgoing now that she can be understood more easily.
	Haylee demonstrates the following percent accuracy in sentence level: • /s/ and /s/ blends 95% all positions with no cues • /l/ 90% all positions with no cues
	Standard articulation therapy techniques, such as modeling and tactile and visual cues, were used throughout treatment.

Case #2

Carlos, 23 months old, is moving to a different city and will be seen in an early intervention program there for continued treatment for receptive and expressive language disorder.

	Utilized modeling and naturalistic cues throughout treatment.
	Carlos' grandmother reported that Carlos is using gestures and some single words and only pointing to things he wants when he clearly doesn't know the name of the object or doesn't have a sign for it.
	Carlos' grandmother has consistently observed every session and reinforced what was taught.
	Carlos now understands simple directions/commands from his mom, grandparents, or dad (e.g., no, up, give me) with 90%.
	Carlos has been referred to Sunny Days Early Intervention Services for continued therapy to address receptive and expressive delays.
	Carlos requests help/assistance with toys, food, book reading, door opening with words and/or gestures with 90%.
	Carlos has responded well in treatment, learning about two to three new signs each week.
	Carlos should continue to receive regular checkups by his pediatrician and otolaryngologist concerning pressure equalization tubes.
	Carlos' grandmother reports a significant decrease in tantrums since he began therapy.
	Teach-back and return demonstration were used with Carlos' grandmother at each session and on the few occasions when one of the parents were present.
	As Carlos begins to talk more, an assessment of his phonological skills should be completed.

Case #3

Ms. Hakashi, 87 years old, has completed short-term intervention for mild cognitive impairment/early dementia. She is accompanied by her daughter, Yadira.

	Used visualization and rehearsal strategies as well as spaced retrieval during treatment.
	Yadira, Ms. Hakashi's daughter, has participated in each session and implemented all requested strategies.
	Reviewed the home practice activities, including the specific software for cognitive activities, with Ms. Hakashi and Yadira.
	Ms. Hakashi reports that she has been looking at the posted daily schedule at home several times a day, and this seems to reduce her frustration.
	Yadira reported that she and her mother are arguing far less now that she has stopped trying to "prove" that her mother should remember something.
	Yadira demonstrated the use of phonemic cues when Ms. Hakashi has word retrieval deficits 95% of trials in recent conversation.
	This short period of intervention has been beneficial to the client and her daughter in coming to grips with the probable progression of the disease.
	Yadira and other family members should continue to encourage the use of daily planners, sticky notes, and other visual cues.
	Ms. Hakashi demonstrated ability to use visualization to recall specific words on 75% of trials.
	Ms. Hakashi should be seen every 6 months for re-evaluation of her cognitive-linguistic skills so that the home program can be adjusted as the disease continues to progress.

Case #4

Abigail, 32 years old with a voice disorder, has successfully completed treatment.

	Abigail is able to sustain front-focus, nasal "ee" for 16 seconds, compared with 7 seconds at baseline.
	Abigail has diligently practiced the vocal function exercises several times per day with noticeable improvement in vocal quality.
	Abigail states that her spouse noted that Abigail is no longer yelling when they attend the hockey games.
	Abigail completes all steps of the vocal function exercises independently, with targets achieved.
	Abigail reports she is able to use her voice throughout her 8- to 9-hour days at work with no feeling of strain or tiredness.
	Abigail reports compliance with decreased caffeine intake and increased water intake.
	Abigail should continue to utilize the audio exercises for vocal function exercises several times per week to help maintain her skills.
	Abigail should ask Emily to continue to monitor for any increase in vocal abuses.
	Abigail is able to use diaphragmatic breathing in standing and sitting 100% in conversation.
	Auditory, visual, and tactile feedback cues used throughout treatment.

Case #5

Mr. Karim, 62 years old, status post-cerebrovascular accident with moderate apraxia, is terminating therapy after only three sessions because he is moving to another state to stay with his daughter, Aisha.

	Treatment is being terminated because the client is relocating to stay with his daughter while he recovers from the stroke.
	Aisha apologized that she had not been able to complete any of the home activities with her father because they have been busy making arrangements for his move.
	Mr. Karim's apraxia is about the same as it was at the start of intervention because he has only attended 3 sessions over the past 10 days.
	During the short course of treatment, articulatory kinematic strategies were employed.
	At the end of treatment, intersystemic facilitation/reorganization strategies were introduced.
	Mr. Karim completes contrastive word activities with bilabials and labiodentals with 70% accuracy.
	Mr. Karim repeats two-syllable words when given maximum cues with 65% accuracy.
	Mr. Karim should continue to receive intensive speech-language therapy at least three times per week to address his moderate apraxia.
	Mr. Karim was provided with some home practice activities that he and Aisha can use until he begins treatment in his new location.
	Mr. Karim has a good prognosis for return to speaking in sentences with only minimal impact from the apraxia.

Appendix 9-A
Discharge Summary

Speech-Language Pathology Discharge Summary

Patient name: Spring Sneeze **DOB:** 1/23/2003 **Patient #:** XXXX
Medical diagnosis/ICD-10: Moderate Oral Dysphagia R13.11; Mild-moderate dysarthria R47.1; Secondary to status postsurgery for malocclusion M26.4; Late effect of complications from that surgery T89.9XXS
Problem areas to be addressed: Drooling, can't drink from cup, difficulty chewing solids; impaired oral phase; impaired articulation. Both are interfering with school performance.
Date treatment initiated/plan established: 2/12/17 **Intervention time frame:** 2/12/17 through 5/1/17
Estimated amount, frequency, and duration of treatment: Individual 1-hour sessions; 2-3x/week for 5 weeks; then 1-2x/week for 6 weeks
Reasonable expectation to meet treatment goals: Guarded given uncertain etiology and probable nerve damage.
Date of report: 2/12/17 **Total # sessions:** 26

Long-term functional goal(s):

1. Spring will be able to eat and drink without difficulty. Current state: Client still eats more slowly than others. Drinks from a cup without anterior loss and able to chew most foods.
2. Spring will be able to correctly articulate all sounds. Current state: Can articulate all sounds at word level, but still imprecise in conversation.

Date Established	Short-Term Goal(s) and Treatment Objectives	Progress/Date 5-2-17
2-12-17	1. Spring will improve lip movement for speech and swallowing, including the ability to:	
	a. Achieve and maintain lip closure for 2 to 3 minutes without visual cues	a. Can approximate lips, but can only hold briefly.
	b. Consistently close lips to produce bilabial phonemes /p,b,m/ in all positions of words at conversational level without visual cues	b. When looking in mirror, can approximate each of these at sentence level. Cannot produce in conversation.
	c. Pucker lips and maintain that position for 30 seconds without visual cues	c. Can maintain loose pucker 14 seconds. For shorter periods, can get tight pucker.
	d. Lateralize pursed lips side to side without visual cues on 10/10 trials	d. Still relies on mirror for visual input and accuracy is 6/10.
	e. Retract top lip to show teeth without visual cues on 10/10 trials	e. Movement is much improved, but still accessory eye movement.
	2. Spring will improve tongue movement for speech and swallowing, including the ability to:	
	a. Protrude tongue and maintain for 10 seconds without visual cues	a. Achieved as of 4-22-17
	b. Lateralize tongue tip to corner of lips bilaterally without visual cues 10/10 times	b. Achieved as of 4-22-17
	c. Lateralize tongue tip into lateral buccal cavity without visual cues 10/10 times	c. Achieved as of 5-1-17

Date Established	Short-Term Goal(s) and Treatment Objectives	Progress/Date 5-2-17
	d. Elevate tongue tip to alveolar ridge and maintain for 10 seconds without visual cues	d. Achieved as of 5-1-17
	e. Forcefully "pop" tongue against roof of mouth 10/10 trials	e. Can "pop" but definitely not forcefully
	f. Elevate back of tongue to produce /k/ with force at beginning and end of words 100%	f. Achieved as of 5-1-17

S: Spring and her mother are pleased with the changes that have taken place, but the drooling is still having a major impact on her participation in school, and she has not been able to return to band, where she played the flute.

A: Exercise, sometimes with resistance, and tactile and visual cues and biofeedback have been used throughout the course of intervention. She rarely drools when in the session, although still carries a rag to wipe her chin. She can now drink from a cup without looking in the mirror. Her speech is acoustically much more accurate, although still has a long way to go on bilabials. Chewing is still problematic with excessive rotary movement. She is being discharged from this facility because her insurance coverage has run out.

P: She will be followed at another facility where she can afford the charge out of pocket. She has also been referred to physical therapy for e-stim for facial muscles but wants to talk to the consulting surgeon before beginning.

Speech-language pathologist signature: ____________

Date: ____________

CC: G. Surgeon, MD; K. Adolespeds, MD; C. Sulting, MD

Date sent: 5-8-17

Appendix 9-B
Example Treatment Plan: Pediatric

Speech-Language Pathology Discharge Summary

Patient name: Malika Fazal **DOB:** 12-3-2016 **Patient #:** XXXX
Medical diagnosis/ICD-10: Oral dysphagia R13.11
Problem areas to be addressed: Noisy sucking with excess gas; refusing spoon feeding
Date treatment initiated: 08-24-17 **Period of treatment:** 8-24-17 to 11-24-17
Estimated amount, frequency, and duration of treatment: Individual 45-minute sessions 1x/week for 6 weeks; then 1x mos for 3 mos
Reasonable expectation to meet treatment goals: Excellent
Date of report: 08-24-17 **At discharge, total # treatment sessions:** 4

Long-Term Goal(s)

1. Child will eat and drink age-appropriate foods and liquids in typical amount of time. Current state: Child is eating more foods than when treatment started but is still far below typical-age peers in variety of foods and in length of time it takes to eat.

Date Established	Short-Term Goals	Progress/Date 10-15-17
08-24-17	1. Infant will increase efficiency with bottle feeding.	
	a. Infant will be provided minimal jaw support by her mother while sucking from bottle without cues.	a. Malika's mother uses jaw support only as indicated at end of feeding when child tires.
	b. Infant will use bottle/nipple that reduces intake of air for 100% of bottle feeds.	b. Malika's mother declined to use the bottle recommended.
	2. Infant will take at least three vegetables, one meat, and one fruit runny pureed foods from spoon.	
	a. Child will be positioned in supported upright position for spoon feeding attempts on all trials.	a. Malika's mother uses a car seat for feeding Malika, and this provides good support.
	b. Food will be placed mid-tongue by feeder with no cues.	b. Malika's mother remembers this about 50% of the trials. Still scraping spoon on upper gums.
	c. Lip closure will be encouraged with physical assist as needed by feeder.	c. Malika's mother uses tactile support to lower lip only occasionally.

S: Malika's mother indicates Malika is still a noisy feeder but admits the feedings take less time. She stated she wanted to keep using the bottle her sister had recommended.

A: Modeling and coaching of the infant's mother were utilized throughout treatment. Malika's attendance was not optimal. She missed four appointments with no advance notification by her mother. Malika is accepting a few vegetables in limited quantities from the spoon. Anterior loss is typical for her developmental level. Malika has missed the last three scheduled appointments, and despite repeated attempts to reach her mother to reschedule, Ms. Fazal does not return calls. Malika is being discharged due to not adhering to the attendance policy.

P: Malika should optimally continue to receive feeding therapy. Her mother has been mailed a packet of information regarding other services available in the community.

Speech-language pathologist signature: ________________

Date: __________

CC: V. Friendly, MD

Date sent: 10-16-17

APPENDIX 9-C

Home Program for Infant Feeding

Speech-Language Pathology Feeding Tips for Nadia

Congratulations! Nadia has made great progress with feeding. As Nadia gets ready to come home, here some suggestions to help her continue to help make her transition smooth.

Bottles: The Dr. Brown's bottle came with a level 1 nipple, which is similar in flow rate to the standard bottle used at the hospital. In about 3 to 4 months, you will want to offer her the level 2 nipple because it is a bit faster.

Breastfeeding: After the next weight check, encourage breastfeeding by moving back to the preemie nipple on the Dr. Brown's bottle. Put Nadia to the breast as often as possible, then offer the bottle as supplement. For example, Nadia may want to breastfeed for 10 minutes, then take a bottle for the remainder of the feed. This will be a balance because you want to try to keep feeding times under 40 minutes total.

If Nadia is taking a while to get organized at the breast, try pumping until letdown (1 to 2 min) before putting Nadia to the breast.

You may consider making an appointment for outpatient lactation evaluation for additional support. Additionally, please feel free to contact Speech-Language Pathology with any questions or concerns.

Appendix 9-D

Home Program Tips for Family of Patient With Myocardial Infarction and Dysarthria

Luis Garcia Home Program

1. When Mr. Garcia starts to have trouble thinking of the word he wants to use, encourage the following word-finding techniques:
   a. Think of a word that means the same thing or is associated with the word.
   b. Try to describe the word:
      i. Describe what it looks like.
      ii. Tell what it is a type of.
      iii. Tell where you might find it.
      iv. Describe what it is used for.
2. Encourage clear speech. See attached list of words and phrases to practice.
   a. *Slow down.* If he is having trouble coordinating this, try tapping each word on the table or even his leg—whatever it takes to slow down his speech.
   b. Talk louder. Projecting our voice makes our speech clearer.
   c. Exaggerate speech sounds. Encourage him to open his mouth more and think "big talk."
3. Responding to yes/no questions: Encourage him to stop and think before he responds to the question.
4. When Mr. Garcia is going to be in social situations with friends or family, rehearse possible conversation topics. The night before the social gathering, discuss conversation starters about each person so that Mr. Garcia can engage in conversations. For example, "Did you watch the game last night?"
5. Encourage eye contact. This is an important part of communication. It also allows the listener to better understand his message.
6. Practice reading the headlines in the newspaper. This not only works on reading, but it allows him to discuss current events.

APPENDIX 9-E

Home Program: Aphasia

Marquis Jackson Home Program

We are working on Mr. Jackson's speech, reading, and writing. I have outlined instructions and techniques for working on these areas at home.

Speech

Our main goal is for Mr. Jackson to be able to utilize word-finding techniques on his own. You can practice word finding using any of the speech handouts I provided. The following are techniques that we have practiced in therapy if he is unable to think of a word:

1. Use gestures or actions to help retrieve the word.
2. Think of something related to or associated the word. For example, if he is having trouble thinking of the word *car*, he can try thinking of the words *drive*, *engine*, *wheels,* etc.
3. Try to put the word in a sentence: "This is a ___________."
4. Think of what the item/word is used for or its purpose. If he is able to, he can describe the item. Tell what it is used for, what it looks like, where you find it, or what it is a type of.
5. Write the word.
6. Draw a picture.
7. If he is still unable to find the word, give him the first sound of the word.

Reading

Mr. Jackson already practices reading every day by reading the newspaper. A good activity to do is to discuss what he read in the paper with someone—telling stories he read or any details he can recall from articles. We are practicing reading at the sentence level to improve his reading comprehension. Practice reading by completing the handouts I provided. If he gets stuck on a word, he should try to read the other words in the sentence to improve comprehension of the sentence. When completing the handouts, use a piece of paper to cover up the other sentences so he isn't distracted by all that is on the page.

Writing

Continue to practice writing name, address, birthday, and family members' names. This will improve not only writing, but also recall of names when he is trying to say them. To practice spelling, continue the program using the letter tiles. See attached sheet. Start by spelling three- and four-letter words. If he is comfortable with these, move to words with more letters. It doesn't have to be the pictures provided; you can try any items around the house.

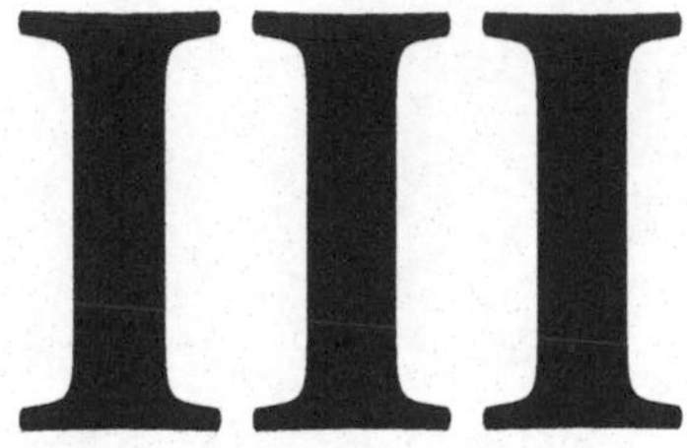

Documentation and Reimbursement in Adult Health Care Settings

The chapters in Section I of this book provided the basics of documentation. Section II described documenting the different types of services, with the focus mostly on health care. Sections III and IV delve into the specifics of documentation and reimbursement in specific settings. Section III addresses the following settings in adult health care:

- Acute care
- Palliative and hospice
- Inpatient rehabilitation
- Skilled nursing facilities
- Home health
- Outpatient (e.g., hospital outpatient departments, clinics, private practices)

Each chapter in this section is authored by speech-language pathologists who have extensive experience practicing in those settings. I've written the chapters on acute care, palliative/hospice, and outpatient, having provided services in those settings through my private practice and then at the hospital for over 30 years. Although I've provided services in inpatient rehabilitation, skilled nursing, and home health, I haven't done so recently, and therefore asked these experts to contribute these chapters.

The chapters will reinforce the basics from Section I and the types of services covered in Section II but will go more in-depth about the particular requirements in that setting. You will find information on the following:

- Documentation requirements in that setting (from evaluation to discharge)
- Tips on how to document efficiently
- Basics of reimbursement for clients/patients in that setting and how reimbursement rules impact documentation in that setting
- Any tips on coding (diagnostic and/or procedural)
- Examples of evaluations, treatment plans (including examples of long- and short-term goals for some typical disorders), progress notes, discharge summaries, and any specific outcomes tools or other forms that have to be filled out
- A case history example(s) from that setting to help you understand the coding, reimbursement, and documentation rules

10

Acute Care
Adult

Nancy B. Swigert, MA, CCC-SLP, BCS-S

Reimbursement in Acute Care

Regardless of the third-party payer, the services in an acute care hospital are almost certainly done on a prospective payment methodology. The payer and the hospital have agreed to a methodology that dictates what amount the payer will reimburse the hospital, either per day of the patient's stay or more likely per diagnosis of the patient. The payer does not assume any of the financial risk because the amount of reimbursement has been predetermined. If the hospital overutilizes services (e.g., performs four chest x-rays when two would suffice, prescribes an expensive drug when a generic drug would work), the hospital loses money.

Medicare Diagnosis-Related Groups: Part A

When a beneficiary with Medicare is admitted to a hospital, Medicare Part A is the payer. The patient has a deductible to meet, but then Medicare covers 100% (for the first 60 days). The beneficiary does not have to pay any coinsurance. When Medicare was originally established, hospitals were reimbursed on a retrospective, cost-based system. Whatever the hospital charged, called *reasonable charges*, Medicare reimbursed. In 1982, the first prospective payment system was established for acute care hospitals. Medicare determined it would pay a rate for a specific type of case, or diagnosis-related group (DRG). There are hundreds of these groups into which a patient can be classified. For example, there is a group for transient ischemia, several different groups for acute ischemic stroke, and several for intracranial hemorrhage or cerebral infarction (U.S. Department of Health & Human Services, 2001).

Therapy services are covered as a part of the payment the hospital receives. Medicare does not care how much therapy is provided because they are not going to reimburse the hospital any more for a patient who gets a lot of services. The hospital, however, may care a great deal. Out of the limited, preset amount the hospital receives, they have to pay for all the services they are providing. Thus, there might be pressure from hospital administration on the therapy departments to scale back the services they provide.

Medicare Part B in a Bed

This DRG-based prospective payment system is the way hospitals are reimbursed for inpatients under their Medicare Part A benefit. One might think that if a Medicare beneficiary is in a bed in a hospital, he or she is an inpatient. However, in order to qualify for inpatient status, the patient must meet two criteria: He or she must have a qualifying diagnosis and he or she must stay in the hospital two

Swigert, N. B.
Documentation and Reimbursement for Speech-Language Pathologists: Principles and Practice (pp. 131-149).

midnights. If the patient does not meet these requirements, even though he or she is in a bed in the hospital, he or she is classified as in observation status, and that is considered to be an outpatient service. Sometimes this patient is referred to as a *B in a bed*, meaning his or her stay is being paid by Medicare Part B. When that happens, the speech-language pathologist must follow all the rules for coding and documentation for Medicare Part B, and the facility is reimbursed as if the patient were an outpatient. This includes functional outcomes reporting, or G-codes. See Chapter 15 for more information on Medicare rules for Part B.

Other Payers

Each state Medicaid plan may differ slightly, but all pay for inpatient stays through a prospective system. This may be a per-stay reimbursement or, more likely, a per-diagnosis reimbursement based on the DRG system (Henry J. Kaiser Family Foundation, n.d.).

Each private insurance company can establish its own rules for what it covers, how much it will reimburse, and how it will reimburse. Each may offer different kinds of plans for an individual to select. Most private insurance plans now are health maintenance organizations, preferred provider organizations, and high-deductible plans, which are all forms of managed care.

As each insurance plan is different, no specific details can be provided here about which companies cover speech-language services in outpatient settings.

Focus on Value and Outcomes Related to Reimbursement

Centers for Medicare & Medicaid Services (CMS) is changing the way it reimburses hospitals so that there are rewards for providing quality services and higher value. Value is described as reaching the needed outcomes at a lower cost. Hospitals are reimbursed for meeting certain goals and penalized if the goals are not met. Several different programs are in place, including the Hospital Readmissions Reduction Program, the Hospital Value-Based Purchasing Program, and the Hospital-Acquired Condition Reduction Program. The speech-language pathology departments at hospitals may be involved in helping the hospitals reach designated targets. For example, the speech-language pathology department might address reducing readmissions by accurately identifying patients admitted with pneumonia who have dysphagia so that the dysphagia can be identified and managed (CMS, n.d.).

Electronic Medical Records in Acute Care

Because of the implementation of *meaningful use* (see Chapter 4), acute care hospitals have moved quickly to implement an integrated electronic medical record (EMR). Documenting in an EMR, if well-designed, should be point-and-click for most documentation. It should reduce duplicative documentation. For example, once goals are selected during the evaluation, those goals should flow to the screen where daily treatment documentation is completed. The speech-language pathologist in acute care is almost certainly documenting on a computer in the patient's room, on a computer immediately adjacent to the patient's room, or on a laptop or tablet taken into the patient's room.

Point-of-Care Charting

As much as possible, the documentation in acute care should be completed during the time the speech-language pathologist spends in the patient's room. This is more challenging during some interactions than others. For example, it is difficult to document during a clinical swallow evaluation because that is such a hands-on procedure. When that is the case, ideally the documentation would be completed in the patient's room immediately after the procedure, discussing the results with the patient and family while documenting. Instrumental swallowing evaluations (i.e., videofluoroscopic swallowing study [VFSS], fiberoptic endoscopic evaluation of swallowing [FEES]) would be impossible to chart while performing the study but should ideally be done soon after. The video of the study likely needs to be reviewed, and perhaps scored, before the results can be documented.

Treatment sessions are a bit easier to chart during the session. A short break can occur between each treatment activity while the clinician takes the time to record the patient's performance.

Hybrid Electronic Medical Record and Paper Record

As hospitals transition to fully integrated EMRs, there may still be occasions when the speech-language pathologist has to handwrite a note in the chart. This might be for all of the speech-language pathologist's documentation if the hospital is not very far along in the transition to the EMR, or might be the note left for the physician in the physician's orders section of the chart. If that is the case, there are ways to streamline this documentation by developing templates for the different types of evaluations completed (see Appendices 10-A and 10-B for examples). The clinician should ensure that his or her handwriting is legible.

> 7-01-17 0915
>
> Telephone order Paul Munology, M.D. to Nancy Swigert
>
> Evaluate for use of tracheostomy speaking valve when patient is on trach collar trial.
>
> Read back and verified
>
> Nancy B. Swigert, M.A., CCC-speech-language pathologist, BCS-S

Figure 10-1. Telephone order with read back.

> 10-9-17 1425
>
> Per Protocol Failed Dysphagia Screen/N. Ternal, M.D.
>
> Speech-language pathology to evaluate swallow. May perform VFSS or FEES as needed.
>
> Nancy B. Swigert, M.A., CCC-SLP,BCS-S
>
> Co-signature: ______________________________

Figure 10-2. Per protocol order.

Orders and Protocol Orders

A provider's (i.e., physician's) order, or an order from a non–physician practitioner such as an advanced practice registered nurse or physician's assistant, is required before the speech-language pathologist can provide services to inpatients. The order will have been entered electronically or written on a physician's orders sheet in the physical chart. It is the responsibility of the speech-language pathologist to verify the order and be sure it has been signed by the provider. The clinician should clarify with the provider anything that is not clear about the intent of the order.

Sometimes the provider gives a verbal or telephone order to the clinician. The Joint Commission states that verbal orders (i.e., the physician and clinician are in the same location) should only be given in emergency situations. If it is not an emergency, the Joint Commission expects the physician to enter her own orders. Therefore, there should be no verbal orders for speech-language pathology services. Any time an order is verbally communicated, there is a chance the information will be entered or written incorrectly (University of Cincinnati School of Medicine, n.d.).

Telephone orders, on the other hand, are allowed when the provider is not physically on the premises. When the speech-language pathologist takes a telephone order, he or she should record:

- Date and time
- Name of provider giving the order
- Name of clinician receiving order
- Exactly what was said
- A phrase indicating that the transcribed order was read back to the provider and verified as accurately transcribed
- The speech-language pathologist's signature (Figure 10-1)

Many hospitals establish approved protocols that help to streamline care. When a protocol is in place, the speech-language pathologist can proceed with certain evaluations and treatments without having to contact the physician. The speech-language pathologist can enter a protocol order that the physician can later cosign. For example, a hospital may have an approved protocol that when a patient fails a nurse-administered dysphagia screening, the speech-language pathologist may evaluate the patient for dysphagia per protocol. There may also be a protocol in place that allows the speech-language pathologist to place an order for, and perform, an instrumental swallowing evaluation based on the results of a screening or clinical evaluation. There should be a full written protocol, typically approved by the physician governing body, that specifies under what conditions the protocol can be implemented.

Protocol orders should clearly indicate that this was a protocol order and which physician will be cosigning the order. The procedure can be performed before the cosignature is obtained. CMS and the Joint Commission have specific requirements regarding the use of protocol orders (Figure 10-2) (Joint Commission on Accreditation of Healthcare Organizations, 2012).

Cognitive-Communication Evaluations in the Inpatient Setting

Evaluation of inpatients takes place at the bedside, creating specific challenges and opportunities. The challenges include the physical environment. Many hospital rooms are semiprivate, with only a curtain separating two patients. This leaves little room for the speech-language pathologist to set up materials for an evaluation. It is not possible to ensure that the patient's roommate does not overhear the conversation. Regulatory agencies recognize that complete privacy cannot be ensured in these situations. Another challenge in inpatient settings is the situation in which the patient is in isolation because of an infectious disease. Sometimes the presence of an infection is not known immediately. Therefore, some speech-language pathology departments decide not to take any materials (e.g., formal tests, therapy objects) into the patient's room. Cleaning such items between patients can be challenging. The result is that many evaluations are informal and completed with the objects that can already be found in the patient's room.

The inpatient setting typically presents an opportunity to interact with the patient's family and engage them in the discussion about the patient's care. Many family members stay with the patient and thus can help implement strategies and compensations. The interactions with the family should be part of the clinician's documentation.

Informal Evaluations of Cognitive-Communication

Patients in acute care are there because they are acutely ill; many could not tolerate a full, standardized assessment. For patients with aphasia, an informal approach is recommended, using items within the room. For example, get-well cards can be used to assess reading and the patient can be asked to tell about the person who sent the card to assess spoken language. Word retrieval can be assessed by having the patient name objects in the room (Holland & Fridriksson, 2001). Many clinicians adapt formalized testing, selecting items from different standardized tests to compile an informal assessment protocol. The Kentucky Aphasia Test was developed with that goal in mind (Marshall & Wright, 2007).

As cognitive-communicative evaluations in this setting are often informal, there are no standard scores to report. The clinician must make a judgement about the client's skills without the benefit of normative data. In addition, the cognitive-communicative and swallowing skills of patients in acute care change quickly, hopefully improving each day, but sometimes declining when the patient has had a setback. This is another reason that trying to administer a full evaluation with testing instruments is not indicated.

However, without the benefit of standardized testing, the speech-language pathologist may be challenged to accurately state the severity of impairment. It will not be possible to document, for example, the percentile level or standard score of a patient's receptive skills. It would be beneficial for the staff in the department to agree on guidelines for what they will describe as a mild, moderate, severe, or profound deficit. Utilizing an outcomes measure like the American Speech-Language-Hearing Association (ASHA) National Outcomes Measurement System Functional Communication Measures scales can be useful in the acute care setting (ASHA, n.d.-b).

The speech-language pathologist can use terms like *appears to present* or *symptoms are consistent with* rather than definitive statements like *patient has a* ______. In the acute care setting, the physician and other members of the care team are not as concerned about a severity level as they are in understanding the impact the cognitive-communication disorder is having on the patient's ability to participate in his or her own care.

In fact, the *International Classification of Functioning, Disability and Health* model can be very helpful in organizing the statements the speech-language pathologist will enter in the record. This puts the results in practical terms that will be helpful to the care team, the patient, and the patient's family. If only results from body structure and function are reported, much important information is excluded that could be useful in the patient's care (Table 10-1).

Current Procedural Terminology Codes for Cognitive-Communicative Evaluations

Because standardized tests are rarely used in acute care, the Current Procedural Terminology (CPT) timed evaluation codes 96105 Assessment of Aphasia and 96125 Standardized Cognitive Performance Testing are not likely to be used. Instead, the two codes that will be used are 92522 Evaluation of Speech Sound Production and 92523 Evaluation of Speech Sound Production with evaluation of language comprehension and expression. If speech sound production is not assessed, modifier -52, indicating that not all components were completed, should be appended to the code. However, in many cases of language impairment in the adult in an acute care setting, it is most appropriate to also assess motor speech skills.

Evaluation of Patients With Tracheostomy Tubes

Patients with tracheostomy tubes are referred for assessment of communication skills. If a patient was deemed not ready to try a speaking valve, this might be an assessment for a non-verbal means of communication, such as a picture communication board or teaching the patient a few gestures. That evaluation would likely be coded with 92523 with modifier -52. If the patient's ability to mouth words (i.e., articulate) was also assessed, perhaps the modifier would not be needed.

Table 10-1

Organizing Cognitive-Communication Evaluation Summary in the *International Classification of Functioning, Disability and Health* Format

Patient	Body Structure and Function	Activity and Participation	Environmental Factors	Personal Factors
R. B.	Appears to present with severely impaired receptive and expressive language skills.	Patient is not able to follow simple directions or answer yes/no questions.	Performs better when background noise is eliminated, lights are on, and you face the patient when talking.	No family has been present so far to help the patient.
L. B.	Appears to present with moderate flaccid dysarthria.	Patient can make himself understood if he talks slowly and sometimes has to add gestures to get his point across.	Patient's cultural background seems to make it hard for him to accept help from others.	Doesn't appear to have good coping skills and becomes easily frustrated.
E. S.	Confusion and memory loss are mild-moderate, and per family, patient is at baseline.	Patient has been maintained at home with significant support for last 6 months. If given written cues and repetition of requests, can comply.	Patient's insurance will not pay for another day of hospitalization so he is being d/c to son's care.	ETOH abuse continues and contributes to mental status.

Abbreviations: d/c = discharged; ETOH = ethanol (alcohol).

If an assessment for the use of a speaking valve is undertaken, the speech-language pathologist will likely collaborate with the nurse and, if the patient is on the ventilator, the respiratory therapist. Essential information to document on the evaluation of a speaking valve is listed in Table 10-2. The CPT code for this evaluation would be 92597 Evaluation for use and/or fitting of voice prosthetic device to supplement oral speech.

Evaluation of Swallowing

By far, the largest percentage of referrals in acute care is for the speech-language pathologist to assess swallowing. The evaluation may be a clinical (bedside) swallow evaluation and/or a subsequent instrumental swallowing evaluation. In any type of swallowing evaluation, the care team needs the speech-language pathologist to use his or her expertise to summarize the findings and make recommendations. It is not necessary to document every bolus presented and the patient's response to every bolus. The other members of the care team would not be able to interpret the impact of this information. What they need from the speech-language pathologist is an analysis of the patient's skills.

Clinical Swallow Evaluation

The clinical swallow evaluation is often the first assessment of the patient's swallowing skills. That is not always the case, of course. Some patients, after failing a nurse-administered dysphagia screening, are immediately referred for an instrumental exam. The essential elements to document from a clinical evaluation are listed in Figure 10-3.

It is not necessary to present food or liquid to the patient in order to complete the evaluation; sometimes it is deemed unsafe. The CPT code 92610 description is Evaluation of oral and pharyngeal swallowing function. This can be completed with a thorough oral motor exam, cranial nerve exam, and assessment of cognitive-communication skills related to the patient's ability to participate in care related to management of the dysphagia. Several examples of summaries of clinical swallow evaluations are included in Appendix 10-C.

Instrumental Swallow Evaluations

All acute care hospitals have the capacity for VFSS, with the patient being transported to the radiology department. The CPT code for the speech-language pathologist's involvement in the study is 92611. Many hospitals also have a FEES program. The CPT code used in most situations

Table 10-2

Things to Include in Documentation for Tracheostomy Speaking Valve

Dates of Intubation	Type of Speaking Valve Used
Any reintubations	Articulation and language skills
Any self-extubations	Whether assessment was completed on vent or trach collar trial
Date of tracheostomy	Respiratory rate before, during, and after assessment
When patient is on and off vent	Heart rate before, during, and after assessment
How often patient is suctioned	Oxygen saturation before, during, and after assessment
Type of secretions (e.g., thick)	Patient's response to trial (e.g., tolerated for how long? Coughing?)
Patient coughing to clear any secretions	Patient's ability to communicate with speaking valve
Any known upper airway obstruction	Education provided about speaking valve and tracheostomy
Size and type of tracheostomy tube	At conclusion of trial, was valve left on or removed? Cuff left deflated or reinflated?
Patient's current method of communication	Recommendations for use (e.g., does speech-language pathologist need to be present?)

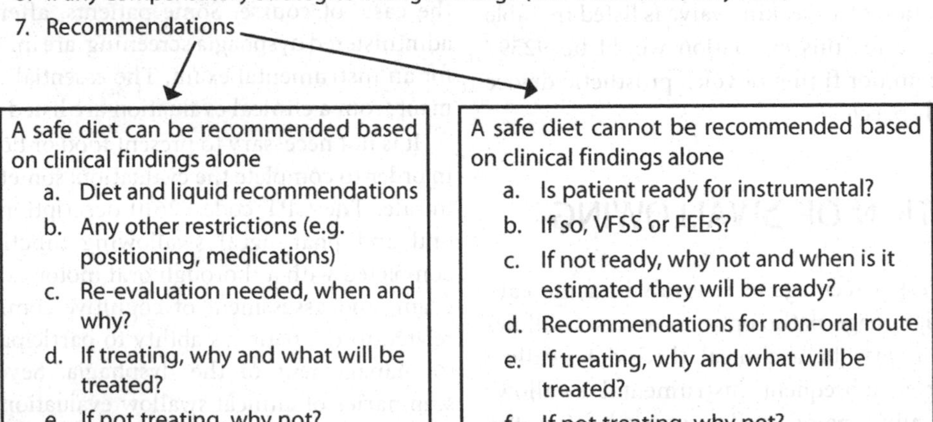

Figure 10-3. Writing cohesive summary of clinical swallow evaluation.

when the speech-language pathologist is passing the scope and interpreting the exam is 92612. When assessing pharyngeal swallow with fiberoptic exam, the speech-language pathologist will observe abnormalities and lesions on the vocal folds. Speech-language pathologists cannot diagnose vocal lesions, so the documentation should include a description of what was observed without making a diagnosis (Figure 10-4). Appropriate referrals should then be made to an otolaryngologist.

As with the clinical swallow exam and the videofluoroscopic exam, documenting each bolus presented is not necessary. The clinician should analyze all of the results and draw conclusions.

If the speech-language pathologist observes what appear to be nodules, the documentation could state:

Bilateral swelling/fullness/lesions on the anterior third of the true vocal folds

If an apparent polyp is observed:

A pendunculated or sessile-based lesion noted on the ______

If paralysis or paresis is observed:

Ⓛ/Ⓡ vocal fold appears fixed in midline/paramedian/lateral position. Movement is absent/sluggish. Bowing/atrophy observed

Figure 10-4. Describing rather than diagnosing vocal lesions.

Writing Cohesive Summaries of Instrumental Assessments

1. How patient presented to you
2. Impaired physiology, including cranial nerve
3. Impact on function of this impaired physiology
4. What consistencies were presented (and if something wasn't tried, why?)
5. Summary statement of severity/phase(s)
6. If any compensatory strategies changed things (and if not tried, why not)
7. Esophageal (VFSS only)
8. Recommendations
   a. Diet
   b. Any other restrictions (e.g. positioning, medications)
   c. Re-evaluation indicated
   d. If treating and why/what?
   e. If not treating, why not?

Figure 10-5. Writing cohesive summaries of instrumental assessments.

For either type of instrumental exam, there are essential elements to report in the summary (Figure 10-5). Examples of summary statements from instrumental exams are included in Appendix 10-D.

Establishing Goals in Acute Care

Patients stay in acute care for a very short period of time. The mean length of stay for adults 65 years and older in 2012 was 5.2 days (Weiss & Elixhauser, 2014). Even if the patient is referred to the speech-language pathology department on the day of admission, that is a very short time in which to have an impact. At least for the first day, the department will be completing necessary evaluations. Treatment delivered in acute care might be better described as management. Data from the ASHA National Outcomes Measurement System database indicate that patients do make progress during these short hospitalizations. Some of this, of course, may be related to spontaneous recovery. These improvements occur not just in swallowing. For example, over 60% of patients demonstrate improvement in receptive and expressive language skills and 70% make progress in motor speech. About one-third of patients seen by speech-language pathologists in the acute care setting need no further intervention after discharge (ASHA, n.d.-a).

Acute-Onset Disorders

The goals set for inpatients related to a new dysphagia are more about managing the disorder and keeping the patient safe from complications like pneumonia. Compensatory and diet changes may comprise the majority of treatment strategies, particularly if the patient is still lethargic and unable to fully participate in active treatment. Educating

Table 10-3

Examples of Goals for Support, Education, and Guidance

Goals for Patients in Early Days After Stroke	Goals for Family in Early Days After Stroke
• Patient will be encouraged to attempt conversation. • Patient will be reassured when experiencing frustration with communication. • Patient will be given information about recovery.	• Family will attend to signs from the patient to indicate when patient is overloaded. • Speech-language pathologist will share information about disorder with family. • Speech-language pathologist will share information about recovery and prognosis with family. • Speech-language pathologist will demonstrate how to engage patient in communication attempts. • Speech-language pathologist will demonstrate how to interpret patient's communication attempts.

the patient and family about dysphagia is an essential role. Some patients will be able to complete swallowing exercises.

The goals set for inpatients with acute-onset cognitive-communication disorders should focus on finding ways to supplement the patient's communication attempts and counseling the patient and family about the deficits and prognosis for return of function. Teaching the family cueing strategies and answering the many questions they have will be time better spent than on a specific language task with the patient. Much of the change that will occur related to a neurological event like a stroke will be due to spontaneous recovery.

For patients with aphasia, the treatment in early stages is conversational, including the following:

- Encouraging the patient to try
- Pointing out changes day-to-day
- Demonstrating how to talk to the patient
- Demonstrating how to interpret responses

Providing support and guidance to the patient and family in the early stages is crucial. Goals can be written to reflect this emphasis (Holland & Fridriksson, 2001; Marshall, 1997; Marshall, 2013). These goals do not meet the rigor of the SMART format (specific, measurable, attainable, realistic, and time bound), and some may not be measurable. However, in acute care situations, the rigorous standards for demonstrating improvement do not apply as they do with Medicare Part B outpatients. More of the goals may apply to the education and counseling the speech-language pathologist will provide to the family (Table 10-3).

Chronic or Progressive Disorders

Patients with acute onset of communication or swallowing disorders are not the only kinds of patients referred to the speech-language pathology department. Patients with chronic or progressive disorders (e.g., dementia, Parkinson's disease) are admitted for other medical reasons. For example, a patient with dementia may suffer a fall and a broken hip and be admitted to the hospital. The speech-language pathologist will be called in to evaluate the patient's status. The clinician must make every attempt to determine the patient's baseline status and document the current status compared with baseline. If this is not done, the patient may receive unnecessary treatment for skills that are at baseline. See Figure 10-6 for examples of statements that can be used in these situations.

Palliative and Hospice Programs in Acute Care

Some hospitals will have palliative and hospice programs and the speech-language pathologist will be consulted on these patients. The speech-language pathologist can provide a valuable service related to swallowing and communication. Obviously, the treatment, or management, plan for patients in palliative or hospice care differs greatly from patients presenting with an acute disorder. Typically, the patient does not need active treatment, but rather counseling and education to help the patient reach his or her goals. The goals at that stage are not to get better but to remain comfortable, participate in his or her care, and maintain a level of independence if possible.

Patient admitted after broken hip with chronic dysphagia from skilled nursing facility

Thank you for the consult. This patient presents with a moderate oral dysphagia related to her dementia. She had an instrumental study at this facility as an out-patient 4 weeks ago and at that time was down-graded to pureed and a few soft foods with thin liquids in small sips. Her condition does not appear to have changed since that time and no further intervention is indicated.

Patient admitted with UTI from home, presents with confusion and memory problems

Thank you for the consult. Discussed patient's current status with her daughter, with whom the patient resides. Her daughter states that the patient has moderate Alzheimer's Disease and that, although the confusion is a bit worse, the memory seems to be at baseline. It is likely the confusion is related to the current UTI. Provided the daughter with strategies for memory to use at home, and encouraged her to contact our OP Memory Clinic periodically as her mother's condition changes. No further intervention needed during this hospitalization.

Figure 10-6. Notes on patients admitted with chronic disorders.

Family Conferences and Rounding

Increasingly, hospitals are conducting rounds and huddles on patients in order to coordinate care, and often to facilitate discharge. Sometimes family case conferences are held on patients with multiple needs and challenges. If the speech-language pathologist has evaluated or is treating that patient, he or she should attend the family conference. Rather than each discipline documenting its involvement in the case conference, there is usually one person assigned to document the results of the conference. Then, each discipline simply notes in its documentation that it attended. There are no appropriate CPT codes to capture the time spent by the speech-language pathologist in these conferences.

It is not possible for the speech-language pathologist to attend each of the rounds and huddles on every floor/unit of the hospital. There is, however, benefit in having a representative of the department attend rounds on certain units. For example, if rounds are held on the neurological unit, it is likely that many of the patients on that unit will be managed by the speech-language pathology department. One member of the department can attend and share information from the treating speech-language pathologist. Documentation of these rounds is cursory, although one member of the team may be assigned to document more detail of the discussion.

Discharge Summaries

Discharge summaries in acute care can be very helpful for the 70% of patients who are going to receive further intervention for their communication or swallowing disorder (ASHA, n.d.-a). The challenge, however, is that many times the patient is discharged without the speech-language pathologist knowing exactly when the discharge will occur. Patients being transferred to another facility (e.g., skilled nursing, inpatient rehabilitation) are often held at the acute care facility until a bed becomes available. That is not always predictable. The quandary, then, is whether the speech-language pathologist should complete a discharge summary in anticipation of pending discharge. The flaw in that method is that the patient's condition and the recommendations might change significantly if he or she is at the acute care facility for several days after the discharge summary was generated. The physician discharge summary is a report on the overall stay, and all too often the details about communication and swallowing are omitted from the summary. Each hospital's speech-language pathology department needs to work with the discharge planners/case managers to determine the most effective way to transmit the information to the facility receiving the patient.

Other Documentation Required by Regulatory Agencies

Accrediting agencies have regulations that may have an impact on documentation. For example, there are specific requirements to chart if a patient is in restraints (The Joint Commission, 2017). There are pain scales that must be completed if applicable (Baker, 2016). The speech-language pathologist should be familiar with these regulations.

Appendix 10-E provides an example of an adult referred for evaluation. A per-protocol order was used.

References

American Speech-Language-Hearing Association. (n.d.-a). The myth about SLP intervention in acute care settings. Retrieved from https://www.asha.org/uploadedFiles/ASHA/NOMS/Adult-NOMS-SLP-Intervention-in-Acute-Care-Settings.pdf

American Speech-Language-Hearing Association. (n.d.-b). National Outcomes Measurement System (NOMS). Retrieved from http://www.asha.org/NOMS/

Baker, D. W. (2016). Joint Commission Statement on Pain Management. Retrieved from https://www.jointcommission.org/joint_commission_statement_on_pain_management/

Centers for Medicare & Medicaid Services. (n.d.). Linking quality to payment. Retrieved from https://www.medicare.gov/hospitalcompare/linking-quality-to-payment.html

The Henry J. Kaiser Family Foundation. (n.d.). Medicaid benefits: Inpatient hospital services, other than in an institution for mental diseases. Retrieved from http://kff.org/medicaid/state-indicator/inpatient-hospital-services-other-than-in-an-institution-for-mental-diseases/?currentTimeframe=0

Holland, A., & Fridriksson, J. (2001). Aphasia management during the early phases of recovery following stroke. *American Journal of Speech-Language Pathology, 10*(1), 19.

The Joint Commission. (2017). Facts about patient safety. Retrieved from https://www.jointcommission.org/facts_about_patient_safety/

Joint Commission on Accreditation of Healthcare Organizations. (2012). New and revised requirements to align with CMS CoPS. *Joint Commission Perspectives, 32*(10), 4-6.

Marshall, R. (2013). *Management of patients with aphasia in acute care.* Presentation made to Baptist Health, Lexington, Kentucky.

Marshall, R. C. (1997). Aphasia treatment in the early postonset period: Managing our resources effectively. *American Journal of Speech-Language Pathology, 6*(1), 5–11.

Marshall, R. C., & Wright, H. H. (2007). Developing a clinician-friendly aphasia test. *American Journal of Speech-Language Pathology, 16*(4), 295–315.

University of Cincinnati School of Medicine. (n.d.). Joint Commission Update. Retrieved from http://med2.uc.edu/libraries/gme_forms/joint_commission_upd_1.sflb.ashx

U.S. Department of Health & Human Services. (2001). Medicare hospital prospective payment system: How DRG rates are calculated and updated. Retrieved from https://oig.hhs.gov/oei/reports/oei-09-00-00200.pdf

Weiss, A. J., & Elixhauser, A. (2014). Overview of hospital stays in the United States, 2012. *Agency for Healthcare Research and Quality.* Retrieved from https://www.hcup-us.ahrq.gov/reports/statbriefs/sb180-Hospitalizations-United-States-2012.pdf

Review Questions

1. Describe the payment methodology used most often for inpatients in acute care hospitals.
2. What are some challenges to completing charting on the computer during a session?
3. Explain a protocol order.
4. What are some advantages and disadvantages to the informal cognitive-communication evaluations that are completed in acute care?
5. Describe some differences between treatment plans developed in acute care and those developed in an outpatient setting.

Activity A

Look at each telephone order below. Note what is missing in each order.

#1

0915
Telephone order Paul Munology, MD to Sam Speech
Evaluate for swallowing problems
Read back and verified
Sam. E. Speech, MA, CCC-SLP

#2

7-01-17
Telephone order Paul Munology, MD to Sam Speech
Evaluate for use of tracheostomy speaking valve when patient is on trach collar trial.
Sam E. Speech, MA, CCC-SLP

#3

7-01-17 0915
Paul Munology, MD
Videofluoroscopic swallow evaluation in the morning
Read back and verified

#4

7-01-17 0915
Telephone to Sam Speech
Clinical swallow evaluation
Read back and verified
Sam E. Speech, MA, CCC-SLP

#5

7-01-17
Telephone order Paul Munology, MD to Sam Speech
Evaluate for confusion
Sue Swallow, MA, CCC-SLP

Activity B

The hospital has approved the following protocol. For each case described, determine whether the speech-language pathologist was following the protocol when writing the order. If not, indicate which criteria was not met.

Protocol

A speech-language pathologist may enter a diet order (including beginning a diet for an NPO [nothing by mouth] patient) after bedside evaluation. The speech-language pathologist should write an order to request consult by dietitian for any patient placed on a dysphagia diet or for any patient not placed on a dysphagia diet who presents with clinical indications for dietary consult.

Criteria for writing diet order after clinical swallow evaluation.

The speech-language pathologist may enter a diet order (including a diet for an NPO patient) after a bedside evaluation if the following criteria are met:

1. No overt signs of pharyngeal dysphagia with recommended diet (including, but not limited to, coughing, choking, throat clearing, multiple swallows when oral cavity is clear)
2. Oral phase adequate to handle recommended diet
3. Patient reliable with compensatory techniques needed for safe swallowing or patient will comply with cues from staff and/or family to use recommended compensatory techniques

Case	Orders Written Per Protocol by Speech-Language Pathologist	Did Order Meet Protocol Guidelines? If Not, What Was Not Met?
Patient presented with thin, nectar, pudding, and cookie. Pocketing with cookie but can clear with cue. No signs of pharyngeal dysphagia.	• Dysphagia diet: Mechanical soft diet with thin liquids • Consult by dietitian	
Patient lethargic and difficult to awaken. Drooling from left side of mouth and loses liquids and pudding from Ⓛ side. Presented with thin and pureed only.	• Dysphagia diet: Soft solids and thins • Consult by dietitian	
Patient awake, alert, and cooperative. Dentures not here. States eats at home without. Presented with thin, solids, and mixed solids. Throat clear noted on mixed solids x3.	• Regular diet	
Patient edentulous. Oral skills mildly impaired with reduced tongue lateralization. Presented with thin, pudding, mixed, and solids. Pocketing with solids and doesn't clear with cues. No pharyngeal signs.	• Dysphagia diet: Pureed and thins	
Patient presented with thin, pureed, mixed, and solids. Handles all but solids well. He will not follow cues to put solids in on Ⓛ side for chewing. Without cues, not safe for solids. No pharyngeal signs.	• Regular diet and thin liquids	

Appendix 10-A

Cognitive-Communication Evaluation Note

Progress Notes	Physician's Orders
Speech-Language Pathology	
Dysphagia and Cognitive/Communication	
Orders received and chart reviewed.	
Dysphagia	
Clinical swallowing diagnosis:	
Pt given: Thin, nectar, honey, pudding, pureed, mixed, solids	
Observation of oral phase swallowing:	
☐ No signs/symptoms of pharyngeal dysphagia	
OR	
☐ Signs/symptoms of possible pharyngeal dysphagia:	
Dysphagia Recommendations:	
Cognitive/Communication Evaluation	
Receptive language skills:	
Expressive language skills:	
Motor speech skills (i.e., dysarthria or apraxia):	
Cognition:	

Progress Notes	**Physician's Orders**
Other:	
Communication Recommendations:	
Anticipate services after discharge _____Y _____N _____n/a	
Speech-language pathologist signature:	Physician signature:
Date: Time:	Date: Time:

Appendix 10-B

Speech-Language Pathologist Bedside Dysphagia Evaluation

Progress Notes	**Doctor's Orders**
Date: Time:	Date: Time:
Speech-Language Pathology	
Bedside/Clinical Dysphagia Evaluation	
Orders received and chart reviewed.	
Clinical Swallowing Diagnosis:	
Pt given: Thin, nectar, honey, pudding, pureed, mixed, solids	
Observation of oral-phase swallowing:	
☐ No signs/symptoms of pharyngeal dysphagia	
OR	
☐ Signs/symptoms of possible pharyngeal dysphagia:	
Coughing/throat clearing	
Wet vocal quality	
Dysarthria	
Multiple swallows	
Other:	
Patient's cognitive-communicative skills:	
Recommendations:	
Speech-language pathologist signature	

Appendix 10-C

Sample Summaries of Clinical Swallow Exams

Case #1: Findings Within Normal Limits

Patient alert and cooperative. Oral motor and cranial nerve exam within normal limits. Presented with thin, pudding, solid, and mixed consistency. Oral phase within functional limits (limited only because patient does not have dentures here at the hospital). No signs of pharyngeal dysphagia.

Recommendations:

1. Mechanical soft diet until daughter brings in dentures
2. Thin liquids
3. Meds whole with liquids
4. Can upgrade to regular texture when the patient has his dentures
5. No treatment indicated

Case #2: Impaired Oral Phase, Signs of Pharyngeal Disorder

Patient somewhat lethargic, but aroused easily when repositioned and lights turned on. Cooperative throughout. May have some damage to cranial nerve (CN) VII, as has difficulty with lip closure on cup at left. Presented thin, nectar, pudding, and solid. Tried mixed consistencies, but due to anterior loss with thins had a hard time. No difficulty with chewing or forming solid bolus. Oral phase mildly impaired with no signs of pharyngeal impairment.

Recommendations:

1. Mechanical soft, no mixed consistencies
2. Thin liquids
3. Use straw and place on right side
4. Patient can supply pressure to lower lip on left to help with closure
5. Place meds on right and use straw to swallow with liquids
6. Upright for all PO (*per os*)
7. Speech-language pathologist to re-evaluate in 2 to 3 days, as expect quick return of function
8. Will see patient once to teach lip exercises and compensatory strategies

Case #3: Impaired Oral Phase, Signs of Pharyngeal Dysphagia

Patient minimally alert and had to be reawakened several times. Could not fully participate for oral motor and cranial nerve exam. Is able to follow a few directions (e.g., stick out tongue—deviates to Ⓡ; pucker lips—symmetrical). After oral care, presented small sip of water with immediate cough response. Patient presenting with signs of both oral and pharyngeal dysphagia. Not able to follow directions for compensatory strategies.

Recommendations:

1. Keep patient NPO (*nil per os*)
2. Short-term alternative nutrition source (e.g., nasogastric)
3. Speech-language pathologist to reassess when patient is more alert
4. No treatment at this time as patient not able to participate

APPENDIX 10-D
Sample Summaries of Instrumental Swallow Exams

Case #1: Normal

Patient was alert and cooperative. Patient presented with thins, pureed, and solid. Patient presented with functional oropharyngeal swallowing skills. Initiation of pharyngeal swallow response was timely for all consistencies for patient's age and gender. No penetration or aspiration was noted during this evaluation. There was no significant residue in the hypopharynx.

Recommendations:

1. Regular diet with thin liquids
2. No treatment indicated

Case #2: Severe Pharyngeal and Patient Is Good Candidate for Treatment

Patient was lethargic but was able to participate in the study. Thin liquids, nectar, and pureed were tested. Solids not presented as patient does not have dentures and also fatigued at end of study.

Patient presents with moderate oral dysphagia and severe pharyngeal dysphagia. Evidence of impairment of CN X and XII. Patient has reduced tongue movement and poor back-of-tongue control. This results in oral residue after the swallow and premature loss of the bolus over the back of the tongue. The patient exhibits severely limited anterior-superior movement of the hyolaryngeal complex and reduced closure at the entrance to the airway, resulting in penetration of thin liquids in 10 cc sizes or less into the upper laryngeal vestibule that is expelled and swallowed with rest of bolus. With larger thin liquid boluses, the patient silently aspirates. The patient also has significant residue in pyriform sinuses and is at risk to later aspirate this material. Chin-down posture did not reduce penetration or aspiration.

Recommendations:

1. Dysphagia diet level III (pureed with one soft)
2. Thin liquids in teaspoon amounts only
3. Positioning precautions (upright for PO)
4. Medications crushed and mixed with pudding
5. Patient should have another instrumental study before discontinuing these recommendations
6. Speech-language pathologist to treat lingual control, hyolaryngeal excursion, and airway closure

Case #3: Severe Pharyngeal Dysphagia and Patient Is Not Good Candidate to Treat

Patient was minimally alert but arousable. Cooperation was minimal. Patient given thin, nectar, and pureed. Solids attempted, but patient spit out.

Patient presents with oral skills adequate for consistencies tested. He presents with a severe pharyngeal dysphagia. He exhibits inconsistent delay in initiation of pharyngeal response with thin liquids of up to 3 seconds with bolus pooling in pyriforms before the pharyngeal response. Possible impairment CN IX. Patient then silently aspirates from the pyriforms as the swallow begins. Response is timely with nectar and pureed, and there is no penetration or aspiration. He also has reduced tongue base and pharyngeal wall movement with significant residue with all materials. Possible involvement of CN X, XI, and XII. Patient doesn't respond to verbal cue to dry swallow to clear residue. Patient cannot maintain postural change (e.g., chin down) and is unable to follow directions for other techniques.

Recommendations:

1. Dysphagia diet level II
2. Nectar-thick liquids, spoon or cup
3. Medications whole with nectar thick liquid
4. Repeat instrumental before discharging any recommendations, but probably not for 4 to 6 weeks. Schedule as outpatient.
5. No treatment is recommended due to patient's reduced cognitive skills and lack of cooperation.

Appendix 10-E

Case Example: Adult Inpatient With Medicare Part A

Date	Actions	Billed and Coded	Documented
2-14-17 0920	Order received to evaluate newly admitted 82-year-old who suffered cerebrovascular accident. Failed dysphagia screening administered by nursing. Hospital has policy that if the speech-language pathologist is ordered to assess swallowing, she can also assess communication because it is within her scope of practice to do so.		
2-14-17 1000	Speech-language pathologist reviews history & physical, neurology consult, and other pertinent records in the EMR. Spends 15 minutes in review.	Nothing can be coded/charged	Nothing documented
2-14-17 1020	Speech-language pathologist performs clinical swallow evaluation. This takes about 20 minutes. Also assesses patient's receptive and expressive language skills and motor speech skills. This takes 25 minutes. No motor speech deficits noted, but patient does present with mild receptive and moderate expressive aphasia.	92610 for clinical swallow evaluation; 92523 for the language and speech production assessment. Neither code is timed.	Documents in speech-language pathologist's flowsheet in the EMR. Selects goals for language. Also places note in physician's section of charting.
2-14-17 1115	Speech-language pathologist places order for VFSS per protocol and flags for physician to cosign.		
2-14-17 1530	Speech-language pathologist performs VFSS in radiology department. Study takes total of 30 minutes, including setup of room and counseling patient. Determines a safe diet for the patient and what treatment will be needed.	92611, an untimed code	Documents in speech-language pathologist flowsheet in the EMR. Selects goals for swallowing. Also places note in physician's section of charting.
2-15-17 0900	Speech-language pathologist sees patient for dysphagia treatment and language treatment.	92526 for swallowing treatment; 92507 for language treatment	Progress note in EMR that addresses both the swallowing goals and language goals.
2-15-17 1515	Speech-language pathologist sees patient for dysphagia treatment and language treatment.	92526 for swallowing treatment; 92507 for language treatment	Progress note in EMR that addresses both the swallowing goals and language goals.
2-16-17 1000	Speech-language pathologist sees patient for dysphagia treatment and language treatment.	92526 for swallowing treatment; 92507 for language treatment	Progress note in EMR that addresses both the swallowing goals and language goals.
2-16-17 1400	Speech-language pathologist sees patient for dysphagia treatment and language treatment.	92526 for swallowing treatment; 92507 for language treatment	Progress note in EMR that addresses both the swallowing goals and language goals.

Date	Actions	Billed and Coded	Documented
2-17-17 1030	Speech-language pathologist finds out patient was discharged yesterday afternoon to the rehabilitation facility sooner than expected as a bed became available. If the department had anticipated the discharge, they could have done a discharge summary. Contacts rehabilitation facility to be sure they got the patient's records and answers any questions.	No charge	Depending on hospital's policy, the chart may still be open to document this conversation. In situations like this, a discharge summary is not usually completed.

11

Inpatient Rehabilitation Facility

Lynne C. Brady Wagner, MA, CCC-SLP; Denise M. Ambrosi, MS, CCC-SLP; and Daniel Meninger, MSPT

Through the continuum of health care, each clinical setting has its own criteria for admission or justification of need for the resources provided in that institution. The Centers for Medicare & Medicaid Services (CMS) define these criteria as *rules of participation*. CMS reimburses for the care delivered to one of its beneficiaries if a hospital or clinic meets these rules of participation. Although not all patients seeking medical care are covered by CMS, most third-party payers follow the criteria required by CMS to justify need for admission and criteria for discharge. This chapter will highlight the documentation needs that reflect and support clinical care in an inpatient rehabilitation facility (IRF).

What Is an Inpatient Rehabilitation Facility?

IRFs provide intensive rehabilitation services in an inpatient setting for persons who need complex medical, nursing, and rehabilitation intervention. Patients admitted to an IRF must be able to fully participate in and benefit from the rigorous nature of the rehabilitation program provided there. They must also require the skilled intervention of two or more therapy disciplines, primarily physical or occupational therapy and speech-language pathology. Those who do not require two or more disciplines may reasonably have their needs met in a less resource-concentrated setting. Additionally, there are specific components of documentation that clinicians must be aware of or contribute to in order to ensure a patient's stay meets the criteria for IRF admission. If these components are not present, the institution risks retrospective denial of payment for the patient's entire stay.

Intensity of Treatment

Rehabilitative services in an IRF setting are demanding. Patients must be able to tolerate and benefit from therapy delivered in a minimum of 3 hours/day, at least 5 days/week, measured in a rolling week (hospital day 1 is date of admission). In certain circumstances, therapy can be delivered in a model of 15 hours/week over a 7-day period but must be supported by documentation from the medical team stating that such a model of delivery is beneficial for the patient. More recently, the delivery of therapy is measured in actual minutes spent with the patient providing direct patient care. Documenting a patient's assessment or treatment note while not in the presence of the patient does not count toward direct patient care time (minutes) and is not billable (CMS, 2010).

Swigert, N. B.
Documentation and Reimbursement for Speech-Language Pathologists: Principles and Practice (pp. 151-165).

Admit to Rehabilitation Order

The patient's medical record must contain an order by the physician to "admit to inpatient rehabilitation." This order presumes that a rehabilitation physician has screened the patient's case and has evaluated the patient's need for IRF level of care. The involvement of the speech-language pathologist in the care of a patient in the IRF begins with an order for speech-language pathology consultation (usually broadly written as "eval and treat") by the patient's physician.

Keeping analytical records is a hallmark of professional work. Documentation is therefore a critical skill for every clinician. Each institution will have its own rules for reporting to meet the standards of regulatory agencies who accredit or license the facility or clinic. Additionally, individual clinical departments will require written protocols that guide clinicians to ensure an effective and safe workflow.

Speech-Language Pathologist's Role

Speech-language pathologists are required to describe professional analysis and interpretation of the facts discerned in medical record review, professional hand-offs, and clinical encounters with their patients. Importantly, the speech-language pathologist is part of a team of professionals who provide intense treatment for patients admitted to the facility. Perhaps more than in any other setting, the speech-language pathologist must work to coordinate care with the interprofessional team members in order to ensure that the patient's stay in the IRF successfully meets criteria. In many IRF institutions, the speech-language pathologist intervention serves as one of these essential 3 hours of therapy, especially for patients with neurological diagnoses and disorders. As mentioned, patients admitted to the IRF must be able to benefit from and participate in 3 hours of therapy, at least 5 days/rolling (or admission) week. The rolling week means that the week of a patient's stay is counted from the first day of her admission. For example, when a patient is admitted on a Tuesday, that patient's rolling week extends from Tuesday through the following Monday.

Individualized Interdisciplinary Plan of Care

The individualized interdisciplinary plan of care is signed off by the rehabilitation physician and includes information from the multidisciplinary rehabilitation treatment team after the completion of the initial evaluations. The plan of care must contain the following information regarding the patient:

- Prognosis
- Treatment interventions
- Anticipated outcomes
- Frequency and duration of therapy services
- Anticipated length of stay and discharge destination

Inpatient Rehabilitation Facility Patient Assessment Instrument

The IRF patient assessment instrument (PAI) contains the data collected for each patient and submitted to CMS. Because working under the rules of participation for Medicare is critical to both the fiscal success and the legal obligations of any IRF institution, these hospitals are likely to have specialists who administrate the requirements for documentation submission (IRF PAI managers). The IRF PAI manager may audit documentation and work with supervisors and staff to ensure that the team is meeting the expectations and capturing the essential clinical features and needs of each patient accurately and within the rules.

We will use a fictitious case of patient Sally O. to demonstrate the nuances of IRF certification and the contribution of the speech-language pathologist to the processes and reporting that will support a patient's admission.

An Inpatient Rehabilitation Facility Case Study

Sally O. is a 67-year-old woman with acute onset of right-sided weakness and word-finding difficulties who was brought to an acute care hospital 1 hour after her symptoms began. She was diagnosed with a large left hemisphere ischemic stroke infarct in the middle cerebral artery territory. The patient's past medical history includes hypertension and hypercholesterolemia. She was previously independent with activities of daily living (ADL) and ambulation and was living with her spouse at home.

Sally O. was treated with tissue plasminogen activator, and her hospital course was complicated by cerebral edema requiring a craniotomy. Mrs. O. was found to have a dense right hemiplegia impacting her ability to mobilize and to perform ADL. She demonstrated a moderate-severe non-fluent aphasia and was unable to communicate basic wants and needs.

Results of a videofluoroscopic swallowing study (VFSS) administered at the acute care facility revealed severe oropharyngeal dysphagia resulting in aspiration of thin liquids and significant pharyngeal residue when swallowing pureed and diced/ground solids due to poor bolus drive. Due to aspiration risk and inefficient swallowing, a percutaneous endoscopic gastrostomy tube was placed for primary nutrition and hydration as the patient's trajectory of recovery of function was anticipated to be gradual.

A patient like Sally O. requires an IRF admission for medical management, daily rehabilitation nursing care, and acute therapy rehabilitation (i.e., physical and occupational therapy, speech-language pathology) to address her functional mobility, ADL, non-fluent aphasia, and dysphagia.

Key Components of Inpatient Rehabilitation Facility Documentation: Assessment, Treatment, and Discharge

Documenting the Admission Assessment

Once a patient is admitted to an IRF, each part of his or her stay necessitates specific reporting. The three primary segments of the stay are the assessment, the treatment phase, and the discharge transition (Table 11-1).

Let's think about some elements of the admission documentation for Mrs. O. On admission to the IRF, she remains generally *nil per os* (NPO), or nothing by mouth, but is able to safely swallow ice chips. She is seen for an evaluation of her swallowing skills and her speech and language abilities. Typically, the swallowing and speech-language evaluations are billed using distinct Current Procedural Terminology (CPT) codes, such as 92610 for the clinical swallow evaluation and either 92523 for the speech-language evaluation or 96105 if a focused aphasia evaluation was completed. A report of these assessments is required either in the same or different templates, including results of standardized testing (e.g., Boston Diagnostic Aphasia Examination), informal measures (e.g. ability to follow conversation and/or commands), plan of care, long- and short-term goals, and the plan for patient and family education. The results of informal assessment and formal standardized testing during initial evaluation and throughout the patient's hospitalization must be retained in the medical record according to state laws. In some facilities, the actual published test booklets that include raw data are kept and must include the patient's name, medical record number, and date(s) of service.

The results of the initial assessments, the plan of care, and the anticipated outcomes are shared with the team within the first 4 days of admission, and in turn with the patient and family. A written scope of service plan must be shared with the patient/family and reflected in the medical record. The patient's case manager is typically the point person for formal patient/family communication and may be the one to complete this task.

Table 11-1

Assessment

1. Chart review and patient interview (e.g., patient goals, cultural and spiritual preferences, language preferences for information sharing)
2. Results of standardized and informal measures
3. FIM scoring, FCM scoring, IMPACT scoring
4. Data analysis
5. Diagnosis
6. Recommendations/plan of care, including:
   a. Intended treatment modalities (e.g., e-stim or other biofeedback) and/or further assessment needed (e.g., VFSS, high-level cognitive assessment)
   b. Frequency and duration of intervention
   c. Long-term goals: Duration of the stay
   d. Short-term goals: Duration of approximately 1 week
   e. Patient and caregiver education plan
   f. Prognosis for improvement

Abbreviations: FCM = Functional Communication Measures; FIM = Functional Independence Measures; IMPACT = Improving Medicare Post-Acute Care Transformation; e-stim = electrical stimulation

Documenting Functional Assessment and Outcomes

IRFs are required by CMS to collect assessment and discharge data for all admissions via the FIM. The patient's medical information and results of the FIM are submitted to CMS for review shortly after a patient is admitted. Based on comparison of this individual's admission information with that of hundreds of thousands of other patients with similar diagnoses and functional impairments, CMS uses a predetermined prospective payment for the Medicare beneficiary and provides an expected length of stay (LOS).

One of the benefits of using nationally compared scales such as the FIM or the American Speech-Language Hearing Association's (ASHA's) National Outcomes Measurement System (NOMS) FCM is the ability to compare the progress of patients in your facility with those in another facility and to understand the differences and share best practices. A challenge is that these numbers do not account for individual patient circumstance and the nuances of disease, illness severity, and patient recovery (Table 11-2).

Table 11-2

The Functional Independence Measure

A person can achieve a total score of between 18 and 126. Scores of patient function are determined by gathering data at admission (within the first 72 hours) and at discharge (within the final 72 hours of the stay).

Motor Subscale (Can Achieve a Score of Between 13 and 91)	Functional Independence Measure Scale Score
• Eating • Grooming • Bathing • Dressing, upper body • Dressing, lower body • Toileting • Bladder management • Bowel management • Transfers: Bed/chair/wheelchair • Transfers: Toilet • Transfers: Bath/shower • Walk/wheelchair • Stairs	1 = Total (100%) assistance from another person 2 = Maximal (75% to 50%) assistance from another person 3 = Moderate (50% to 25%) assistance from another person 4 = Minimal (25% to 0%) assistance from another person 5 = Supervision or setup assistance from another person 6 = Modified independence (e.g., using devices or medications) with no assistance from another person 7 = Complete independence with no assistance from another person
Cognition Subscale (Can Achieve a Score of Between 5 and 35)	
• Comprehension • Expression • Social interaction • Problem solving • Memory	

Functional Independence Measure

The FIM is a tool used to describe a patient's performance in ADL, mobilization, and communication and is used to measure the burden of care (i.e., how much assistance is required by the patient). It is completed at both admission and discharge and, in some facilities, at intervals during the patient's care. The FIM has been adopted by Medicare as the primary measure used across facilities to quantify functional outcomes in rehabilitation (Chumney et al., 2010; Linacre, Heinemann, Wright, Granger, & Hamilton, 1994). Although the FIM is widely criticized as having poor specificity, it is the most widely collected data set in the field of rehabilitation medicine and is used as a quality outcome measure for IRFs.

The FIM is a standardized tool, and, in order to maintain the validity of its scoring, clinicians complete a certification examination to ensure inter- and intrarater reliability. Although the individual 18 items of the FIM naturally correspond with the expertise of specific rehabilitation disciplines (e.g., locomotion with physical therapy, Grooming with occupational therapy, and bowel and bladder with nursing), the FIM may be scored by any certified clinician.

The ability to collect data and compare patterns of recovery in similar patients with similar diagnoses is important. Doing so helps us advance our understanding of the natural course of illness, as well as the general effectiveness of our intervention programs. It is important to emphasize, however, that the FIM and other tools like it are disability ratings. These measures describe how much assistance or care a person needs in order to accomplish a functional task (e.g., eating, communicating), but they do not purport to measure impairment level improvement.

In order to capture improvement in a person's ability, which may be where specific speech-language pathology treatments are directed, clinicians should use outcome measures that target these areas. Just as it is important to systematically capture functional outcome data across a health care continuum, it is critical that we assess impairment level gains in a similar standardized manner to support the effectiveness of our intervention. Completing and documenting results of standardized tools, such as the Western Aphasia Battery-Revised (Kertesz, 2006) or the

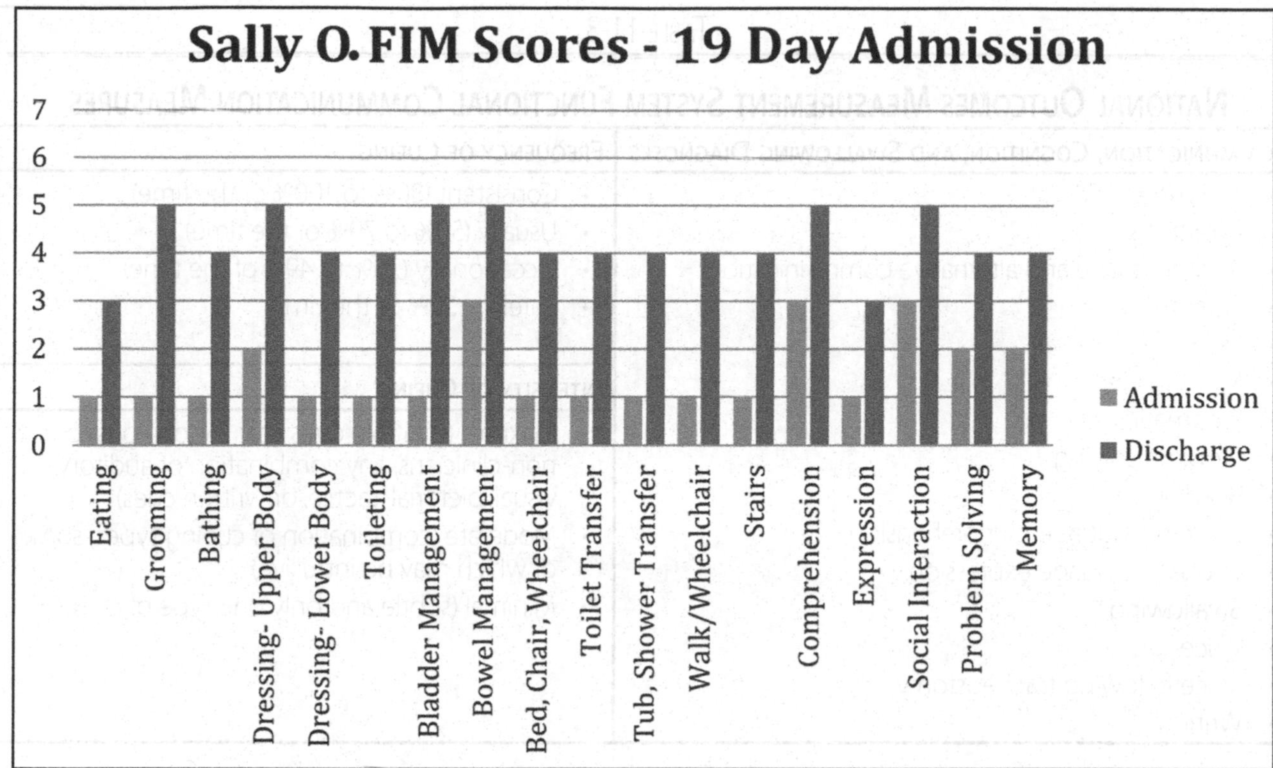

Figure 11-1. Admission and discharge FIM scores for Sally O. during an episode of inpatient rehabilitation.

Modified Barium Swallow Impairment Profile (Martin-Harris, 2010), at periodic intervals in a patient's intervention can describe progress in specific aspects of mobility or ability impacted by the patient's stroke. Speech-language pathologists should work with their departments and institutions to determine the consistent measures they will use to assess patient progress and the efficacy of the interventions and protocols used in treatment.

Figure 11-1 reflects information for our fictional Sally O. These data describe her admission and discharge FIM scores for each functional item. The visual display depicts the patient's improvement in all areas of her functioning. For example, Mrs. O.'s initial FIM for eating was assessed as a 1 because she was NPO and required total assistance, whereas her discharge FIM for eating was scored as a 3 because she improved to the point of needing moderate assistance by the end of her IRF stay. Graphic representation of patient change can be useful for educating patients, families, other professionals, and stakeholders about the patient's outcomes.

Functional Communication Measures

The NOMS (ASHA, 2013) is a data collection system developed by ASHA to illustrate the value of speech-language pathology services provided to individuals with cognitive, communication, and/or swallowing disorders. For this reason, it is recommended that speech-language pathologists use FCMs in the IRF setting. FCMs are a series of disorder-specific, seven-point rating scales, ranging from least functional (Level 1) to most functional (Level 7), designed to describe the change in an individual's functional communication and swallowing abilities over the course of speech-language pathology intervention. The FCMs are scored by a speech-language pathologist on admission and at discharge to represent the amount of change in the patient's communication and/or swallowing skills, thereby reflecting the benefits of treatment and the outcome of rehabilitation. The FCMs are determined only by a speech-language pathologist who has passed the scoring reliability test for NOMS.

When scoring the FCMs, the speech-language pathologist takes into account the frequency and intensity of cueing and the use of compensatory strategies that are needed to facilitate a patient's functional communication and swallowing skills. Like the FIM, FCMs are not dependent upon administration of any particular formal or informal evaluation tool but are scored based on the clinical observations made by the speech-language pathologist. The speech-language pathologist selects the FCMs that are pertinent to the primary areas of deficit that will be addressed in treatment for any given patient. When scoring the swallowing FCM, the speech-language pathologist also takes into consideration the dietary levels/restrictions and the need for a feeding tube, in addition to the frequency and intensity of cues.

Table 11-3 outlines the ASHA FCMs and associated cueing descriptors. Table 11-4 illustrates the admission and discharge FCMs for Sally O. based on the case study in this chapter.

Table 11-3

National Outcomes Measurement System Functional Communication Measures

Communication, Cognition, and Swallowing Diagnoses	Frequency of Cueing
• Alaryngeal • Attention • Augmentative and alternative communication • Fluency • Memory • Motor speech • Pragmatics • Problem solving • Reading • Spoken language comprehension • Spoken language expression • Swallowing • Voice • Voice following tracheostomy • Writing	• Consistent (80% to 100% of the time) • Usually (50% to 79% of the time) • Occasionally (20% to 49% of the time) • Rarely (< 20% of the time) **Intensity of Cueing** • Maximal (multiple cues that are obvious to non-clinicians; any combination of auditory, visual, pictorial, tactile, or written cues) • Moderate (combination of cueing types, some of which may be intrusive) • Minimal (subtle and only one type of cue)

Table 11-4

Functional Communication Measures Outcome Measures for Sally O.

Functional Communication Measure	Admission Functional Communication Measure Score Days 2 and 3	Discharge Functional Communication Measure Score Day 18
Swallowing	1	4
Spoken language comprehension	3	5
Spoken language expression	1	3
Motor speech	1	4
Attention	3	5
Memory	2	4

- Swallowing Level 1: Individual is not able to swallow anything safely by mouth. All nutrition and hydration are received through non-oral means.
- Swallowing Level 4: Swallowing is safe but usually requires moderate cues to use compensatory strategies, and/or the individual has moderate diet restrictions and/or still requires tube feeding and/or oral supplements.
- Spoken Language Expression Level 1: The individual attempts to speak, but verbalizations are not meaningful to familiar or unfamiliar communication partners at any time.
- Spoken Language Expression Level 3: The communication partner must assume responsibility for structuring the communication exchange, and with consistent and moderate cueing, the individual can produce words and phrases that are appropriate and meaningful in context.

These shifts in Sally O.'s ability during her hospitalization indicate significant change in her functioning in specific areas of cognition, communication, and swallowing.

Improving Medicare Post-Acute Care Transformation Act

As of this writing, the Improving Medicare Post-Acute Care Transformation (IMPACT) Act of 2014 is a functional assessment newly required by CMS (implemented in October 2016). The goal of the IMPACT tool is to allow comparison of outcomes in treatment and quality for similar diagnoses over a variety of levels of care and potentially to develop a more uniform Medicare payment for diagnosis specific care regardless of where the care is delivered (IMPACT Act, 2014). After an initial data collection period, the information will be analyzed and future recommendations and requirements will be developed.

Developing and Documenting Patient Goals

As in other levels of care, the speech-language pathologist must create long- and short-term goals for patients as part of the plan of care in an IRF. Long-term goals are usually written for the duration of the estimated stay for the patient, and short-term goals are written for incremental improvement toward the long-term goals. Short-term goals are written for a time period proportional to a shorter segment of the LOS. The short-term goal period may correlate to the expected LOS for a particular diagnosis. For example, if the average LOS for a patient with a stroke is 3 weeks, the short-term goals will likely be written for a 1-week period. If the average LOS for a patient who is in the IRF to manage debility after a flare of multiple sclerosis is 10 days, the short-term goals may be written for 5 days. Many hospital speech-language pathology departments develop protocols that standardize the length of time for which short-term goals are set. Long-term goals are generally created for the patient's LOS in the IRF, whereas short-term goals are for each 7-day period, therefore corresponding with weekly progress documentation.

Goals should always be individualized based on the patient's unique impairments and personal aspirations. Goals must be clearly stated and measurable. Many clinicians use the acronym SMART to guide clear and understandable goal writing:

S = Specific: Clearly defines the task, activity, or ability

M = Measurable: Delineates the unit by which the goal is described (e.g., percentage of correct trials)

A = Agreed upon: In all cases, goals should be created with the patient based on her priorities.

R = Realistic: The measurement should be attainable based on the patient's diagnosis and other factors.

T = Time based: The goal should state the time frame in which it will be achieved. Conversely, the expected time for completion of short- and long-term goals may be established by protocol.

Goals should also be created in the context of the interprofessional assessment of the patient's needs and reflect a good understanding of the patient's discharge environment. In addition to addressing specific deficit areas, rehabilitation goals are typically functional in nature in the IRF setting.

Possible goals for Sally O. are shown here. Long-term goals are set to be achieved in a 3-week period (by the end of the stay), and short-term goals are set to be achieved in a week's time:

- Verbal Expression
    - Long-term goal: Patient will produce short phrases to express her basic needs, wants, and feelings with minimum to moderate cues.
    - Short-term goals: Patient will produce high-frequency single words given maximum phonemic and written cues.
    - (Later in the stay) Short-term goal: Patient will produce high-frequency, personal single words given minimal cues and self-initiation of an augmentative communication tool (written words reference).
- Swallowing
    - Long-term goal: Patient will safely and efficiently swallow basic soft solids and nectar-thick liquids using compensatory strategies with moderate cues.
    - Short-term goal: Patient will safely and efficiently swallow ice chips using compensations given maximum cues.
    - (Later in the stay) Short-term goal: Patient will safely and efficiently swallow trials of pureed solids using compensatory strategies with maximum cues (Table 11-5).

TABLE 11-5

THE TREATMENT PHASE

1. Daily note to describe patient performance and justify treatment charge. Every charge code must have corresponding documentation.
2. Weekly progress note to define overall movement toward goals and observations regarding patient recovery
    a. Progress toward achievement of goals
    b. Need to adjust plan of care
    c. In some institutions, update FIM scoring or complete other standard measures to systematically assess patient progress throughout the stay

Daily and Weekly Progress Notes

Once treatment has begun, daily documentation is needed after each session to describe patient performance toward long- and short-term goals and to justify the care provided and the charge submitted to the patient's account. Goals are modified as needed based on changes in the patient's clinical presentation.

Daily documentation may take the form of a note or may be entered in the form of a flow sheet or other specific format but must be descriptive enough to support the plan

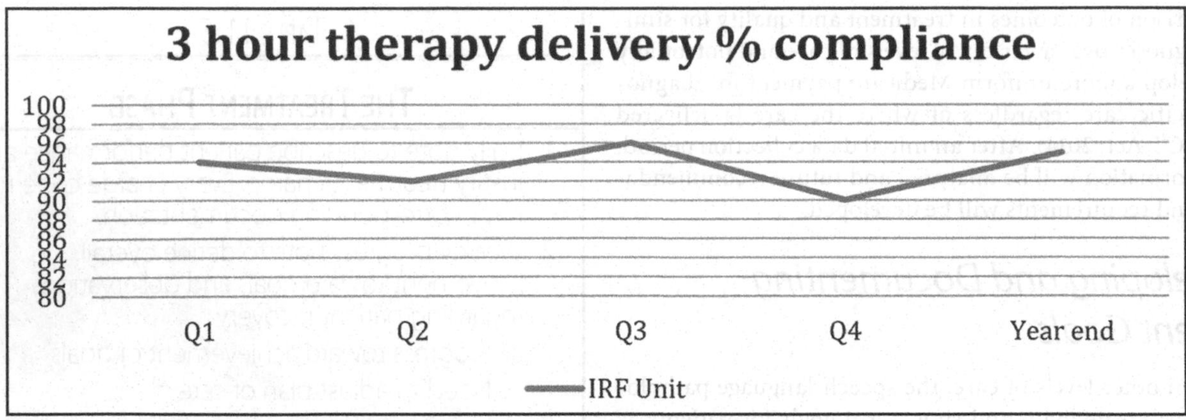

Figure 11-2. Compliance with three-hour therapy rule as measured on a quarterly basis.

of care and charges. These notes must be understandable by many stakeholders, including other clinicians, patients, and third-party payment administrators.

A weekly progress note that summarizes the patient's progress in therapy is also warranted at least every 7 days from the initial evaluation during the inpatient hospitalization. Short-term goals are addressed in the weekly progress note. Description of patient change related to these goals is included, and the speech-language pathologist must state clearly whether the goals were met. If goals are not met, the clinician indicates whether the goal will be continued, modified, or discontinued. If a goal is modified or discontinued, the speech-language pathologist reports whether the corresponding long-term goal will be altered as well.

As the patient advances toward the estimated discharge date, the team members meet regularly (at least once weekly) to discuss patient progress and barriers to discharge that impact return to home and/or the next level of care. The case manager typically documents these regular discussions and includes a statement of the patient's progress toward her individualized plan of care in each clinical area.

In the case of Mrs. O., who has a 19-day hospital stay, the speech-language pathologist would write two weekly progress notes and a discharge summary prior to leaving the IRF.

The Three-Hour Rule

Compliance with the three-hour rule is measured and reported based on participation with scheduled therapy and is tracked at regular intervals. Additionally, reasons that therapy services were missed and instances of noncompliance are tracked to allow for process and quality improvement programming to occur. It is important to track performance because denial of payment for the entire IRF stay can be imposed if all criteria for IRF admission are not met (Figure 11-2 and Table 11-6).

Missed Treatment Algorithm

It is important to have a system in place if therapy minutes are missed to assist with meeting the requirement for delivery of services. The process here outlines one way to address missed minutes when a patient does not receive the full scheduled treatment session. Interprofessional teams may develop an internal tracking method to respond quickly and remain compliant for that day. For example, if a patient misses a significant amount of time in physical therapy due to required nursing care, and if no other physical therapist was available to see this patient later, a speech-language pathologist who has a schedule opening may be asked to work with the patient to facilitate rehabilitation intensity that day. To remain compliant, therapy services must be delivered by two separate disciplines during a treatment day; not all of the therapy minutes (180 minutes) can be delivered by one discipline during 1 day (Figure 11-3 and Table 11-7).

Discharge Documentation

At discharge, the speech-language pathologist is required to complete a re-evaluation of the patient's skills, score and interpret formal and informal measures, complete functional rating scales, update status of short- and long-term goals, plan for the patient's post-discharge needs, and complete patient and family education.

The documentation essential at the end of the patient's stay summarizes the diagnosis and patient change during the course of the stay in the IRF. This note should be comprehensive in nature and objectively compare initial ability with patient status at the end of the stay. Outcome measures are scored, and the patient's attainment of expected goals and education are described.

Our patient, Sally O., made good improvements in the IRF level of care. Many IRFs contract with health care organizations that collect aggregate follow-up information after patients leave the hospital. These data can help the IRF track effectiveness and understand patterns of improvement

Table 11-6

Commonly Documented Reasons for Missed Minutes of Therapy

Reason for Missed Treatment	Explanation
Patient refused	No specified reason for refusal given by the patient. Despite education and encouragement, patient refuses to engage in treatment session.
Patient refused due to fatigue	Patient refused to participate due to fatigue despite efforts to modify treatment session or schedule.
Nursing care required	Patient is requiring intervention from nursing staff that is not able to be rescheduled.
Conflict with scheduling due to outside appointment	Patient requires follow-up outside of IRF unit and, due to travel and/or wait times at appointment, has missed part or all of session.
Patient placed on medical hold	Medical staff have deemed that patient is not safe for treatment and have placed on a medical hold.
Patient refusing and reporting feeling unwell	Patient presents with specific or non-specific complaints regarding illness and not agreeable to modification to treatment.
Patient demonstrating a change in mental status	Patient is showing a change in baseline status observed since admission.
Patient is showing decreased arousal or is unarousable	Patient is showing known or increased difficulty in maintaining arousal and/or attention, either inhibiting participation in treatment session or requiring medical assessment and intervention.
Conflict with scheduling due to inside appointment	Patient is requiring an intervention in the IRF by a member of the treatment team that was not scheduled.
Patient missed all or part of session due to toileting needs	Patient has immediate toileting needs that prohibit participation in scheduled session and that cannot be incorporated into treatment session.
Patient not safe for treatment due to an increase or demonstration of new agitation	Patient is demonstrating unsafe behaviors toward self or others that limit ability to safely participate in treatment session at the scheduled time, possibly requiring medical assessment and intervention.
Patient refusing treatment due to increased or new pain	Patient is refusing to participate in treatment session due to pain despite efforts to intervene with medications or other modalities to alleviate pain.
Other	Any interruption that limits the patient's ability to participate in treatment must be specified by clinician in documentation.

and quality at periodic intervals post-discharge. In Sally's case, the IRF was able to share with Sally and her family the percentage of patients who indicated they are able to manage their own care needs 3 months after discharge, despite a majority of patients continuing to need some level of assistance at the end of their IRF stay.

Additional Considerations

Efficiency

Efficiency in completion of documentation is an important component of work-life balance, work satisfaction, and effectiveness (U.S. Department of Health & Human Services, 2014). Over the years, clinicians have developed several tools to help them manage the challenges of completing paperwork.

Productivity requirements for therapists in an IRF are estimated to be an average of 6 billable hours in an 8-hour work day. Although completion of clinical records is necessary, the time spent with one's patient aiding her in behavioral change is the most important activity a clinician provides.

There are currently three types of medical records used in an IRF setting:

1. Paper-only medical charts
2. Electronic medical records (EMRs) and electronic health records (EHRs)
3. EHR with some paper records preserved, such as billing or patient-signed forms

Speech-language pathology departments should have adequate training and orientation for all new staff members to help them successfully navigate which forms and what parts of the medical record must be completed and

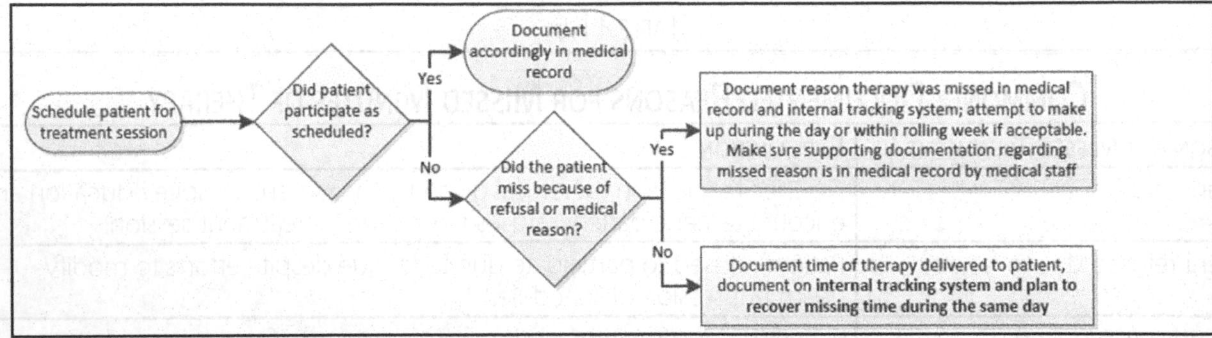

Figure 11-3. Decision-making process for documentation of patient participation with therapy.

Table 11-7
Discharge
1. Re-evaluation results of standardized and informal measures 2. Discharge FIM, FCM, and IMPACT scoring 3. Summary and analysis of patient progress and change during the stay, including comprehensive description of objective performance in education and functional goal areas 4. Discharge diagnosis 5. Recommendations/plan of care, including: a. Need for further skilled therapy b. Frequency and duration of intervention c. Long-term goals d. Your contact information for patient and clinician follow-up e. Warm handoff to next care provider recommended

when. The use of a workflow checklist can be a valuable aid in consistent documentation of accurate documentation completion.

Templated Documents

Long before the advent of the EHR, clinicians developed templates for their documentation. Templates help capture the essential diagnostic information and streamline the documentation process. The formatted note can also help the reader know where to find the specific information he or she is looking for. The challenge with a template note is that it may lend itself to generalized description. To guard against this, the clinician should provide a descriptive analysis of the data and an individualized patient care plan.

Point-of-Care Documentation

There has been an emphasis on increasing point-of-care documentation since the advent of the EMR and use of portable documentation devices. Clinicians struggle with documenting in the presence of a patient and are concerned about the impact on face-to-face communication and rapport. Speech-language pathologists are accustomed to scoring tests and noting behavioral observations during assessments and treatment sessions, and use of the EMR for this purpose feels less connected than writing on a piece of paper. When a speech-language pathologist has access to a documentation device (portable or stationary) and/or is able to interact with a patient in a configuration that does not require his or her back to be turned to a patient for any notable period of time, he or she may be able to incorporate documentation observations and brief remarks of analysis while providing assessment or treatment. The speech-language pathologist can engage with a patient throughout the session and, in the context of education, summary, and support, describe to the patient his or her performance while making note of it directly into the record. Talking with your patient about why you are documenting your interaction and the importance of recording daily changes can eliminate awkwardness in the interaction or can reveal individual patient discomfort with the arrangement. Clinicians should always be mindful of a patient's individual needs and interact accordingly. Capturing real-time information in the medical record decreases the risk that observations are recorded inaccurately. It also allows other care providers to act on the information in a timely manner.

Documentation of the Shared Decision-Making Process

Although it is not in the scope of this chapter to explore thoroughly, it is important to note that there will occasionally be disagreements in patient care that speech-language pathologists will need to reflect in their documentation. The speech-language pathologist makes recommendations for treatment, and a patient who has decision-making capacity has the right to accept or refuse those recommendations. When a patient has a cognitive-communication disorder caused by neurological impairment, it can be difficult to assess his or her decision-making capacity (Tunzi, 2001). When there is disagreement between a decisionally capable adult patient and clinician recommendations, we typically defer to the patient's autonomous choice. These conversations with patients or their proxies should involve informed consent and voluntary choice. When documenting such a clinical decision point, the speech-language pathologist should include the following:

- The rationale for the clinical recommendation (e.g., non-oral nutrition and hydration)
- The patient's capacity for decision making (Tunzi, 2001)
- The patient's response (e.g., questions, concerns), preferences, and reasons (e.g., rejects NPO because eating gives her great joy and she fears being socially isolated)
- As needed, the patient's desires for continued treatment and for how potential complications of his or her condition will be managed (e.g., the patient will eat trial portions of pureed foods with use of safest strategies and will use the oral suction at the end of the meal)
- The follow-up plan (e.g., that the speech-language pathologist will check in with the patient weekly to maximize safety and re-evaluate the plan of care)

Hand-Off Communication

Adequate interprofessional communication is a critical and primary component of the milieu of IRF level of care. Treatment team members are expected to work together in a patient-focused approach to help the patient and/or caregivers develop achievable goals for the near term.

It is important for all clinicians to recognize that patient recovery and care extends beyond the intervention they provide. For example, most patients who are admitted to the IRF setting will continue to need speech therapy for weeks, months, and sometimes years after the onset of their illness. In order to use the resources of the health care system wisely, it is beneficial for the patient's clinicians to view their colleagues in the patient's care across the continuum as team members.

It is good practice for speech-language pathologists to create relationships with colleagues from all levels of the care continuum in their area. Hand-off communication avoids redundancies in high-cost care when not needed (e.g., a patient presenting with dysphagia who has had a VFSS the day prior to discharge from the acute care hospital should not need a new VFSS in the initial part of an IRF stay unless there are notable clinical changes). It also facilitates smooth transitions when clinicians are informed about the nuances of a patient's needs, and patients and families feel there is continuity of care. To think of it another way, although medical record documentation is available, a speech-language pathologist would unlikely go on vacation without talking with the team member who will cover his or her patients during the time off. Why would we not offer the same consideration when a patient is transferred to an entirely new team? A hand-off is an important patient-centered quality and safety practice.

Coding

As mentioned in Chapter 5, CPT codes are regularly used for billing of outpatient services as prescribed by CMS for purposes of reimbursement. Services are carefully coded according to the National Correct Coding Initiative (CMS, 2017) and Outpatient Code Editor (CMS, 2010) Edit Tables, which denote whether certain codes can be billed on the same day for patients with Medicare Part B. Speech-language pathologists working in an inpatient acute rehabilitation hospital setting (i.e., IRF) may be asked to enter charges and associated CPT codes for specific services delivered, but this is mainly for internal tracking and productivity purposes, because Medicare Part A reimburses inpatient care through the prospective payment system and not based on specific CPT codes. Nevertheless, inpatient settings generally follow the Correct Coding Initiative coding guidelines.

Conclusion

All rubrics of expertise, competence, and evidence-based practice apply to the work of the speech-language pathologist in the IRF setting. IRF rules of participation as a specialty level of care necessitate that the speech-language pathologist and all clinicians work together to ensure that any regulatory requirements are met. Individualized assessment and treatment are the hallmarks of a patient-centered approach and must be reflected in the standardized documentation elements. Speech-language pathologists can practice at the top of their ability when they know the needs for reporting in the IRF level of care and when they work with their departments and interprofessional teams to develop practices to meet these obligations.

References

American Speech-Language-Hearing Association. (2013). National Outcomes Measurement System (NOMS): Adult speech-language pathology user's guide. Retrieved from https://www.asha.org/NOMS/

Centers for Medicare & Medicaid Services. (2010). CMS Manual Pub 100-02 Medicare Benefit Policy, Transmittal 119. Retrieved from https://www.cms.gov/Medicare/Coding/OutpatientCodeEdit/Index.html

Centers for Medicare & Medicaid Services. (2017). NCCI Policy Manual for Medicare Services–Effective January 1, 2017. Retrieved from https://www.cms.gov/Medicare/Coding/NationalCorrectCodInitEd/Downloads/NCCI-Policy-Manual-2017.zip

Chumney, D., Nollinger, K., Shesko, K., Skop, K., Spencer, M., & Newton, R. A. (2010). Ability of Functional Independence Measure to accurately predict functional outcome of stroke-specific population: Systematic review. *Journal of Rehabilitation Research & Development, 47*(1), 17–29.

Improving Medicare Post-Acute Care Transformation (IMPACT) Act of 2014, Pub. L. No. 113-18 (2014).

Kertesz, A. (2006). *Western Aphasia Battery-Revised* [Screening tool]. San Antonio, TX: Pearson Education Inc.

Linacre, J. M., Heinemann, A. W., Wright, B. D., Granger, C. V., & Hamilton, B. B. (1994). The structure and stability of the Functional Independence Measure. *Archives of Physical Medicine and Rehabilitation, 75*(2), 127–132.

Martin-Harris, B. (2010). *Modified Barium Swallow Impairment Profile* [Assessment tool]. Gaylord, MI: Northern Speech Services.

Tunzi, M. (2001). Can the patient decide? Evaluating patient capacity in practice. *American Family Physician Journal, 64*(2), 299–308.

U.S. Department of Health & Human Services. (2014). What are the advantages of electronic health records? Retrieved from https://www.healthit.gov/providers-professionals/faqs/what-are-advantages-electronic-health-records

Review Questions

1. What is the nationally required outcome measure used by clinicians in the IRF setting?
2. What documentation is required for admission to fulfill criteria for IRF level of care?
3. Why is it important for speech-language pathologists to document standardized outcome measures for their patients?
4. Why should the speech-language pathologist be a regular part of meeting the three-hour rule for patients who need speech-language or swallowing treatment?
5. What components of documentation should the speech-language pathologist include in the following phases of IRF care?
   a. Assessment
   b. Treatment
   c. Discharge
6. What should the speech-language pathologist include in documentation of disagreement between clinician recommendations and patient preferences?
7. What acronym is used by many clinicians to guide adequate goal development?

Activity A

1. Given the description of Sally O. at her evaluation, write three SMART long-term goals for the period of a 3-week stay in an IRF.
2. Take one of the long-term goals in the previous question and write two sequential short-term goals related to it.
3. Describe a plan for completing your daily reporting with a combination of point-of-care documentation and documentation outside of the session with a patient.
   a. How would you discuss your actions with patient and caregiver if you document with the patient present? What would you say specifically?
   b. What kinds of information are reasonable or easier to document during the patient's session?
   c. What would need to be written outside of the patient's session?
4. Achieving the required number of therapy minutes per 5 days of a rolling week can be a challenge given all the human factors we encounter. Describe how you can envision working with the team to ensure this goal is met each day.

Appendix 11-A

Timeline and Summary of Documentation and Billing in the Inpatient Rehabilitation Facility Setting for Patient Sally O.

	Visit	Actions (Evaluation and Treatment)	Billing/ Coding	Speech-Language Pathologist Documentation
Rolling Week 1	Day 1 Tuesday	Admission to IRF		
	Day 2 Wednesday	Swallowing evaluation completed in a 60-minute session	92610	Swallowing evaluation report Admission FIM ratings: Day 2 FIM Admission NOMS FCM rating (swallowing)
	Day 3 Thursday	Speech-language evaluation completed in a 60-minute session	92523	Speech-language evaluation report Admission FIM ratings: Day 3 FIM Admission NOMS FCM ratings (speech/language)
	Day 4 Friday	Swallowing treatment and speech-language treatment completed in a 60-minute session (30 minutes each segment)	92526 92507	Daily treatment documentation reflecting patient performance Patient/family education
	Day 5 Saturday	Swallowing treatment and speech-language treatment completed in a 60-minute session (30 minutes each segment)	92526 92507	Daily treatment documentation reflecting patient performance Patient/family education
	Day 6 Sunday	No treatment scheduled		
	Day 7 Monday	Swallowing treatment completed (30 minutes) and VFSS completed (45 minutes)	92526 92611	Daily documentation of treatment session and VFSS evaluation template
Rolling Week 2	Day 8 Tuesday	Swallowing treatment: Begins PO trials and speech-language treatment completed in a 60-minute session (30 minutes each segment)	92526 92507	Daily treatment documentation reflecting patient performance Patient/family education Completion of weekly note
	Day 9 Wednesday	Speech-language treatment completed in a 60-minute session	92507	Daily treatment documentation reflecting patient performance
	Day 10 Thursday	Swallowing treatment and speech-language treatment completed in a 60-minute session (30 minutes each segment)	92526 92507	Weekly note reflecting patient performance over first week since initial evaluations
	Day 11 Friday	Swallowing treatment and speech-language treatment completed in a 60-minute session (30 minutes each segment)	92526 92507	Daily treatment documentation reflecting patient performance Patient/family education
	Day 12 Saturday	Patient refuses all NPO; wants to begin eating full PO diet		Document shared decision discussion

	Visit	Actions (Evaluation and Treatment)	Billing/ Coding	Speech-Language Pathologist Documentation
	Day 13 Sunday	No treatment scheduled		
	Day 14 Monday	Swallowing treatment and speech-language treatment completed in a 60-minute session (30 minutes each segment)	92526 92507	Daily treatment documentation reflecting patient performance
Rolling Week 3	Day 15 Tuesday	Swallowing treatment completed (30 minutes) and speech-language individual and group treatments (60 minutes each)	92526 92507 92508	Daily treatment documentation reflecting patient performance in all sessions Completion of weekly note
	Day 16 Wednesday	Swallowing treatment completed (30 minutes) and speech-language individual and group treatments (60 minutes each)	92526 92507 92508	Daily treatment documentation reflecting patient performance in both sessions Patient/family education
	Day 17 Thursday	Swallowing treatment completed (30 minutes) and speech-language individual and group treatments (60 minutes each)	92526 92507 92508	Daily treatment documentation reflecting patient performance in both sessions Patient/family education
	Day 18 Friday	Swallowing treatment/informal re-evaluation completed (30 minutes) Speech-language re-evaluation completed in a 60-minute session	92526 92523	Complete documentation of: • Speech-language discharge summary • Discharge FIM ratings • Discharge NOMS ratings • Patient/family discharge instructions
	Day 19 Saturday	Discharge		

12

Skilled Nursing Facility

Renee Kinder, MS, CCC-SLP, RAC-CT

Skilled Nursing Facility Medicare Part A Coverage Criteria

Services provided to a Medicare beneficiary in the skilled nursing facility (SNF) setting must be skilled in nature and may include nursing or rehabilitation services or a combination of both. SNF Part A benefits include coverage for up to 100 days in a benefit period. The benefit period begins on the day an individual is admitted as an inpatient and ends when the beneficiary has not had any inpatient hospital care (or skilled care in an SNF) for 60 days in a row. If an individual is admitted into a hospital or SNF after one benefit period has ended, a new benefit period begins.

In order for a beneficiary to be eligible for SNF services under Medicare Part A, the Medicare beneficiary must have days available in the benefit period. The Medicare beneficiary must also have a 3-day qualifying stay in an acute hospital or be transferred to the SNF within 30 days of discharge from an acute hospital.

Once a beneficiary is eligible for an SNF Medicare Part A stay, there are certain factors that must be met for Medicare to cover the beneficiary's care in the SNF. Medicare Part A provides coverage for SNF care only when the following criteria are met:

- Patient requires skilled nursing services or skilled rehabilitation services
- Services must be ordered by physician
- Services are rendered for condition for which patient was seen in hospital or for a condition that arose while receiving care in an SNF for which patient received hospital services
- Requires these services daily
- The services can only be provided on an inpatient basis in an SNF
- Services are reasonable and necessary for the condition
- Duration and quantity of services is reasonable and necessary

When the criteria are met and services are provided for skilled Medicare Part A patients, services are reimbursed based on the amount and frequency of therapy services across all disciplines, including physical, occupational, and speech therapy and are captured in a Resource Utilization Group category. Under the SNF prospective payment system (PPS), payment is made based on the Resource Utilization Group category that a beneficiary falls into based on the amount of skilled therapy that the beneficiary needs and receives. The categories for rehabilitation services are Rehab Ultra High (RU), Rehab Very High (RV), Rehab High (RH), Rehab Medium (RM), and Rehab Low (RL) (Table 12-1) (Centers for Medicare & Medicaid Services [CMS], 2017a, 2017b).

Swigert, N. B.
Documentation and Reimbursement for Speech-Language Pathologists: Principles and Practice (pp. 167-198).

Table 12-1

Rehabilitation Resource Utilization Groups

RU	Rehabilitation Rx 720 minutes/week minimum *and* at least 1 rehabilitation discipline 5 days/week *and* a second rehabilitation discipline 3 days/week
RV	Rehabilitation Rx 500 minutes/week minimum *and* at least 1 rehabilitation discipline 5 days/week
RH	Rehabilitation Rx 325 minutes/week minimum *and* at least 1 rehabilitation discipline 5 days/week
RM	Rehabilitation Rx 150 minutes/week minimum *and* 5 days any combination of 3 rehabilitation disciplines
RL	Rehabilitation Rx 45 minutes/week minimum *and* 3 days any combination of 3 rehabilitation disciplines

Medicare Coverage for Speech-Language Pathology Services

Per the Medicare Benefit Policy Manual, Chapter 15, Section 230.3, "speech-language pathology services are those services provided within the scope of practice of speech-language pathologists and necessary for the diagnosis and treatment of speech and language disorders, which result in communication disabilities and for the diagnosis and treatment of swallowing disorders (dysphagia), regardless of the presence of a communication disability" (CMS, 2017b).

For program coverage purposes, a qualified speech-language pathologist meets one of the following requirements:

- "The education and experience requirements for a Certificate of Clinical Competence in (speech-language pathology) granted by the American Speech-Language-Hearing Association (ASHA); or
- Meets the educational requirements for certification and is in the process of accumulating the supervised experience required for certification."

Services of speech-language pathology assistants are not currently recognized by Medicare (CMS, 2017b).

Establishing a Therapy Plan of Care

In order for a patient to receive skilled rehabilitation care, certain conditions must be met. Per the Medicare Benefit Policy Manual, Chapter 15, Section 220.2: Reasonable and Necessary Outpatient Rehabilitation Therapy Services, conditions for skilled care include the following:

- "Services must be directly and specifically related to an active written treatment plan that is based on an initial evaluation performed by a qualified therapist after admission to the SNF that is approved by the physician after any needed consultation with the qualified therapist.
- Services must be of a level of complexity and sophistication, or the condition of the patient must be of a nature that requires the judgment, knowledge, and skills of a qualified therapist.
- The services must be provided with the expectation, based on the assessment made by the physician of the patient's restoration potential, that the condition of the patient will improve materially in a reasonable and generally predictable period of time; or, the services must be necessary for the establishment of a safe and effective maintenance program; or, the services must require the skills of a qualified therapist for the performance of a safe and effective maintenance program.
- The services must be considered under accepted standards of medical practice to be specific and effective treatment for the patient's condition.
- The services must be reasonable and necessary for the treatment of the patient's condition; this includes the requirement that the amount, frequency and duration of the services must be reasonable." (CMS, 2017b)

Identifying Patients Who Can Benefit From Skilled Rehabilitation Care

Collaboration with all members of the interdisciplinary team is key for the success of a speech-language pathologist in the SNF setting. One key member of the interdisciplinary team is the Minimum Data Set (MDS) Coordinator. The MDS Coordinator is responsible for completing the Resident Assessment Index (RAI), which includes the MDS, Care Area Assessments (CAA), and the working Care Plan (Figure 12-1).

Minimum Data Set

The MDS is a screening tool that provides information about the resident's functional status. The MDS is the first step in the RAI process used to identify functional changes

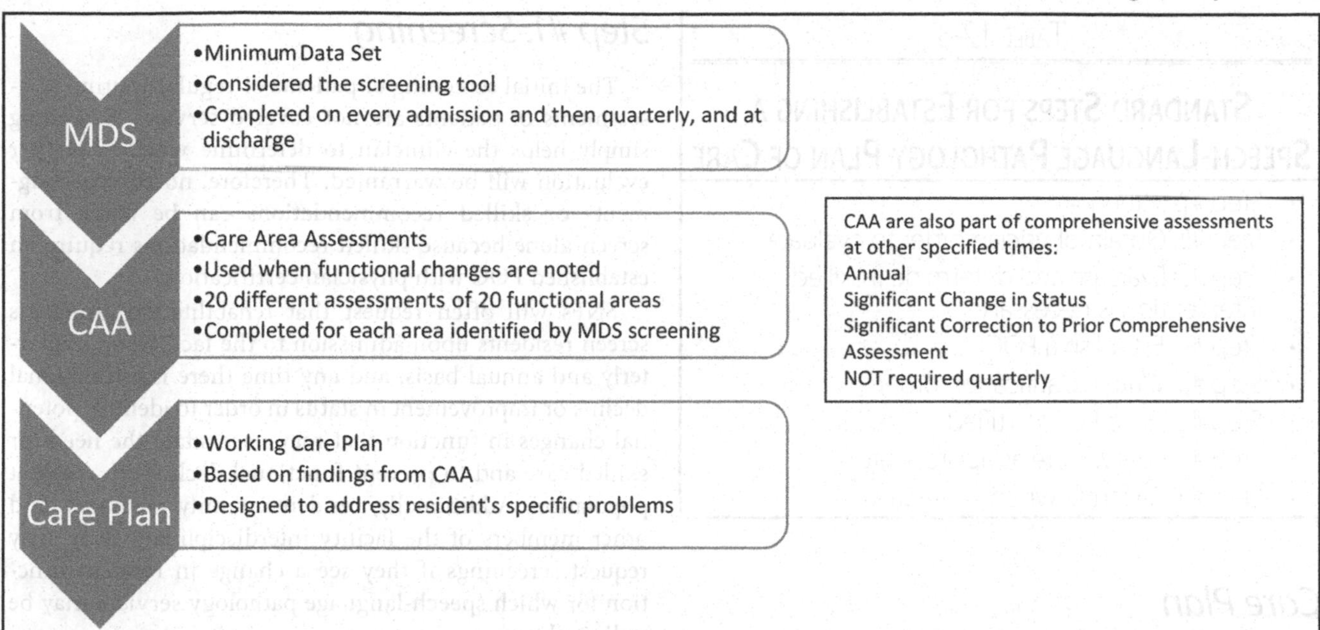

Figure 12-1. Resident assessment steps.

Table 12-2

Care Area Assessments

1. Delirium	11. Falls
2. Cognitive loss	12. Nutritional status
3. Visual function	13. Feeding tube(s)
4. Communication	14. Dehydration/fluid maintenance
5. ADL: Functional status	15. Dental care
6. Urinary incontinence and indwelling catheter	16. Pressure ulcer(s)
7. Psychosocial well-being	17. Psychotropic medication use
8. Mood state	18. Physical restraints
9. Behavioral symptoms	19. Pain
10. Activities	20. Return to community referral

Abbreviation: ADL = activities of daily living.

in an individual resident's status. MDS clinical screenings are completed upon every admission to an SNF and every quarter following the admission. MDS screenings are also completed upon discharge from the facility. As the MDS itself is merely a screening tool, when functional changes are noted, the entire interdisciplinary team should move the patient to the next level of assessment via CAAs. Refer to Appendix 12-A for the sections of the MDS.

Care Area Assessments

CAAs are a set of 20 different assessments that are further in-depth evaluations of specific functional areas. A CAA must be completed for each care area that is identified as a possible problem, or triggered, as a result of the MDS assessment. After completing the CAA, a clinical decision is made based on the results as to whether the possible problem is in fact a real problem. When a problem is identified, the next step is to determine the root causes and contributing factors, risk factors for the resident related to the problem, and the need for referrals to other disciplines.

CAAs are also included in comprehensive assessment periods throughout the resident's stay, including Admission assessment, Annual assessment, Significant change in status assessment, and Significant correction to prior comprehensive assessment. They are not required in the Quarterly assessments and the Significant correction to prior quarterly assessment (Table 12-2).

TABLE 12-3

STANDARD STEPS FOR ESTABLISHING A SPEECH-LANGUAGE PATHOLOGY PLAN OF CARE

- Step #1: Screen
- Step #2: Obtain physician order to evaluate
- Step #3: Evaluate and determine if skilled intervention is necessary
- Step #4: Establish a POC
- Step #5: Write a clarification order
- Step #6: Have POC certified
- Step #7: Re-evaluate as appropriate
- Step #8: Recertify when necessary

Care Plan

The working action plan that is developed based on the findings that result from the CAAs is called a *care plan*. The development of an individualized, interdisciplinary care plan designed to address the resident's specific problems, strengths, preferences, risk factors, and complications is the primary purpose of the RAI process.

ESTABLISHING A SPEECH-LANGUAGE PATHOLOGY PLAN OF CARE/TREATMENT PLAN

Development and certification of treatment plans requires that a speech-language pathologist completes a true hands-on assessment, which is then followed by timely certification of the plan of care (POC). POC requirements as outlined in Chapter 15, Section 220 of the Medicare Benefit Policy Manual (CMS, 2017b) require that:

- The speech-language pathologist provide a clear distinction between screening, evaluation, and re-evaluation
- The beneficiary's history and the onset or exacerbation date is clear in conjunction with current symptoms
- Prior level of function (PLOF) and baseline abilities are provided
- Recommended frequency and duration of care follow acceptable standards of practice for the patient's specific condition

Following the development of a comprehensive POC, continued documentation is required to support skilled levels of care, including progress reports, daily notes, and discharge summaries (Table 12-3).

Speech-language pathologists typically initiate or receive referrals for resident needs in two ways: Either they receive a direct order from a physician or they recognize the need for evaluation during a screening process.

Step #1: Screening

The initial screening of patients or regular routine reassessments of patients are not covered services. Screening simply helps the clinician to determine whether further evaluation will be warranted. Therefore, no clinical judgments or skilled recommendations can be made from screen alone because skilled recommendations require an established POC with physician certification.

SNFs will often request that rehabilitation clinicians screen residents upon admission to the facility, on a quarterly and annual basis, and any time there is a functional decline or improvement in status in order to identify potential changes in function that may necessitate the need for skilled care and to prevent functional declines in resident population. Additionally, residents, family members, and other members of the facility interdisciplinary team may request screenings if they see a change in resident function for which speech-language pathology services may be indicated.

The process of screening does not have the same requirement as an evaluation in that a hands-on assessment is not required. Therefore, sources for obtaining information often include the following:

- Resident observation and interview
- A thorough review of the medical record, including:
  - Physician progress reports
  - Nursing daily and weekly notes
  - Dietary records
  - Physical and occupational therapy documentation
- Review of admission, annual, and quarterly MDS records, which can be extremely beneficial for deriving documentation related to functional changes in status

Refer to Appendices 12-B and 12-C for more detail on potential areas for obtaining information specific to swallowing, language, cognition, motor speech, and voice.

Step #2: Obtaining Physician Orders

Evaluation Orders

After completion of a screen, if the speech-language pathologist sees the need for further evaluation, request for an evaluation order should be made to the beneficiary's physician. The order or referral for the evaluation and any specific testing in areas of concern should be designated by the referring physician in consultation with the therapist. After the signed order is received, the speech-language pathologist can complete an evaluation specific to the patient's needs.

Clarification Orders

Following completion of the evaluation, the speech-language pathologist should provide the physician with the completed comprehensive POC document and request a signature. Subsequently, the physician's signature on the

POC acts as certification/clarification of services after evaluation. Many SNFs will also request that the speech-language pathologist complete a clarification order outlining target area(s), anticipated frequency and duration of care, and planned skilled interventions because orders are often used as the facility's guide for any changes in a resident's care that should be transferred over onto the individualized care plan.

Additional Orders

Additional orders may be needed after initiation of the initial POC. Cases where this may occur include the following:

- Any significant updates to POC affecting a long-term goal, which will also require a recertification or re-evaluation
- Addition of new interventions not included on initial plan (e.g., speech-language pathologist begins services for dysphagia alone; as resident progresses with laryngeal function, further evaluation is warranted for voice and motor speech)
- Recertification of a POC (often be accompanied by clarification orders)

Discharging Orders

On occasion, a speech-language pathologist may receive an order for services that are not warranted or for one specific area of function when another is clinically indicated. In these cases, orders should be discharged, and, if deemed necessary, orders for the appropriate clinical area should be requested.

For example, in some SNFs, all Medicare Part A PPS patients who are admitted to the facility will have standing order as follows: "Physical, occupational, and speech therapy to eval/treat as indicated." This form of an order is often built into the facility's policies and procedures or a portion of the electronic medical record (EMR); however, this does not require that an evaluation be completed in the absence of need. Therefore, a speech-language pathologist can always screen the resident first and complete an order request such as, "Please discharge speech therapy order to eval/treat as not clinically indicated at this time."

Additionally, if a speech-language pathologist requests orders for one target area and needs orders for an additional area, an order request should be made.

For example, if a speech-language pathologist receives an order such as, "Speech therapy to evaluate and treat for dysphagia," but needed orders for language, he or she would request a change such as, "Speech therapy order to evaluate and treat for dysphagia received; however, order needed for language; therefore, request evaluation and treatment orders for language alone."

Additionally, if a speech-language pathologist receives an order for only one needed area and needs multiple, he or she would request a change such as, "Speech therapy received order to evaluate and treat for dysphagia alone; requesting additional evaluation and treatment order for language" (Table 12-4).

Step #3: Evaluating and Determining the Need for Skilled Care

Evaluation

Per the Medicare Benefit Policy Manual, Section 220 (CMS, 2017b), an evaluation helps the clinician with determining the need for skilled service. They are separately payable, comprehensive, hands-on services provided by a clinician, and therefore require professional skills to make clinical judgments about conditions for which services are indicated.

Evaluations may be warranted for a new diagnosis following screening when there has been an evidenced change from PLOF, or when an individual shows an increased desire or ability to participate in skilled intervention whereas they were limited prior.

Evaluation judgments are essential to the development of the POC, including goals and the selection of interventions.

Key elements of the evaluation document include the following:

- Clear documentation related to onset date in conjunction with current symptoms
- Inclusion of objective and subjective measures
- Established baseline measures in comparison to prior level of function
- Realistic, functional, measurable short-term objectives and long-term goals

Following completion of these elements, the need for skilled care is determined.

To begin, the evaluation should address the beneficiary's history in conjunction with the onset or exacerbation date of the current symptoms or conditions. The onset/exacerbation date refers to the date of the functional change that, as a result of diagnosis, indicated the need for skilled care. For individuals with chronic conditions, the onset date may not be the date of diagnosis for condition but relate to the exacerbation date of the disease process. Alternatively, for new conditions, such as new-onset cerebrovascular accident (CVA) or a traumatic brain injury, the onset date will be date of new insult. These onsets should be documented in conjunction with current symptoms in order to provide a correlation of why the new onset has resulted in symptoms requiring your unique skilled services.

The following are some examples:

- Mrs. Adams presents with medical diagnosis of Parkinson's disease with recent exacerbation, resulting in an acute care stay from 5-15-16 to 5-20-16 and noted reduction in vocal intensity.

Table 12-4

Sample Speech-Language Pathology Physician Orders

Dysphagia	
Evaluation/ treat order	• Speech-language pathology to evaluate/treat as indicated • Speech-language pathology to complete bedside swallow evaluation and treat as indicated secondary to reported decline in swallow function • Speech-language pathology to complete bedside swallow evaluation and treat as indicated due to noted decreased ability to tolerate current diet per recent screening
Clarification orders	*Speech-Language Pathology Clarification* • Please add R13.12 Oropharyngeal Dysphagia to dx list • Please change diet to puree with nectar-thick liquids, continue with therapeutic recs per RD • Patient to participate in skilled services 5 times/week for 8 weeks, which may include compensatory swallow strategies, oral motor exercises, NMES, and patient caregiver education in order to treat oropharyngeal dysphagia
Cognitive/Language	
Evaluation/ treat order	• Speech-language pathology to evaluate/treat as indicated due to reports of declines in cognitive status affecting ability to follow commands • Speech-language pathology to evaluate/treat as indicated due to presentation of recent falls secondary to suspect reduced safety awareness
Clarification orders	*Speech-Language Pathology Clarification* • Please add R48.8 Symbolic Dysfunction and R47.01 Aphasia to dx list • Patient to participate in skilled services 4 times/week for 6 weeks, which may include language therapy, cognitive therapy, and patient/caregiver education
Voice/Dysarthria	
Evaluation/ treat order	• Speech-language pathology to evaluate/treat as indicated due to reports of declines in speech intelligibility affecting her ability to communicate with staff • Speech-language pathology to evaluate/treat as indicated due to presentation of recent decline in vocal function associated with progression of Parkinson's disease
Clarification orders	*Speech-Language Pathology Clarification* • Please add R47.1 Dysarthria to dx list • Patient to participate in skilled services 5 times/week for 4 weeks, which may include motor speech therapy, compensatory training, and patient/caregiver education in order to treat dysarthria secondary to Parkinson's disease
Cerebrovascular Accident	
Evaluation/ treat order	• Speech-language pathology to evaluate/treat as indicated due to declines related to recent CVA
Clarification orders	*Speech-Language Pathology Clarification* • Please add I69.391 Dysphagia following cerebral infarction and I69.820 Aphasia following other cerebrovascular disease to dx list • Patient to participate in modified barium swallow study in order to determine severity of dysphagia and establish appropriate treatment • Patient to participate in skilled services 5 to 7 times/week for 12 weeks, which may include oral motor exercises, compensatory swallow strategies, language therapy, and patient/caregiver education

Abbreviations: dx = diagnosis; NMES = neuromuscular electrical stimulation; RD = registered dietician; recs = recommendations.

- Mr. Lee has significant medical diagnosis of dementia of Alzheimer's type with recent declines in cognitive function, as evidenced by cognitive testing completed by his primary care physician during his annual wellness visit.

Determining the Need for Skill

Following completion of the evaluation, the therapist will establish the POC and determine the need for skilled services. Skilled services per the Medicare Benefit Policy Manual, Chapter 15, Section 220.2 (CMS, 2017b), must adhere to the following key criteria:

- Services must follow evidence-based practice
- Services must be at such a level of complexity and sophistication that only a skilled clinician can provide the care
- Determinations cannot be made solely on diagnosis alone
- Established frequency and duration of care must be individualized

Evidence-Based Practice

The services shall be considered under accepted standards of medical practice to be a specific and effective treatment for the patient's condition. Medicare acceptable practices are found in Medicare manuals, contractors' Local Coverage Determinations and National Coverage Determinations, and guidelines and literature of the profession of speech-language pathology.

Complexity and Sophistication

Skilled services should be provided at a level of complexity and sophistication or the condition of the patient shall be such that the services required can be safely and effectively performed only by a qualified therapist. Subsequently, the services that do not require the performance or supervision of a therapist are not skilled and are not considered reasonable or necessary therapy services, even if they are performed or supervised by a qualified professional.

Therefore, if the Medicare contractor determines the services furnished were of a type that could have been safely and effectively performed only by or under the supervision of such a qualified professional, it shall presume that such services were properly supervised when required.

Medical Diagnoses

Determinations on whether skilled interventions are warranted should not be made on diagnosis alone. Medicare clarifies that although a beneficiary's particular medical condition is a valid factor in deciding whether skilled therapy services are needed, a beneficiary's diagnosis or prognosis should never be the sole factor in deciding that a service is or is not skilled. The key issue is whether the skills of a qualified therapist are needed to treat the illness or injury or whether the services can be carried out by nonskilled personnel.

Individualized Frequency and Duration

Established frequency and duration of care should never be static in nature, meaning that each patient should have established frequency and duration of care individualized to his or her specific clinical needs. Additionally, Medicare states that there must be an expectation that the patient's condition will improve significantly in a reasonable (and generally predictable) period of time or the services must be necessary for the establishment of a safe and effective maintenance program required in connection with a specific disease state. The amount, frequency, and duration of the services must be reasonable under accepted standards of practice.

Step #4: Establishing the Plan of Care

Following establishment of medical diagnoses, clarification of current symptoms, and completion of objective and subjective measures, the clinician will develop the formal treatment plan. Key elements of the POC include the following:

- Clearly defined PLOF
- Diagnostic and assessment testing services that ascertain the type and causal factor(s) identified during the evaluation
- Baseline abilities for all target areas
- Goals (i.e., realistic, long-term, functional)
- Established duration and frequency of therapy, and definition of the type of service
- Clarification on whether the plan is anticipated to be rehabilitative/restorative or maintenance based

To begin, PLOF should be clearly defined. PLOF is the level of functional status at which the individual was functioning prior to the onset of functional decline that necessitated the need for skilled care. Additionally, the initial assessment establishes the baseline data necessary for evaluating expected rehabilitation potential, setting realistic goals, and measuring communication status at periodic intervals. Methods for obtaining baseline function should include objective or subjective baseline diagnostic testing (standardized or non-standardized), followed by interpretation of test results and clinical findings. Therefore, goals should not be created for areas that do not have documented baseline measures; hence, the use of EMR measures such as "DNT [did not test]" or "Will not be addressed during POC" should not be used for target areas.

The clinician should then use PLOF in comparison to baselines in order to establish the basis for the therapeutic interventions (Figure 12-2). The difference between baseline and PLOF measures should assist the therapist with determining appropriate frequency and duration of care. Greater changes may require more intensive interventions.

As the space between baseline and PLOF decreases, preparations for discharge planning should begin and

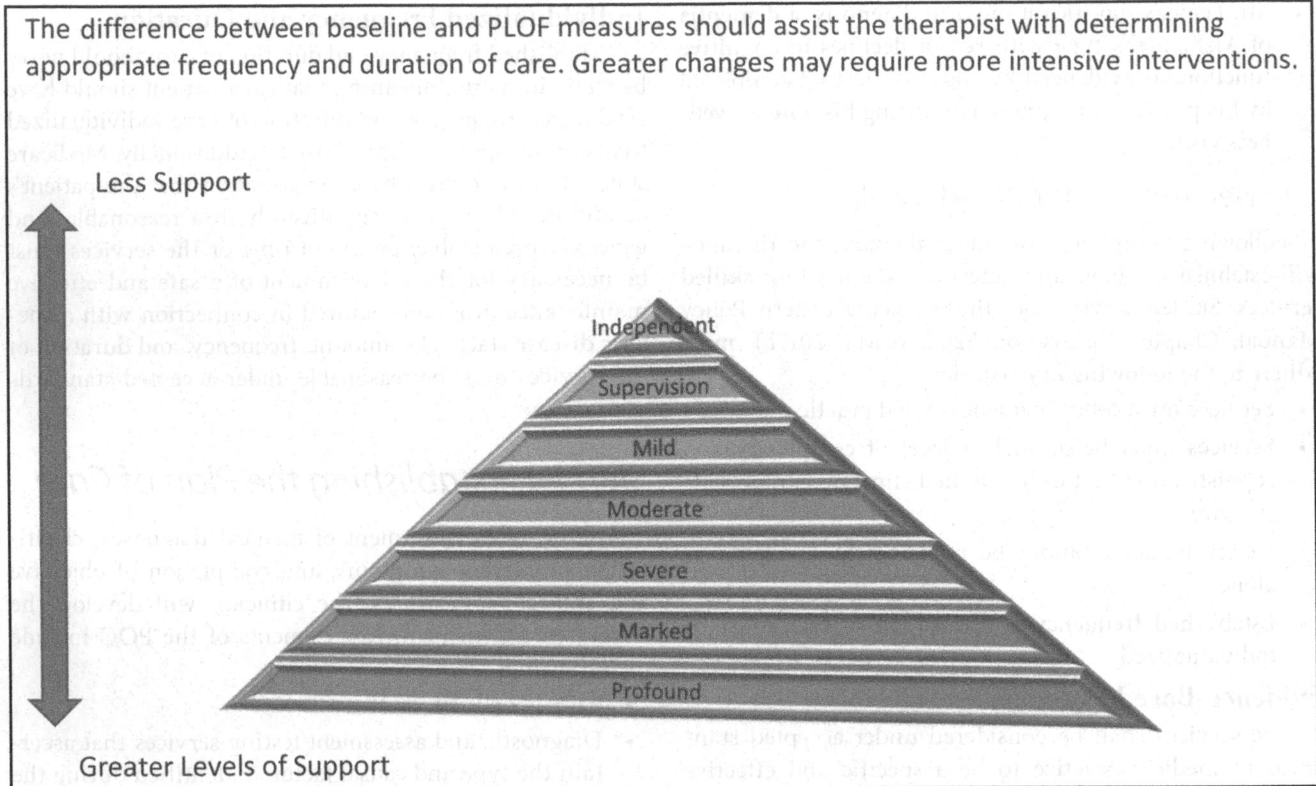

Figure 12-2. Comparing baseline and PLOF.

frequency should be tapered in order to promote carry-over of newly learned skills and promote the highest level of independence upon discharge from skilled care.

An example of using PLOF to establish goals follows: Ms. Jones is referred for bedside swallow evaluation. Baseline measures reveal moderate oropharyngeal dysphagia with significant impairments in oral processing and coughing/wet voice after the swallow with regular textures and thin liquids. PLOF was independent. The speech-language pathologist determines initially frequency and duration of 5 times/week for 4 weeks is essential to increase swallow function, allow for LR PO (*per os:* by mouth) diet, and prevent aspiration risks.

Goals/Treatment Measures

Treatment goals should be established based on clinical findings with *minimal* requirements for completion of realistic, long-term, functional targets. All targets should be established with the expectation of measurable functional improvement in a reasonable and generally predictable period of time. To strengthen plans, short-term goals should be included by sub-tasking the functional impairment area and clarifying steps needed to achieve each long-term goal target.

For example, an overall long-term goal target area for auditory comprehension could be, "Patient will demonstrate auditory comprehension of simple conversation with 100% accuracy and no cues in order to improve receptive communication skills (goal target 4 weeks)."

Short-term goals to help attain the long-term goal would be the following:

- Within 2 weeks, patient will follow one-step commands with 100% accuracy in order to enhance patient's ability to follow directions for activities and ADL.
- Within 2 weeks, patient will understand yes/no questions with 100% accuracy in order to communicate basic wants/needs.

Measurable components of goals can be created using a percentile (e.g., 50%) or number of clinical trials (e.g., 5/10 trials) and needs to be attached to all short- and long-term goals.

Functional components of goals are the "in order to" statements that needs to be attached to all short- and long-term goals to clarify true functional outcome for each target area.

Frequency and Duration

The frequency refers to the number of times per week or number of visits over a specific time frame the type of treatment is provided. The duration is the number of weeks, or the number of treatment sessions, for the POC. If the episode of care is anticipated to extend beyond the 90-calendar-day limit for certification of a plan, it is desirable, although not required, that the clinician also estimate the duration of the entire episode of care in this setting.

Frequency and duration should be patient specific, related to level of functional decline, and appropriate based on evidence-based practice patterns. Frequency and duration alone may not be used to determine medical necessity, but they should be considered with other factors, such as condition, progress, and treatment type, to provide the most effective and efficient means to achieve the patient's goals (Figure 12-3).

For example, it may be clinically appropriate, medically necessary, and most efficient and effective to provide short-term intensive treatment for some patients or longer-term and less frequent treatment for others, depending on the individual's needs. Additionally, Medicare recommends that therapists taper the frequency of visits as the patient progresses toward an independent level or reaches maximum benefit with need for a caregiver-assisted self-management program upon discharge from care.

Restorative/Rehabilitative Plans

Following updates to Chapter 15 of the Medicare Benefit Policy Manual after the *Jimmo v. Sebelius* ruling, which challenged the Medicare improvement standard, therapists are now required to clarify from the start of care whether services will be restorative/rehabilitative or maintenance based in nature (ASHA, 2016). Therefore, evaluation, re-evaluation, and assessment documented in the progress report should describe objective measurements that, when compared, show improvements in function, decrease in severity, or rationalization for an optimistic outlook to justify continued treatment.

Rehabilitative/restorative therapy is defined as intervention aimed at addressing recovery or improvement in function and, when possible, restoration to a previous level of health and well-being (i.e., PLOF).

Maintenance-based plans are programs established by a therapist that consist of activities and/or mechanisms that will assist a beneficiary in maximizing or maintaining the progress he or she has made during therapy or to prevent or slow further deterioration due to a disease or illness.

Individuals with chronic conditions can benefit from either level of care. Per the Medicare Benefit Policy Manual, rehabilitative therapy may be needed, and improvement in a patient's condition may occur, even when a chronic, progressive, degenerative, or terminal condition exists.

For example, a terminally ill patient may begin to exhibit self-care, mobility, and/or safety dependence requiring skilled therapy services. The fact that full (i.e., full movement from baseline to PLOF) or partial recovery is not possible does not necessarily mean that skilled therapy is not needed to improve the patient's condition or to maximize his functional abilities. The deciding factors are always whether the services are considered reasonable, effective treatments for the patient's condition and require the skills of a therapist, or whether they can be safely and effectively carried out by non–skilled personnel. Appendix 12-D provides examples of documentation in maintenance cases.

Question: How do I set my duration of care in EMR to appropriate date? The system wants to auto-set to 100 days.

Answer: When the document is created in the EMR the date ranges will have to be pulled back to the range appropriate for individual's clinical need. Certification dates must match anticipated duration of care in order for system to require recertification documents in a timely manner. Otherwise clinicians run the risk of providing skilled care outside of certification window.

Figure 12-3. Frequently asked question.

Step #5: Obtaining Certification for Plan of Care

The certification of the POC is the physician's/non–physician practitioner's approval of the POC. Certification requires that a signature must be from the physician or non–physician practitioner in a timely manner, occurring within 30 days. A dated signature must be located on the POC or some other document that indicating approval for the POC. When initial certification expires, a recertification must then be completed certified within 30 days.

Step #6: Re-Evaluate as Appropriate

A re-evaluation is not a routine, recurring service but is focused on evaluation of progress toward current goals, making a professional judgment about continued care, modifying goals and/or treatment, or terminating services. Re-evaluations may be covered if necessary because of a change in the beneficiary's condition. They are usually focused on the current treatment and might not be as extensive as initial evaluations. Continuous assessment of the patient's progress is a component of ongoing therapy services and is not payable as a re-evaluation. Additionally, re-evaluations are covered only if the documentation supports the need for further tests and measurements after the initial evaluation.

Indications for a re-evaluation include new clinical findings, a significant change in the patient's condition, or failure to respond to the therapeutic interventions outlined in the POC. They may be appropriate prior to planned discharge for the purposes of determining whether goals have been met, or for the use of the physician or the treatment setting at which treatment will be continued.

Step #7: Recertify When Necessary

The maximum time range for which a certification can be written is 90 days; however, the speech-language pathologist should always write his or her initial certifications for the medically necessary time frame specific to the patient's needs. When initial certification expires, a written recertification must then be completed and certified within 30 days.

Goal Writing

Goals, as the foundation of a treatment plan, should paint a clear and distinct picture of anticipated outcomes of skilled speech-language pathology services. Goals serve as clinical roadmaps for the patient and the speech-language pathologist in addition to providing clear, functional, objectively measurable target areas that serve as a guide to payers for outcomes achieved during intervention. Finding a happy medium between creation of objective measures and remaining focused on function can be a difficult task.

The key components of goal creation require clinicians to take into account the following considerations:

- What is the patient's PLOF?
- What are the patient's and family's desired long-term outcomes, including preferred discharge setting?
- What specific evidence-based practice interventions are available to address the patient's specific functional impairments?
- Should I use percentiles or clinical trials as measurable aspects for my goals?
- Are cues clinically indicated either as a reducible clinical measure to promote functional independence or as a static measure when creating functional maintenance plans?

The Anatomy of Goal Building

There are two primary forms of goals included on treatment plans: Long-term goals and short-term goals. Long-term goals should reflect the highest level of desired function anticipated upon discharge. In most cases, these targets will be reflective of the patient's PLOF. Short-term goals are the stepping stones, targeting specific areas that are used to increase overall function in order to achieve long-term goals (Figure 12-4).

Consider an individual receiving skilled speech-language pathology care for receptive language abilities following new-onset of acute CVA.

- Target area: Auditory comprehension
  - "Patient will demonstrate auditory comprehension of..."
- Specific short-term objective level:
  - Biographical yes/no, environmental yes/no, simple yes/no, complex yes/no, common ADL objects, association objects/items, simple questions, simple instructions/commands, complex questions, simple conversation, complex conversation, various levels of functional communication, specific medications
- Measurable aspect:
  - Accuracy can be measured in percentile level (e.g., 80%, 100%) or therapeutic clinical trials (e.g., 8/10, 10/10).
- Functional outcome:
  - The functional outcome allows the clinician to tie-in an "in order to" statement for clarification of what the patient will be able to do as a functional outcome of skilled services. For example, for auditory comprehension we could say, "in order to improve receptive communication skills."

Goals should also include the reason that the speech-language pathologist is addressing that specific goal. Appendices 12-E and 12-F provide examples of goals for cognitive-communication and dysphagia.

Inclusion of Cues in Goals

The use of verbal, visual, and tactile cues are additional measurable components that can be included in the creation of goal targets. Additionally, for patients with cognitive impairment, a level of cues may be necessary to document success and ability to learn per Medicare criteria, and use of a cueing hat/hierarchy is considered to be a skilled service.

Clinicians should remain mindful, however, that although the use of cues is considered a skilled service, use of repetitive cues will limit our ability to show and justify skilled care. Consistent levels of cues, once established with subsequent caregiver training, can be utilized as a tool for the establishment of functional maintenance programs.

Functional maintenance programs are established to train nursing assistant staff on the use of cue cards, with competency verified via initial verbal understanding of the patient's needs from nursing assistants followed by return demonstration of tasks. Once competency is verified and the patient has reached his or her highest practicable level of function, skilled speech-language therapy services are discharged.

Progress Reports and Discharge Summaries

Following the completion of a comprehensive POC with timely certification from the supervising physician, continued documentation is required to support the skilled therapy need during the course of care. Few specific documentation guidelines are found in Chapter 8 of the Medicare Benefit Policy Manual, which contains guidelines for Part A. Per Chapter 15 of the Medicare Benefit Policy Manual (CMS, 2017b), which is for Part B, the minimum

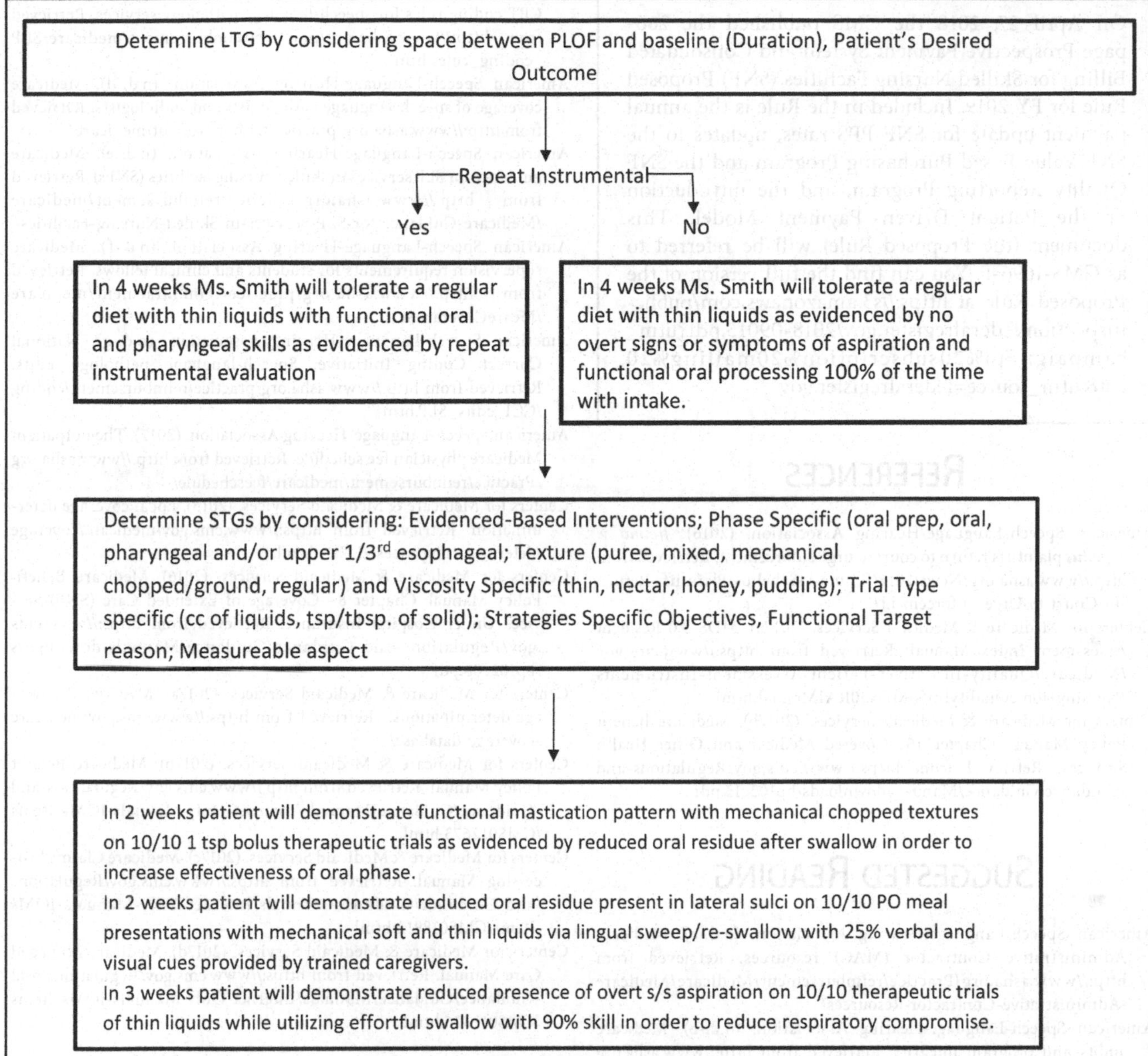

Figure 12-4. Dysphagia goal-building decision tree. (LTG = long-term goal; STG = short-term goal)

progress report period shall be at least once every 10 treatment days or once every 30 days, whichever comes first. The day beginning the first reporting period is the first day of the episode of treatment, regardless of whether the service provided on that day is an evaluation, re-evaluation, or treatment. Progress reports are required to show a clinician's active participation to provide justification for the medical necessity of treatment. Many facilities and agencies in long-term care have clinicians follow the more stringent Part B guidelines.

The discharge summary, also referred to as the *discharge note*, should be a progress report written by a clinician that covers the reporting period from the last progress report to the date of discharge. In the case of a discharge unanticipated in the plan or previous progress report, the clinician may base any judgments required to write the report on the treatment notes.

On April 27, 2018 the CMS published the 266-page Prospective Payment System and Consolidated Billing for Skilled Nursing Facilities (SNF) Proposed Rule for FY 2019. Included in the Rule is the annual payment update for SNF PPS rates, updates to the SNF Value-Based Purchasing Program and the SNF Quality Reporting Program, and the introduction of the Patient Driven Payment Model. This document (the Proposed Rule) will be referred to as CMS-1696-P. You can find the full version of the Proposed Rule at https://s3.amazonaws.com/public-inspection.federalregister.gov/2018-09015.pdf?utm_campaign=pi%20subscription%20mailing%20list&utm_source=federalregister.gov

References

American Speech-Language-Hearing Association. (2016). *Jimmo v. Sebelius* plaintiffs return to court to urge enforcement. Retrieved from http://www.asha.org/News/2016/Jimmo-v-Sebelius-Plaintiffs-Return-to-Court-to-Urge-Enforcement/

Centers for Medicare & Medicaid Services. (2017a). MDS 3.0 Resident Assessment Index Manual. Retrieved from https://www.cms.gov/Medicare/Quality-Initiatives-Patient-Assessment-Instruments/NursingHomeQualityInits/MDS30RAIManual.html

Centers for Medicare & Medicaid Services. (2017b). Medicare Benefit Policy Manual: Chapter 15—Covered Medical and Other Health Services. Retrieved from https://www.cms.gov/Regulations-and-Guidance/Guidance/Manuals/downloads/bp102c15.pdf

Suggested Reading

American Speech-Language-Hearing Association. (n.d.-a). Medicare Administrative Contractor (MAC) resources. Retrieved from http://www.asha.org/Practice/reimbursement/Medicare/Medicare-Administrative-Contractor-Resources/

American Speech-Language-Hearing Association. (n.d.-b). Medicare audits and program integrity. Retrieved from http://www.asha.org/Practice/reimbursement/medicare/Medicare-Audits-and-Program-Integrity/

American Speech-Language-Hearing Association. (n.d.-c). Medicare CPT coding rules for speech-language pathology services. Retrieved from http://www.asha.org/practice/reimbursement/medicare/SLP_coding_rules.htm

American Speech-Language-Hearing Association. (n.d.-d). Medicare coverage of speech-language pathologists and audiologists. Retrieved from http://www.asha.org/practice/reimbursement/medicare/

American Speech-Language-Hearing Association. (n.d.-e). Medicare guidance for SLP services in skilled nursing facilities (SNFs). Retrieved from http://www.asha.org/Practice/reimbursement/medicare/Medicare-Guidance-for-SLP-Services-in-Skilled-Nursing-Facilities/

American Speech-Language-Hearing Association. (n.d.-f). Medicare supervision requirements for students and clinical fellows. Retrieved from http://www.asha.org/practice/reimbursement/medicare/McareCoverageSLP

American Speech-Language-Hearing Association. (n.d.-g). National Correct Coding Initiative: Speech-language pathology edits. Retrieved from http://www.asha.org/practice/reimbursement/coding/CCI_edits_SLP.htm

American Speech-Language-Hearing Association. (2017). The outpatient Medicare physician fee schedule. Retrieved from http://www.asha.org/Practice/reimbursement/medicare/feeschedule/

Centers for Medicare & Medicaid Services. (2015). Local coverage determination. Retrieved from https://www.cms.gov/medicare/coverage/determinationprocess/LCDs.html

Centers for Medicare & Medicaid Services. (2016). Medicare Benefit Policy Manual: Chapter 8—Coverage of Extended Care (SNF) Services Under Hospital Insurance. Retrieved from https://www.cms.gov/Regulations-and-Guidance/Guidance/Manuals/downloads/bp102c08.pdf

Centers for Medicare & Medicaid Services. (2017a). MAC local coverage determinations. Retrieved from https://www.cms.gov/medicare-coverage-database/

Centers for Medicare & Medicaid Services. (2017b). Medicare Benefit Policy Manual. Retrieved from http://www.cms.gov/Regulations-and-Guidance/Guidance/Manuals/Internet-Only-Manuals-IOMs-Items/CMS012673.html

Centers for Medicare & Medicaid Services. (2017c). Medicare Claims Processing Manual. Retrieved from https://www.cms.gov/Regulations-and-Guidance/Guidance/Manuals/Internet-Only-Manuals-IOMs-Items/CMS018912.html

Centers for Medicare & Medicaid Services. (2017d). Medicare Managed Care Manual. Retrieved from https://www.cms.gov/Regulations-and-Guidance/Guidance/Manuals/Internet-Only-Manuals-IOMs-Items/CMS019326.html

Review Questions

1. If you wanted to find more information in the Medicare Benefit Policy Manual about acceptable practices for therapy, what sections would be helpful?
2. What are some considerations you should consider when demonstrating that the services are reasonable and necessary?
3. How does Medicare define an evaluation in the SNF setting?
4. Discuss the difference between a screening and an evaluation, both in terms of what is done and how each is reimbursed.
5. What are some good reasons for using cues in goal writing?

Activity A

Case Study

Mr. Jones was admitted for a 3-day acute care stay secondary to progressive decline associated with Parkinson's disease. He was admitted to your long-term care facility for skilled rehabilitation services.

His prior functional status includes the following: he lived in an assisted living facility; he was able to voice wants, needs, and ideas with others in a structured setting free of environmental noise; and he consumed a regular diet with thin liquids without signs of oral or pharyngeal phase dysphagia.

His baseline status includes moderate dysarthria with functional communication at the word level; moderate oral-phase dysphagia with anterior loss of textured materials; and instrumental assessment of swallow revealing moderate-severe pharyngeal dysphagia with frank aspiration of thin liquids via uncontrolled cup during swallow, but no aspiration with small controlled cup sips.

Complete the following POC requirements for Mr. Jones.

1. Justification for Skilled Services Statement (tip: compare baseline to PLOF; include evidence-based practice considerations and impact of current medical history)

   ____

   ____

   ____

   ____

2. Write two long-term goals and three to five short-term goals that are SMART for Mr. Jones.

   Long-term goals:

   a.

   b.

   c.

   d.

   e.

   Short-term goals:

   a.

   b.

   c.

   d.

   e.

Activity B

True or False: Skilled Nursing Medicare Part A Prospective Payment System

Please answer True or False of each statement and also state why you answered that way.

1. ______ Skilled therapy services are any services that are delivered by a therapist.
   Why?____
2. ______ Skilled speech-language pathologist services can be provided by sleep-language-pathology assistants to Medicare beneficiaries.
   Why?____
3. ______ Frequency and duration of care under a Medicare Part A PPS benefit should be provided for 100 days.
   Why?____
4. ______ Diagnostic and assessment testing services to ascertain type and causal factor(s) should be identified during the evaluation.
   Why?____
5. ______ Rehabilitative/restorative therapy includes services designed to address recovery or improvement in function and, when possible, restoration to a previous level of health and well-being.
   Why?____

Activity C

Using Skilled Language to Describe Your Services

Select five skilled words from the bank, and use them to describe your services for the case scenarios below.

Skilled Words Bank

- Activity advanced
- Activity graded
- Altered modified
- Analyzed
- Assessed
- Caregiver education with verbal understanding and return demonstration
- Educated
- Facilitated
- Provided developed
- Provided retraining
- Trained

1. Mr. Smith presented with mild cognitive impairment, and you are providing caregiver training for use of calendar assistance for recall and tracking of daily events.
2. Ms. Adams presents with a moderate oral-phase dysphagia, and you are providing resistance-based lingual exercises.
3. Mr. Pitman was referred for a maintenance-based plan for visual signage, and you are educating him on the use of visual signage to facilitate ability to follow three-step directives during completion of dressing tasks.
4. Mrs. Apple presents with a moderate hypokinetic dysarthria following a new-onset CVA, and you are targeting strategies to increase clarity at the word level.

Appendix 12-A

Sections of the Minimum Data Set

Section B: Hearing, Speech, and Vision

B0100: Comatose
B0200: Hearing
B0300: Hearing aide
B0600: Speech clarity
B0700: Makes self understood
B0800: Ability to understand others
B1000: Vision
B1200: Corrective lenses

Section C: Cognitive Patterns (Often Completed by Social Services)

C0100: Should brief interview for mental status be conducted?
C0200-C0500: Brief interview for mental status (BIMS)
C0200: Repetition of three words
C0300: Temporal orientation (year, month, day)
C0400: Recall
C0500: Summary score
C0600: Should the staff assessment of mental status (C0700-C1000) be conducted?
C0700-C1000: Staff assessment of mental status item
C0700: Short-term memory
C0800: Long-term memory
C0900: Memory/recall ability
C1000: Cognitive skills for daily decision making
C1300: Signs and symptoms of delirium
C1600: Acute onset of mental status change

Section D: Mood

D0100: Should resident mood interview be conducted?
D0200: Resident mood interview (PHQ-9)
D0300: Total Severity score
D0350: Follow-up to D0200I
D0500: Staff assessment of resident mood (PHQ-9-OV)
D0600: Total severity score
D0650: Follow-up to D0500I

Section E: Behavior

E0100: Potential indicators of psychosis
E0200: Behavioral symptom—presence and frequency
E0300: Overall presence of behavioral symptoms
E0500: Impact on resident
E0600: Impact on others
E0800: Rejection of care—presence and frequency
E0900: Wandering—presence and frequency
E1000: Wandering—impact
E1100: Change in behavioral or other symptoms

Section F: Preferences for Customary Routine and Activities

F0300: Should interview for daily and activity preferences be conducted?
F0400: Interview for daily preferences
F0500: Interview for activity preferences
F0600: Daily and activity preferences primary respondent
F0700: Should the staff assessment of daily activity preferences be conducted?
F0800: Staff assessment of daily activity preferences

Section G: Functional Status

G0110: Activities of daily living assistance
G0120: Bathing
G0300: Balance during transitions and walking
G0400: Functional limitation in range of motion
G0600: Mobility devices
G0900: Functional rehabilitation potential

Section H: Bladder and Bowel

H0100: Appliances
H0200: Urinary toileting program
H0300: Urinary continence
H0400: Bowel continence
H0500: Bowel and toileting program
H0600: Bowel patterns

Section I: Active Diagnoses

Active Diagnoses in the last 7 days

Section J: Health Conditions

J0100: Pain management (5-day look back)
J0200: Should pain assessment interview be conducted?
J0300-J0600: Pain assessment interview
J0300: Pain presence (5-day look back)

J0400: Pain frequency (5-day look back)
J0500: Pain effect on function (5-day look back)
J0600: Pain intensity (5-day look back)
J0700: Should the staff assessment of pain be conducted? (5-day look back)
J0800: Indicators of pain (5-day look back)
J0850: Frequency of indicator of pain or possible pain (5-day look back)
J1100: Shortness of breath (dyspnea)
J1300: Current tobacco use
J1400: Prognosis
J1550: Problem conditions
J1700: Fall History on admission/entry or reentry
J1800: Any falls since admission/entry or reentry or prior assessment (Omnibus Budget Reconciliation Act [OBRA] or scheduled PPS)
J1900: Number of falls since admission/entry or reentry or prior assessment (OBRA or scheduled PPS)

Section K: Swallowing/Nutritional Status

K0100: Swallowing disorder
K0200: Height and weight
K0300: Weight loss
K0310: Weight gain
K0510: Nutritional approaches
K0700: % intake by artificial route

Section L: Oral/Dental Status

L0200: Dental

Section M: Skin Conditions

M0100: Determination of pressure ulcer risks
M0150: Risks of pressure ulcers
M0210: Unhealed pressure ulcers
M0300: Current number of unhealed pressure ulcer at each stage
M0300A: Number of stage 1 pressure ulcers
M0300B: Stage 2 pressure ulcers
M0300C: Stage 3 pressure ulcers
M0300D: Stage 4 pressure ulcers
M0300E: Unstageable pressure ulcers related to non-removable dressing/device
M0300F: Unstageable pressure ulcers related to slough and/or eschar
M0300G: Unstageable pressure ulcers related to suspect deep tissue injury
M0610: Dimensions of unhealed stage 3 or 4 pressure ulcers or unstageable pressure ulcer due to slough or eschar

Section N: Medication

N0300: Injections
N0350: Insulin
N0410: Medications received

Section O: Special Treatment, Procedures, and Programs

O0100: Special treatments, procedures, and programs
O0250: Influenza vaccine
O0300: Pneumococcal vaccine
O0400: Therapies
O0450: Resumption of therapy
O0500: Restorative nursing programs
O0600: Physical examinations
O0700: Physician orders

Section P: Restraints

P0100: Physical restraints

Section Q: Participation in Assessment and Goal Setting

Q0100: Participation in assessment
Q0300: Resident's overall expectation
Q0400: Discharge Plan
Q0490: Resident's preference to avoid being asked question Q0500B
Q0500: Return to community
Q0550: Resident's preference to avoid being asked question Q0500B again
Q0600: Referral

Section V: Care Area Assessment Summary

V0100: Items from the most recent prior OBRA or PPS assessment
V0200: CAAs and care planning

Appendix 12-B

Speech-Language Pathology Screen Administration Instructions

Screening Area	Screening Triggers Identifying Need for Assessment	Resources/Tools
Dysphagia		
Oral-phase dysphagia	• Oral holding of food or liquid • Anterior loss of food or liquid • Pocketing or stasis present in cavity after oral swallow • Labored repetitive chewing at meals • Weight loss • Aversions with intake, spitting during meals • Oral hygiene, presence of, complaints related to dry mouth • Functional dentition; adequate fit of dentures/partials	• Patient, family, and nursing interview • Patient observation • MDS Section K: Swallowing/nutritional status • Registered dietician notes • Nursing notes: Weekly and monthly weights • Daily PO intake logs
Pharyngeal-phase dysphagia	• Delayed initiation of swallow; may present as oral holding of food/medications	• Patient, family, and nursing interview • Patient observation • MDS Section K: Swallowing/nutritional status • Registered dietician notes • Nursing notes: Weekly and monthly weights • Daily PO intake logs
Esophageal-phase dysphagia upper one-third	• Fullness in throat during meals (i.e., globus sensation) • Regurgitation during meals • Heartburn/discomfort during or after meals • Weight loss • Difficulty swallowing pills (crushed meds required?)	• Patient, family, and nursing interview • Certified nursing assistant interview regarding med administration • Patient observation • MDS Section K: Swallowing/nutritional status • Registered dietician notes • Nursing notes: Weekly and monthly weights • Daily PO intake logs

Screening Area	Screening Triggers Identifying Need for Assessment	Resources/Tools
Language		
Expressive language	• Ability to name objects in environment • Ability to complete automatic tasks (e.g., greetings, counting, naming days of week and months of year) • Ability to effectively communicate wants, needs, and ideas with caregivers/family members	• Patient, family, and nursing interview • Patient observation • MDS Section B0700: Makes self understood
	• Use of communication boards/augmentative and alternative communication (AAC) speech-generating and non–speech-generating devices	
Receptive language	• Ability to understand yes/no, multiple choice, and open-ended questions • Discrimination of body parts, objects, and pictures. Is patient able to identify during ADL tasks? • Ability to follow commands	• Patient, family, and nursing interview • Patient observation • Consultation with physical/occupational therapy: Can patient follow commands during tasks? • MDS Section B0800: Ability to understand others
Cognition		
Attention	• Can patient attend to task during ADL routines? • Is patient noted to be easily distracted in environments with increased background noise? Does patient become agitated?	• Patient, family, and nursing interview • Patient observation • MDS Section E0900: Wandering—presence and frequency • MDS Section E1000: Wandering—impact
Memory	• Orientation to place, time, purpose, caregivers • Ability to formulate sentences with adequate semantic memory (i.e., word-finding skills). Does patient "block" during interactions? Have complaints regarding "losing my words"? • Can patient recall facts from personal history (i.e., declarative memory) such as significant dates and family history? • Does patient require use of visual cues, calendar assist, and written log to recall daily events and routines including meals, activities, and visitors?	• Patient, family, and nursing interview • Consultation with physical/occupational therapy: Can patient recall steps for ADL, transfers, appropriate use of assistive device? • Patient observation • MDS Section C: Cognitive patterns

Screening Area	Screening Triggers Identifying Need for Assessment	Resources/Tools
Executive function	• Ability to complete functional sequencing, problem-solving tasks, judgment, and reasoning during familiar and new situations • Does patient appropriately use environmental tools such as call bell and adaptive equipment and appropriate process for completing of transfers and ADL tasks?	• Patient, family, and nursing interview • Consultation with physical/occupational therapy regarding safety and judgment during ADL, ambulatory, transfer tasks • Patient observation
Motor Speech		
Apraxia	• Does patient appear to have groping/effortful behaviors when attempting to communicate?	• Patient, family, and nursing interview • Patient observation • MDS Section B0600: Speech clarity
Dysarthria	• Does patient appear to fatigue during communication? • Does patient present with reduced O_2 saturations during communication with others?	• Patient, family, and nursing interview • Patient observation • MDS Section B0600: Speech clarity
Voice		
	• Does patient present with adequate intensity to express needs? • Social isolation: Have we noted withdrawal due to reduced ability to communicate with others?	• Patient, family, and nursing interview • Patient observation • Activities participation notes

Appendix 12-C
Speech-Language Pathology Screening Form

Patient name: ______________________________ Room: ______________

Referred by: ______________________________

Current symptoms/problems:

_______ Coughing or choking with PO intake
_______ Shortness of breath at meals
_______ Complaints of pain when swallowing
_______ Decreased ability to follow directions during ADL
_______ Decreased ability to communicate wants, needs, and ideas
_______ Reduced loudness of voice
_______ Reduced speech clarity or slurring of words

Current changes/improvements:

_______ Increased desire for PO intake or diet advance
_______ Increased motivation to participate in rehab
_______ Increased alertness, ability to attend to tasks

Supportive documentation: ______________________________

____

____

____

Therapist signature: ______________________________

_______ Evaluation to be completed _______ Evaluation not currently indicated

APPENDIX 12-D
Maintenance-Based Case Examples

The following case examples demonstrate how documentation is used in maintenance-based cases.

Motor Speech/Voice

Skilled speech-language pathology services may be deemed reasonable and necessary in order to maintain vocal clarity and intensity for an individual with Parkinson's disease to continue training via use of Lee Silverman Voice Therapy techniques for maintenance. Note: Transition from therapy services aimed at increasing function to maintenance therapy should occur following therapist/resident determination that maximum benefit has been achieved at a particular communication level (i.e., word, phase, sentence, structured conversation, spontaneous conversation), with maintenance interventions being aimed at continued communication success (pending modifications that may be warranted secondary to typical declines with disease progression) at this level at a decreased intensity from prior services.

Why Can These Services Not Be Transitioned to a Non–Skilled Professional Such as a Certified Nursing Assistant or Nurse for Restorative/Maintenance?

Example of how this might be documented: Due to the progressive nature of vocal and motor speech system changes, the skilled eye of a speech-language pathologist is needed to develop and continue vocal function protocol and conduct differential diagnosis when changes occur across various systems of communication with disease progression.

Auditory Comprehension/Cognition

Skilled speech-language pathology services may be deemed reasonable and necessary in order to maintain auditory comprehension skills in the case of an individual status post–new neurological insult following a period of intensive skilled speech-language pathology interventions aimed at increasing abilities to comprehend language and perform cognitive tasks (e.g., sequencing, problem solving) at the highest level possible continued services for maintenance may be warranted to continue skilled therapeutic tasks for high-level tasks in order to prevent functional declines in preparation for discharge to prior living environment while continued services are being provided by physical/occupational therapy. Interventions provided as maintenance vs rehabilitation in nature are to be provided at a decreased intensity from initial services.

Why Can These Services Not Be Transitioned to a Non–Skilled Professional?

Example of how this might be documented: Skilled interventions for high-level auditory comprehension tasks, including the ability to follow multistep ADL/instrumental ADL (IADL) commands, comprehend conversational interactions, sequence during tasks, and complete functional problem solving with others, requires administration of tasks that cannot be performed or conducted by a non–skilled professional. In addition, these tasks will require periodic modification secondary to anticipated increased success with physical/occupational therapy sessions, which will change task segmentation and progression of ADL and IADL. Remember: Cases such as those described may also move from rehabilitative in nature to maintenance and return to rehabilitative in nature secondary to increased physical abilities necessitating the need for higher-level cognitive and language learning.

Dysphagia

Skilled therapy services may be deemed reasonable and necessary in order to maintain adequate swallow functions for pleasure feeding regiment, which is clearly defined and agreed upon by members of the interdisciplinary team in conjunction with the resident and family members.

Why Can These Services Not Be Transitioned to a Non–Skilled Professional?

Per the Medicare Benefit Policy Manual, swallowing assessment and rehabilitation are highly specialized services. The professional rendering care must have education, experience, and demonstrated competencies. Competencies include, but are not limited to, identifying abnormal upper aerodigestive tract structure and function; conducting an oral, pharyngeal, laryngeal, and respiratory function examination as it relates to the functional assessment of swallowing; recommending methods of oral intake and risk precautions; and developing a treatment plan employing appropriate compensations and therapy techniques.

These competencies cannot be performed by a non–skilled professional in an individual presenting with dysphagia severity that would warrant pleasure feedings.

Note: The need for pleasure feedings must be necessitated by a dysphagia secondary to oral, pharyngeal, and/or upper one-third of the esophageal phase. Services for maintenance in end-stage dementia secondary to the presence of tongue thrust as root cause or esophageal impairments/strictures/blockages in the lower two-thirds of the esophagus would not warrant services because they are not covered for the Medicare beneficiary.

APPENDIX 12-E
Goal Bank

Receptive Language

TARGET AREA	GOAL
Receptive language: Understanding across complexity of tasks	Patient will demonstrate auditory comprehension of (choose: biographical yes/no, environmental yes/no, simple yes/no, complex yes/no, common ADL objects, association objects/items, simple questions, simple instructions/commands, complex questions, simple conversation, complex conversation, various levels of functional communication, specific medications) with 100% accuracy and no cues in order to improve receptive communication skills.
Follows commands	
One- or two-step commands	Patient will follow one-step commands with 100% accuracy in order to enhance patient's ability to follow directions for activities and ADL.
Multistep directions	Patient will follow multistep verbal commands with 100% accuracy and 25% verbal cues in order to enhance patient's ability to increase ability to participate in ADL.
Discriminate objects or pictures	Patient will discriminate objects (choose Field Choice 1-8) FC times 6 with 100% accuracy in order to improve receptive communication skills.
Understands yes/no or open-ended questions or sentences	Patient will understand yes/no questions with 100% accuracy in order to communicate basic wants/needs.
Conversation	Patient will comprehend conversations with 100% accuracy (choose: non-structured contexts with non-familiar listeners, structured contexts with non-familiar listeners, structured contexts with familiar listeners, or non-structured contexts with familiar listeners) during structured contexts with non-familiar listeners in order to participate in meaningful interactions.

Verbal Expression

TARGET AREA	GOAL
Automatic speech	
Component tasks	Patient will produce automatic speech (e.g., greetings, chains) with 100% of attempts to increase ability to communicate basic wants/needs.
Repetition	Patient will repeat (choose: vowels, syllables, automatics, CVC (consonant-vowel-consonant) stimuli, core functional, or fill in the blank) CVC stimuli with 100% to improve patient's ability to improve expressive communication. Note: Use this target only when treating patients in whom evidence-based practice warrants interventions where repeating yields greater success/outcomes, because Medicare may otherwise view this as a non-skilled task; also build in a level of cues that will classify as cueing, which is a skilled service, as needed to increase success. Here we have options for verbal, visual, or semantic cues.
Naming objects or pictures	Patient will name objects with 100% accuracy to increase ability to communicate basic wants/needs.
Picture description	Patient will complete picture-description tasks with 100% accuracy to increase ability to improve expressive communication.

Target Area	Goal
Singing	Patient will increase verbal language/expression during singing tasks with 100% accuracy to increase ability to improve expressive communication. Think here: Patient noted to increase function with melodic intonation.
Making needs known	Patient will increase ability to make needs known with 100% of attempts to increase ability to participate in meaningful interactions.

Motor Speech

Target Area	Goal
Intelligibility Compensatory strategies	Patient will articulate (choose: complex conversation, simple conversational tasks, paragraphs, complex/long sentences, simple/short sentences, phrases, polysyllabic words/phrases, multisyllabic words/phrases, 10 functional words, words, automatics/chains, sounds/phonemes) with 100% intelligibility using (choose: decreased rate, increased volume, overarticulation, pacing, phrase monitoring, breath support and control, intonation patterns, intonation variances, phrase control with visual markers, environmental modifications, relaxation techniques, or easy-onset techniques) using increase volume and overarticulation in order to participate in meaningful interactions.
Verbal agility	Patient will accurately perform verbal agility/diadokokinesis tasks 100% in order to increase speech intelligibility to 100% at (choose communication level) paragraphs level.
Sustained phonation	Patient will increase ability to sustain phonation for (choose time) 10 secs in order to (choose: increase coordination between respiration and phonation, improve vocal quality during speech production, facilitate laryngeal/pharyngeal functioning, facilitate self-monitoring of vocal quality and pitch during speech production, or fill in the blank).
Coordination of respiration/phonation	Patient will increase use of breath support and control strategies to 100% accuracy during production of (choose level) simple/short sentences to increase (choose: speech intelligibility, voice quality, vocal intensity)

Voice

Target Area	Goal
Endurance	Patient will increase ability to sustain phonation for (insert 1-15 secs) in order to (choose: increase coordination between respiration and phonation, improve vocal quality during speech production, facilitate laryngeal/pharyngeal functioning, or facilitate self-monitoring of vocal quality and pitch during speech production). Patient will demonstrate adequate vocal endurance for (choose: 1-3 mins, 3-5 mins, or 5-10 mins) with (insert percentile) of opportunities during (choose: word, phrase, sentence, structured conversation, spontaneous conversation) in order to (choose: increased vocal intensity, decrease vocal hoarseness, decrease vocal harshness, reduce vocal abusive behaviors, increase vocal hygiene, increase functional communication skills, decrease embarrassment during interactions, and increase confidence during interactions).

TARGET AREA	GOAL
Intensity	At (build for 1-3 feet, 4-7 feet, or 8-10 feet) from conversational partner, patient will demonstrate vocal intensity of (choose: 5-10 decibels (dB), 11-20 dB, 21-40 dB, or 41-60 dB) (insert percentile) of opportunities during (choose: word, phrase, sentence, structured conversation, spontaneous conversation) in order to (choose: increase vocal intensity, decrease vocal hoarseness, decrease vocal harshness, reduce vocal abusive behaviors, increase vocal hygiene, increase functional communication skills, decrease embarrassment during interactions, and increase confidence during interactions).
Quality	Patient will decrease presence of (choose: aphonia or breathy voice) on (insert percentile) of opportunities during (choose: word, phrase, sentence, structured conversation, spontaneous conversation) in order to (choose: increase vocal intensity, decrease vocal hoarseness, decrease vocal harshness, reduce vocal abusive behaviors, increase vocal hygiene, increase functional communication skills, decrease embarrassment during interactions, and increase confidence during interactions).

Pragmatics

TARGET AREA	GOAL
Initiate/maintain eye contact	Patient will initiate/maintain eye contact during contact during structured (or non-structured) tasks on 100% of therapeutic opportunities in order to participate in meaningful interactions.
Inhibition	Patient will demonstrate functional inhibition during structured (or non-structured) tasks with 100% in order to allow for increased socialization.
Regulating social exchanges	Patient will appropriately regulate social exchanges during structured (or non-structured) tasks 100% of therapeutic opportunities.
Requesting information	Patient will request information during structured (or non-structured) tasks 100% of therapeutic opportunities.
Self-correction	Patient will independently self-correct during structured (or non-structured) tasks 100% of opportunities in order to increase functional communication skills.
Self-monitoring	Patient will independently self-correct during structured (or non-structured) tasks 100% of opportunities in order to increase functional communication skills.
Topic maintenance	Patient will exhibit functional topic maintenance during structured (or non-structured) tasks 100% of opportunities in order to participate in meaningful interactions.
Turn taking	Patient will demonstrate functional turn taking during structured (or non-structured) tasks 100% of therapeutic opportunities.

Executive Function

TARGET AREA	GOAL
Budgeting	Patient will safely perform financial management/budgeting tasks with independence and the task broken down in two steps for compensatory tech due to cognitive-communicative impairments.
Medication management	Patient will safely and efficiently manage medications with independence and the task broken down into 0 steps in order to facilitate community reintegration.
Alertness	Patient will respond to various forms of sensory stimulation 10/10 opportunities to increase alertness for functional task performance.
Insight	Patient will demonstrate increased insight into deficits with 100% of opportunities (choose quality of life reason which for insight includes language reasons).

Target Area	Goal
Problem solving	Remember with problem-solving tasks in order to increase specificity of measures, initiate targets at most basic level of function (e.g., simple problem solving) and then advance targets as appropriate to higher levels of functioning (e.g., problem solving multiple solutions and complex problem solving). Patient will demonstrate adequate categorization and association skills 100% of opportunities in order to facilitate decision-making skills/care/needs. Patient will exhibit safe reasoning skills during new situations. OR Patient will demonstrate functional problem solving during new situations with 100% in order to (see choices above). Additional areas: abstract reasoning, categorization/association, cause/effect, complex verbal problem solving, deductive reasoning, general problem solving, judgment/inferencing, multiple solutions, safety awareness, and simple verbal problem solving.
Memory: Short-term with parameters Declarative: Episodic memory Non-Declarative: Procedural memory	Patient will recall (choose: daily events, using visual aids as needed, new information up to three elements, new information up to five elements, new information after 30-minute delay of presentation, concrete/abstract story/news information) with 100% in order to promote independence. Patient will demonstrate increased long-term memory during daily life tasks 100% of opportunities (choose: given environmental modifications implemented by trained caregivers, using visual aids as assisted by trained caregivers, using visual and auditory aids, or fill in the blank) in order to facilitate ability to live in environment with least amount of supervision/assistance. Patient will demonstrate increased procedural memory during daily life tasks 100% of opportunities (choose: given environmental modifications implemented by trained caregivers, using visual aids as assisted by trained caregivers, using visual and auditory aids, or fill in the blank) in order to facilitate ability to live in environment with least amount of supervision/assistance.
Selective attention Attention: Decrease agitation Attention subtasks	Patient will exhibit decreased anxiety/agitation via increased selective attention to (choose: conversation, functional tasks, procedural tasks, or fill in the blank) (choose time) (choose: using environmental modifications established by caregivers, given occasional cues, using augmentative communication book/device, or fill in the blank). Patient will selectively attend to tasks for (choose time) for 1-3 mins in order to enhance patient's ability to follow directions for activities and ADL.

Augmentative and Alternative Communication

Target Area	Goal
Communication topics	Patient will communicate (choose: yes/no responses, basic wants and needs, needs/wants/desires, simple thoughts/ideas, basic information, basic/detailed information, medical needs, complex thoughts/ideas, complex safety and social needs, detailed/complex information, abstract concepts, social responses/interactions, conversational responses/exchanges, or complex/detailed information) then (choose: using speech-generating AAC system or using non–speech-generating AAC system) (choose level of assist).

Tracheostomy/Ventilator-Dependent Populations

TARGET AREA	GOAL
Electrolarynx	Patient will demonstrate proper activation/deactivation with (insert percentile) for use of electrolarynx in (choose: word, phrase, simple sentence, structured conversation, unstructured conversation). Patient will demonstrate proper placement of electrolarynx with (insert percentile) accuracy during (choose: word, phrase, simple sentence, structured conversation, unstructured conversation). Patient will use electrolaryngeal speech with (insert percentile) accuracy in (choose: word, phrase, simple sentence, structured conversation, unstructured conversation) without audible stoma noise. Patient will demonstrate proper placement of electrolarynx on (insert percentile) of trials for increased overall speech intelligibility skills.
Leak Speech	Patient will demonstrate the ability to restrict airflow through the glottis on inspiration (maintaining peak inspiratory pressure of > 25 cm H_2O) with (insert percentile) accuracy given (insert percentile) visual cue from ventilator and (insert percentile) verbal cue from clinician. Patient will demonstrate adduction technique during (choose communication level such as one-way word responses) to (choose communication level such as yes/no or open-ended questions) with 80% accuracy.
Cuff Deflation Targets	Patient will demonstrate the ability to deflate cuff and apply speaking valve prior to oral intake to improve airway protection skills during the swallow with 80% accuracy. (Note: This should be used only if treating an underlying cognitive impairment that affects ability to deflate cuff and apply valve.) Patient will demonstrate (insert percentile) ability to independently deflate and inflate tracheostomy tube cuff for increased airway protection. (Note: This should be used only if treating an underlying cognitive impairment that affects ability to deflate and inflate.) Patient will demonstrate (insert percentile) ability to speak on exhalation in a (choose: word, phrase, sentence) task given (insert percentile) visual cues. Patient will independently demonstrate proper (insert number) steps with (insert percentile) toward cuff deflation in order to increase verbal communication abilities. (Note: This should be used only if treating an underlying cognitive impairment that affects ability to deflate cuff.) Patient will tolerate cuff deflation with (insert percentile) accuracy (choose requirements such as > 90 oxygen saturation and/or respiratory rate of) for (insert time in seconds/minutes). Patient will tolerate a minimal cuff technique for (insert time) with (insert percentile) as determined by cervical auscultation to determine upper airway patency.
Speaking Valve	Patient will achieve voicing with Passy Muir speaking valve at (choose: syllable, word, phrase, sentence) with (insert percentile) accuracy. Patient will tolerate one-way speaking valve with (insert percentile) accuracy and (choose requirements such as > 90 oxygen saturation and/or respiratory rate of) for (insert time limit). Patient will tolerate a Passy Muir valve with (insert percentile) and (choose requirements such as > 90 oxygen saturation and/or respiratory rate of while on the ventilator) for (insert time). Patient will phonate (choose: vegetative sounds, vowels, one-syllable words, sentences) with (insert percentile) while wearing Passy Muir valve.

Appendix 12-F
Dysphagia Goal Bank

Long-Term Goal

Patient will increase ability to safely and efficiently swallow oral intake to independence as evidenced by minimal to absent oral residue, oral spillage, coughing, and/or wet vocal quality post-swallows on 100% of opportunities in order to safely consume highest level of oral intake.

Short-Term Goals

Oral Phase

1. **Patient will exhibit minimal pocketing/stasis as evidenced by clear oral cavity 100% of attempts while consuming __________ consistencies and __________ liquids.**
2. **Patient will increase oral motor control of swallow musculature to __________ to increase ability to safely swallow __________ textures and __________ liquids as evidenced by no signs/symptoms of dysphagia.**
3. **Patient will decrease oral transit time to __________ following stimulation in order to enhance patient's ability to efficiently consume __________ textures and __________ liquids.**

Pharyngeal Phase

1. **Patient will demonstrate clear vocal quality post-swallows 100% of the time while consuming __________ textures and __________ liquids to enable patient to protect airway.**
2. **Patient will decrease throat clearing, coughing, and choking to 0% of intake attempts of __________ textures and __________ liquids.**

Swallow Strategies

1. **Patient will utilize tongue sweep, reswallow when consuming __________ textures and __________ liquids with no cues in order to effectively clear pocketing/stasis from oral cavity 10/10 therapeutic attempts.**
2. **Patient will safely swallow successive amounts of __________ consistencies and __________ liquids using finger or utensil sweep, alternation of liquids/solids with 0% cues without signs/symptoms of aspiration.**
3. **Patient will increase ability to produce hard throat clear/reswallow 100% of the time when consuming __________ textures and __________ liquids to improve airway protection abilities.**

Appendix 12-G
Sample Daily Notes

Ms. Smith was referred to speech therapy services on January 3 after nursing assistants noted reduced ability to complete dressing sequences with morning routines. Her primary medical diagnosis is dementia of Alzheimer's type, and she was admitted to the long-term care environment from an assisted living setting 2 weeks prior. Speech-language pathologist determines that Ms. Smith presents with increased abilities to complete three-step directives when she is provided with visual cue cards for completion of tasks. Receptive language skills appear moderately impaired at the sentence level limiting her ability to understand communication exchanges with caregivers.

Ms. Smith will demonstrate ability to complete three-step commands with 100% skill while utilizing visual cue cards in order to promote success with ADL and promote functional independence.

Ms. Smith will demonstrate ability to respond to open-ended questions on 9/10 therapeutic clinical trials from trained caregivers utilizing use of slow and simple speech in order to improve receptive language abilities and participate in meaningful interactions.

January 3 daily note:

Ms. Smith was seen in room for skilled speech therapy. Evidenced decreased ability to follow multistep commands present during functional ADL and during completion of standardized assessment. Skilled analysis of the environment revealed increased success for completion of dressing when patient is provided with step-by-step instructions and use of simple language from caregiver as evidenced by increased ability to follow a two-step command from 0% initially to 50% with implementation of slow, simple speech.

January 5 daily note:

Ms. Smith was seen in therapy gym for skilled speech therapy. Daughter was present and engaged alongside speech-language pathologist for completion of cognitive stimulation therapy aimed at morning ADL. Speech-language pathologist was able to analyze variances in Ms. Smith's morning routines in home environment in comparison to current long-term care environment in order to determine most effective sequencing of morning tasks. Verbal rehearsal strategy was reviewed for dressing, toileting, and oral hygiene, with evidenced increased success when tasks were broken down into two steps max.

January 7 daily note:

Ms. Smith was seen in room with speech-language pathologist in conjunction with nursing assistant for completion of oral hygiene regiment following AM meal. Speech-language pathologist analyzed initial breakdowns in sequencing of tasks and noted Ms. Smith was able to demonstrate increased success when provided with verbal rehearsal strategy prior to completion of each ADL. Certified nursing assistant was noted to demonstrate verbal understanding of verbal rehearsal prior to dressing task with increased success from 50% initially during three-step verbal sequence for dressing to 75% accuracy following verbal rehearsal with Ms. Smith.

January 9 daily note:

Ms. Smith was seen in group setting during activities this date with three other residents in order to promote functional abilities during conversational exchanges and increase ability to respond to questions. Speech-language pathologist educated activities staff on best practices for engaging Ms. Smith in group settings and promoting receptive language abilities when asking her open-ended questions. Increased success was noted from 20% initially to 50% when staff allowed increased response time for question reply when facilitating and activity discussion related to gardening tasks.

Following the January 9 session, it was determined that the patient had met maximum potential and was discharged from therapy.

13

Home Health

Rebecca Skrine, MS, CCC-SLP, CHCE, COS-C

Medicare Conditions of Participation

The Home Health Conditions of Participation (HHCoPs) are published by the Centers for Medicare & Medicaid Services (CMS) and outline the requirements that home care agencies must meet to participate as Medicare and Medicaid home care service providers. CMS periodically sends surveyors to each enrolled agency to ensure compliance with each of the conditions of participation. If the surveyor finds that an agency fails to meet any of the HHCoPs, they may be subject to sanctions, including the possibility of termination from the Medicare and Medicaid programs (CMS, 2012).

It All Starts With the Assessments

CMS provides specific guidance on the required assessments in the Medicare HHCoPs.

There are three primary types of assessments: The initial assessment, the comprehensive assessment, and the Outcome and Assessment Information Set (OASIS) assessment. The discipline-specific assessment is considered part of the comprehensive assessment (Table 13-1).

Understanding the order and use of the assessments can be very confusing. Although the HHCoPs describe each type of assessment independently, more than one assessment is often completed in a single visit to the home. The initial assessment is required to be completed on the first visit to establish eligibility for the Medicare home health benefit. If the patient meets the criteria for home care, the comprehensive assessment and the OASIS assessment must be completed. These assessments may be completed at the same time as the initial assessment or no later than 5 days after the start of care. The HHCoPs specify that the comprehensive assessment incorporate use of the most current version of the OASIS without any alterations. If the patient does not qualify for home care services, no further assessments are required (CMS, 2014).

Speech-language pathologists are qualified to complete all of the types of assessments, but many agencies have admission nurses or teams who perform all of the initial and comprehensive assessments. In other agencies, the speech-language pathologist would be responsible for all of the assessments. It is important that the speech-language pathologist receive adequate training and education in the specific requirements for each assessment. It is the responsibility of the speech-language pathologist to request training from the agency if he or she does not feel competent in

Swigert, N. B.
Documentation and Reimbursement for Speech-Language Pathologists: Principles and Practice (pp. 199-211).

Table 13-1

Types of Assessments in Home Health

Type of Assessment	Purpose/Notes	Completed by Speech-Language Pathologist?	Completed by Another Member of Assessment Team?
Initial assessment	Must be completed on first visit to establish eligibility for home health services	Might be for some agencies. Definitely if speech-language pathology is the only services ordered	Usually a nurse unless rehabilitation is the only service ordered
Comprehensive assessment	If patient meets criteria, this is done. Can be done same day as initial visit, but no later than 5 days after start of care	Might be for some agencies Definitely if speech-language pathology is the only service ordered	Usually a nurse Can be physical therapist or speech-language pathologist if rehabilitation service is only service ordered
Discipline-specific assessment	Considered a part of the comprehensive assessment	Yes	No
Outcome and Assessment Information Set (OASIS)	Must be used as part of the comprehensive assessment	If speech-language pathology only or therapy only including speech-language pathology, the speech-language pathologist can complete	If nursing is ordered, the registered nurse will complete. If therapy only, physical therapist or speech-language pathologist can complete. Only one discipline completes the OASIS assessment.

any aspect of the required assessments. The home health agency is responsible for insuring the competency of all skilled professionals who perform the assessments.

Reimbursement can be denied if all the elements of each assessment are not performed and the results documented according to guidance provided by CMS.

For purposes of clarification, a detailed description of the required elements and processes for each assessment follows.

Initial Assessment to Establish Eligibility for Services

The initial assessment is conducted on the initial visit to meet the immediate care and support needs of the patient and to determine whether the patient meets the criteria for eligibility for the Medicare/Medicaid home health benefit. Eligibility for home care is based on homebound status and the medical necessity of intermittent skilled care, such nursing, physical or occupational therapy, or speech-language pathology. The visit must be completed within 48 hours of the referral or 48 hours of the patient's return home unless there is a specific physician ordered date for the start of care.

If there are nursing orders at the start of care, the HHCoPs dictate that a registered nurse conduct the initial assessment. If there are no nursing services ordered but there are therapy services ordered, the initial assessment can be performed by a physical therapist or a speech-language pathologist as determined by the orders. The need for occupational therapy is not recognized by CMS as an initial qualifying skill. Therefore, the initial assessment and eligibility for the Medicare home health benefit in a therapy-only case are established by physical therapy or speech-language pathology.

Determining Homebound Status for Eligibility

Establishing that the patient is homebound for purposes of CMS is one of the required elements of the initial

- Patient has left-sided paralysis following a recent cerebrovascular accident. He is unable to bear weight on the left side. He is currently wheelchair-dependent and unable to maneuver the wheelchair without assistance. He presently requires the assistance of two persons to enter and exit his home.
- Patient is currently undergoing chemotherapy for a recurrence of her osteomyelitis. She exhibits severe weakness and fatigue and becomes exhausted with minimal activity.
- Patient's current weight is 378 pounds. Ambulation within the home is minimal due to shortness of air and need for frequent rest breaks.
- There are 12 steps to enter/exit the home. There are no rails present. The patient refuses to exit the home due to fear of falling and injury.

Figure 13-1. Documentation examples of homebound status.

assessment. CMS requires that both Criteria 1 and Criteria 2 are met to indicate homebound status.

- Criteria 1: *Either*
    - Because of illness or injury, to leave home the patient needs:
        - Assistive device(s)
        - Special transportation
        - Assistance of another person

    or

    - Leaving home is medically contraindicated

  and
- Criteria 2: *Both*
    - Normally patient is unable to leave home
    - Leaving home requires considerable and taxing effort

Patient can still be homebound if he leaves home:

- Frequently for:
    - Doctor's appointments or medical care
    - Certified adult day care
- Infrequently and for short duration for:
    - Faith-based services
    - Haircuts/beauty parlor

Documentation must clearly indicate that these trips outside the home require considerable and taxing effort (CMS, 2013).

Some reasons that persons are homebound include functional impairments, such as the following:

- Ambulation and transfer deficits
- Impaired vision
- Frailty
- Shortness of breath
- Postoperative restrictions
- Pain interfering with activity
- Cognitive deficits, such as dementia or Alzheimer's disease
- Mental health issues, such as extreme anxiety when outside of familiar situations and fear of leaving home
- Structural barriers to enter and/or exit the home, such as multiple steps without rails

If the documentation does not explicitly define the homebound status of the patient, it is highly likely that payment for the visit will be denied. See Figure 13-1 for examples of documenting homebound status.

It is important to note that the homebound requirement must be met for eligibility on the initial visit, but that is not the only time. Homebound status must be detailed throughout the clinical record. Further discussion of the ongoing need to document medical necessity will be found in the routine visit note section.

When a patient is no longer homebound but has continuing medical or therapy needs, the patient should be transitioned to outpatient care.

Medically Reasonable and Necessary and Skilled Care

The medical necessity of intermittent skilled care (e.g., nursing, physical or occupational therapy or speech-language pathology) is the other requirement to establish eligibility for the Medicare home health benefit. A physician order for a service does not inherently make the service medically necessary.

CMS provides very clear guidance about medical necessity as found in the Medicare Benefit Policy Manual. Skilled therapy must require the skills of a qualified therapist and must be reasonable and necessary for the treatment of the patient's illness or injury (CMS, 2017a).

A qualified speech-language pathologist is defined as one who has a master's or doctoral degree in speech-language pathology and who meets either of the following requirements:

1. Licensed in the state where the individual provides services
2. If the state does not require licensing, the individual must have:
    a. Completed 350 clock hours or supervised clinical practice or is in the process of accumulating supervised clinical experience
    b. Performed not less than 9 months of supervised full-time speech-language pathology services after

Table 13-2

Questions to Ask to Help Determine Medical Necessity and Skilled Intervention

Yes or No	
	Do the services meet the Medicare definition of skilled services?
	Are the services inherently complex that they can only be provided safely and effectively by a qualified therapist?
	Does the patient's condition require the specialized skills of a qualified therapist to achieve the treatment goals?
	Are the planned treatments consistent with the patient's condition?
	Are the services reasonable for the patient's medical condition?
	Are the services necessary to meet the standard of care?

obtaining a master's or doctoral degree in speech-language pathology or a related field

c. Successfully completed a national examination in speech-language pathology approved by the Secretary of Health and Human Services

The Medicare Benefit Policy Manual clearly defines skilled therapy services as follows:

- The service must be inherently complex enough that it can be performed safely and/or effectively by or under the general supervision of a skilled therapist.
- The skilled services must also be reasonable and necessary to treat the patient's illness or injury or to restore or maintain function affected by the patient's illness or injury.

If the specialized skills, knowledge, and judgment of a therapist are needed to manage and periodically re-evaluate the appropriateness of a maintenance program, services would be covered, even if the skills of a therapist were not needed to carry out the activities performed as part of the maintenance program (CMS, 2017a).

Coverage is not determined based on the presence or absence of an individual's potential for improvement, but rather on the beneficiary's need for skilled care. Although a patient's diagnosis, prognosis, or medical condition is a valid factor in deciding whether skilled therapy services are needed, that alone does not indicate that a service is or is not skilled. The key question is whether the skills of a therapist are required to treat the illness or injury or whether the services can be carried out by unskilled personnel.

Services are considered reasonable and necessary for the treatment of the illness or injury when:

- They are consistent with the nature and severity of the illness or injury and the patient's particular medical needs, including services that are reasonable in amount, frequency, and duration
- They are a specific, safe, and effective treatment for the patient's condition under accepted standards of medical practice (CMS, 2017a).

The home health record must specify the purpose of the skilled service provided.

The following are examples of reasons that services are medically necessary:

- New-onset or exacerbation of an existing diagnosis: Include new signs and symptoms and the date of onset or exacerbation
- Acute change in condition: Be specific. Include physician contact and the ordered changes to the plan of care
- Family's or caregiver's lack of knowledge of the care required for the patient: For example, patient is on a modified diet and the family has had no instruction
- Complexity of services required to carry out the plan of care: The services could only be performed by a skilled professional speech-language pathologist
- Complicating factors: For example, unreliable caregivers, need for community resources

Although the determination and documentation of medical necessity for skilled services is an essential component of the initial visit, documentation must describe the evidence for medical necessity on each encounter throughout the episode of care from the initial assessment visit to the discharge visit. Information about the patient's prior level of function compared with his or her current status is needed to support why skilled speech-language pathology services are required.

Patient progress toward goals does not justify medical necessity. Patients often make progress without the services of a skilled therapist. Documentation must clearly show how the skilled interventions provided by the speech-language pathologist are critical to the patient's progress or lack of decline. There must be a defined link between the skilled intervention and the outcomes (Table 13-2).

Third-party payers, most often Medicare, review documentation during audits and regulatory visits. The reviewer may be a skilled professional, but often that is not the case. Reviewers may be other skilled professionals, such as registered nurses, but often the first level of reviews are performed by non–health care workers using a list of key words and measurements. The more patient-specific detail provided about the medical necessity of the services, the more likely that the documentation will be accepted by the reviewer. If there is not clear documentation of medical necessity beginning with the initial assessment visit, one or more visits or the entire episode may be deemed not medically necessary and payment denied.

Skilled Intermittent Care

Home care is designed to provide skilled intermittent care. The CMS Medicare Benefit Policy Manual describes intermittent service with regard to skilled nursing and home health aide service but not with regard to therapy services. The industry has routinely assumed that the intermittent standard is applicable to all home care services. Medically necessary treatment can be provided daily if parameters are defined and there is a specific end date.

Comprehensive Assessment

Once eligibility for the Medicare home health benefit is established, each home health patient must receive a comprehensive assessment that includes all of the following patient-specific information:

- Current health status
- Need (or continuing need) for home care
- Medical needs
- Social needs
- Nursing needs
- Rehabilitative needs
- Discharge planning needs
- Eligibility for home care services, including homebound status and medical necessity
- OASIS data

The comprehensive assessment must be completed in a timely manner, no later than 5 calendar days after the start of care. The Outcome Assessment and data items determined by the U.S. Secretary of Health & Human Services must be incorporated into the home health agency's own assessment and must include the following:

- Clinical record items
- Demographics and patient history
- Living arrangements
- Supportive assistance
- Sensory status
- Integumentary status
- Respiratory status
- Elimination status
- Neuro/emotional/behavioral status
- Activities of daily living
- Medications
- Equipment management
- Emergent care
- Data items collected at inpatient facility admission or discharge only

If nursing services are ordered, a registered nurse must complete the comprehensive assessment.

If physical or occupational therapy or speech-language pathology is the only service ordered by the physician, a physical or occupational therapist or speech-language pathologist may complete the comprehensive assessment. The occupational therapist may complete the comprehensive assessment only if the need for occupational therapy establishes home health eligibility.

The comprehensive assessment should be completed within 5 days after the start of care date. The comprehensive assessment may be repeated if there is a significant change in the patient's condition, a hospitalization of more than 24 hours, discharge, or the patient dies while a patient of the agency.

Review of Medications

The HHCoPs require that the comprehensive assessment include a review of all medications the patient is currently using in order to identify any potential adverse effects and drug reactions, including ineffective drug therapy, significant side effects, significant drug interactions, duplicate drug therapy, and non-compliance with drug therapy. This element may be problematic for speech-language pathologists, who have had little or no training in pharmacology. However, the completion of the drug regimen review is appropriate for speech-language pathologists in accordance with the American Speech-Language-Hearing Association's multiskilling policy. It is the responsibility of the speech-language pathologist to seek out knowledge about pharmacology, including how to assess for interactions. It is the responsibility of the home care agency to provide education and training and assess the competency all qualified therapists regarding the drug regimen review. Often, the home health electronic medical record will include prompts and alerts for drug interactions, side effects, and duplicate drug therapy.

Outcome Assessment and Information Set Documentation

CMS mandates the collection of OASIS data elements on all Medicare and Medicaid patients of a Medicare certified home health agency, with the exception of pediatric and maternity patients. OASIS data are used to determine reimbursement and measure patient outcomes for quality and pubic reporting purposes.

OASIS data collection and transmission began in 1999 for adult skilled Medicare and Medicaid patients. Since that time, there have been many revisions to the OASIS data set and its use for quality measurement and payment. At the time of this writing, additional revisions are underway to increase standardization with assessment item sets for other post-acute care settings and to enable calculation of standardized, cross-setting quality measures, pursuant to the provisions of the Improving Medicare Post-Acute Care Transformation (IMPACT) Act of 2014.

Time Points for Collecting Data With Outcome Assessment and Information Set Documentation

OASIS data are collected at the following time points:

- Start of care
- Resumption of care following inpatient facility stay
- Recertification within the last 5 days of each 60-day recertification period
- Other follow-up during the home health episode of care
- Transfer to inpatient facility
- Discharge from home care
- Death at home

All of these assessments, with the exception of transfer to inpatient facility and death at home, require the clinician to have an in-person encounter with the patient during a home visit. The transfer to an inpatient facility requires collection of limited OASIS data (most of which may be obtained through a telephone call). Not all OASIS items are completed at every assessment time point. Some items are completed only at start of care, some only at discharge. The table *Items to Be Used at Specific Time Points*, included at the beginning of the OASIS data set, allows the home health agency to integrate the necessary OASIS items at each time point into clinical documentation forms or an electronic health record (CMS, 2014).

Outcome Assessment and Information Set Documentation: Tips for Completing

Use the following tips to enhance your OASIS accuracy:

- Know the time period under consideration for each item. Report results observed on the day of assessment unless a different time period has been indicated in the item or related guidance. Day of assessment is defined as the 24 hours immediately preceding the home visit and the time spent by the clinician in the home.
- Report the patient's usual status or what is true greater than 50% of the assessment time frame, unless the item specifies differently if the patient's ability or status varies on the day of the assessment.
- Minimize the use of *N/A* and *Unknown* responses.
- A dash (–) response indicates that no information is available and/or an item could not be assessed. The dash would be used when the patient is unexpectedly transferred, discharged, or dies before assessment of the item could be completed.
- Independent observation of the patient's condition and ability at the time of the assessment without referring back to prior assessments drives the response on the OASIS assessment. Follow rules included in the Item-Specific Guidance.
- Look for item-by-item guidance for any exceptions.
- Utilize direct observation to assess physiologic or functional health status.
- References to assistance relate to assistance from another person and include physical contact, verbal cues, and/or supervision.
- Stay current with evolving CMS OASIS guidance updates. CMS may post updates to the guidance manual up to twice per year.
- Only one clinician may take responsibility for accurately completing a comprehensive assessment.

The Plan of Care

The home health agency must be acting upon a physician plan of care (POC) that meets the requirements of this section for home health services to be covered. Following the initial assessments, the speech-language pathologist or other skilled professional will discuss the patient's current condition with the physician and collaborate to establish the POC. The POC includes information obtained in the initial assessment, the comprehensive assessment, and the discipline specific assessments. It is a summary of the patient's current status and the planned interventions for a 60-day episode of care.

The POC must include the following:

- All pertinent diagnoses
- Patient's mental status
- Types of services, supplies, and equipment required
- Frequency of the visits to be made
- Prognosis
- Rehabilitation potential
- Functional limitations
- Activities permitted
- All medications and treatments

- Safety measures to protect against injury
- Instructions for timely discharge or referral
- Any additional items the home health agency or physician chooses to include

The POC for therapy should include the following:

- Measurable, time-specific therapy treatment goals that align with the patient's illness or injury and the patient's resultant impairments
- Expected duration of therapy services
- Description of treatment that is consistent with the assessment of the patient's function
- Type of services to be provided to the patient, the professional who will provide them, the description of the individual services, and the frequency of the services (e.g., ST 3x 2 wk, 2x 1 wk (speech therapy 3/per week for 2 weeks followed by 2 times/week for 1 week) for patient/caregiver education and dysphagia therapy

Other things to consider regarding the POC include the following:

- The POC may indicate a specific range in the frequency of visits such as 2–3x 2 wk (2 to 3 times/week for 2 weeks) to ensure that the most appropriate level of services is provided during the 60-day episode to home health patients. When a range of visits is ordered, the upper limit of the range is considered the specific frequency.
- *As needed*, or *PRN*, treatment orders require a description of the patient's medical signs and symptoms that would trigger a visit and a specific limit on the number of those visits.
- If the POC is altered, including changes in frequency and/or duration of any discipline, supplemental orders must be obtained from the physician and submitted for signature.
- Evaluate and treat orders only cover one visit (the evaluation). The therapist must obtain a verbal order for the treatment plan, document the order, and send it to the physician for signature.
- The POC and all verbal orders include a legible physician signature and date.
- The POC should be signed and dated prior to billing the end of episode claim.

See Appendix 13-A for components of the POC.

Documenting the Plan of Care

The POC is a physician's order and must be followed. In the event you are not able to follow the POC, the physician must be notified. Notify the physician in the following cases:

- Every missed visit (If you scheduled a visit on Tuesday, you can still make it up on any other day until Sunday and will not have breached the physician order.)
- A missed visit if you were unable to follow the frequency
- When you are unable to perform the intervention due to patient refusal
- When there is a change in patient's condition that requires new orders

Routine Visit Documentation

Documentation of a routine visit, often called a *daily*, *treatment*, or *progress note*, documents the implementation of the POC. Documentation of a visit or encounter should include the following:

- Patient/client or family/caregiver report
- Interventions performed and the patient's and/or caregiver's response
- Progress toward goals
- Description of any patient/caregiver education, including, but not limited to, details of the home program
- Statement of ongoing homebound status
- Evaluation of the POC and need for any modifications
- Communication/collaboration with the patient, physician, other team members, and other significant parties
- Discussion of any factors that require changes to the POC or influence progress toward goals
- Plan for next visit(s), including interventions or justification for discharge

The documentation of each visit must substantiate that the interventions performed require the skill of a qualified speech-language pathologist. Documentation is considered incomplete if it is only a listing of treatments. Document the type and level of skilled assistance given to the patient, his or her response, and progress toward goals. Document the rationale for the interventions. Describe functional progress and any barriers to achieving progress.

When maintenance therapy is provided, document why the interventions require the skills of a qualified speech-language pathologist and cannot be performed by a family member or caregiver. Provide details about why the ongoing skilled intervention is medically necessary and appropriate for the patient's condition.

Documenting Changes in Patient Status

Document the patient's current status compared with his or her prior status from one visit to the next. Include references to the status at the time of the initial evaluation.

Note any assessments or reassessments provided on the visit and any updates to the POC resulting from those assessments.

Required Reassessments

In late 2015, CMS clarified the Medicare requirement for ongoing therapy reassessments. The patient must be reassessed at least every 30 days by a qualified therapist (not an assistant) to re-establish the need for skilled therapeutic intervention. This pertains to each discipline. The functional reassessment must be performed using objective tests and measures and accepted standards of clinical practice. The reassessment must include functional tasks such as activities of daily living. Progress from one assessment to the next should be compared to determine the effectiveness of therapy provided to date. The measures used and the results of the reassessment must be documented in the patient's record (IMPACT Act, 2014).

If a test or measure is not standardized on the home health population, it is not an appropriate standardized tool. If the tool requires modification to be used in home care, it is no longer standardized. This is challenging because there are not many assessment tools standardized on the home health population. If you are unable to find an appropriate tool, use the tools commonly used for the patient's diagnosis and cite that there is no other standardized tool for the home health population.

Describe the patient's performance on the tool. Compare performance with the initial assessment and the prior reassessments. Clearly justify ongoing medical necessity and reaffirm homebound status. Determine what changes to the POC are needed in the next 30 days and obtain the appropriate physician orders.

Documenting Transfer to an Inpatient Facility

Sometimes home care patients will have a change in status that requires admission to an impatient facility, or there may be a planned readmission for specific care needs. The following are specific assessment requirements for these transfers:

- If the patient is admitted for less than 24 hours or is in observation status, a transfer OASIS is not required.
- A transfer OASIS must be completed if the patient is admitted for more than 24 hours and then returns home within the current episode; the *Transfer to an inpatient facility—patient not discharged from agency* OASIS would be completed within 2 days of the transfer date.
- If the patient is admitted for more than 24 hours but will not return home before the current home health episode ends, the *Transfer to an inpatient facility—patient discharged from the agency* OASIS assessment is completed within 2 days of the discharge date.
- A speech-language pathologist can complete any of these transfer OASIS assessments.
- The transfer OASIS assessments may be completed without a visit to the home.

Discharge Documentation

Discharges can occur at various time points and for very different reasons. If the patient is no longer homebound, he or she no longer meets eligibility for the Medicare home health benefit and must be discharged. Complete OASIS discharge assessment along with the agency's discharge paperwork.

If the patient meets his or her goals for speech-language pathology but remains homebound and needs continuing services from another discipline, complete the speech-language pathology discharge paperwork required by the agency. No OASIS assessment is required.

If care is no longer medically necessary, complete a *Discharge from the agency not to inpatient facility* OASIS assessment and follow the agency policies for discharge.

When the discharge is unanticipated (e.g., patient refuses further services, moves out of the coverage area) and is not a transfer to an inpatient facility, complete a *Discharge from agency not to inpatient facility* assessment along with required agency discharge paperwork. If a patient dies at home, a *Death at home* OASIS should be documented within 2 calendar days of the death or the agency's notification of the death. This The *Discharge from agency* OASIS assessment is not required if the death occurs in an emergency room or inpatient facility. Utilize data from the most recent home visit to complete the OASIS assessment.

An illustration of how a patient progresses through the assessment, treatment, reassessment, and discharge time points is found in Appendix 13-B.

Documentation Audits for Fraud and Abuse

Home care is under increasing scrutiny due to verified cases of fraud and abuse. CMS now employs Recovery Audit Contractors, Zone Program Integrity Contractors, Supplemental Medical Review Contractors, and Medicare Fee-for-Service Recovery Contractors to uncover inappropriate billing and visit utilization and to request repayment. Insurance companies, including those participating in the Medicare Advantage Program, may also request records for audit to determine whether there are reasons for denial of payment. Any encounter with the patient and/or his or her representative is subject to review (CMS, 2017b). Reviewers come from many different sources (Figure 13-2).

The reader/reviewer look for the following:

- Documentation of eligibility for the home health benefit
- Comprehensive assessment of the patient
- Specific medically necessary therapy needs that justify the skills of a speech-language pathologist
- Identified problems with corresponding measurable, time-specific goals

- Appropriate interventions and details about the patient's response to those interventions
- Timely reassessments
- Communication with the physician and all other care team members
- Discharge planning and appropriate transfer or discharge documentation

The reviewer only knows what you did from reading your documentation. Make sure your documentation will support reimbursement:

- Know the reimbursement rules.
- Understand and follow the guidance in the Medicare Conditions of Participation.
- Stay up to date on regulatory changes.
- Comply with insurer reimbursement requirements. (When is additional documentation needed to continue coverage? Every visit? Every three visits? Every 30 days?)
- Detail homebound status and medical necessity on every visit.
- Document all interactions with the physician and other care team members.

Who Reads the Documentation

- Physicians
- Patients, caregivers, and responsible parties
- Home care team members
- Quality assessment and performance improvement team
- Accreditation surveyors
- Medicare/Medicaid surveyors
- Reimbursement reviewers
- Attorneys
- Risk management and compliance staff

Figure 13-2. Documentation is reviewed to assess for quality, payment and regulatory compliance purposes.

Conclusion

Home care is one of the most gratifying practice settings for a speech-language pathologist. It provides a golden opportunity to make therapeutic intervention truly functional for the patient and those caring for him or her. The documentation requirements are very specific and often subject to regulatory changes as in other practice settings. Provide the detailed documentation required for reimbursement and enjoy making a difference as a home care speech-language pathologist.

References

Centers for Medicare & Medicaid Services. (2012). Home health agencies. Retrieved from https://www.cms.gov/Medicare/Provider-Enrollment-and-Certification/GuidanceforLawsAndRegulations/HHAs.html

Centers for Medicare & Medicaid Services. (2013). CMS Manual Pub 100-02 Medicare Benefit Policy, Transmittal 172. Retrieved from http://www.cms.gov/Regulations-and-Guidance/Guidance/Transmittals/Downloads/R172BP.pdf

Centers for Medicare & Medicaid Services. (2014). CMS Manual Pub 100-07 State Operations Provider Certification, Transmittal 125. Retrieved from https://www.cms.gov/Regulations-and-Guidance/Guidance/Transmittals/downloads/R125SOMA.pdf

Centers for Medicare & Medicaid Services. (2017a). Medicare Benefit Policy Manual: Chapter 7—Home Health Services. Retrieved from https://www.cms.gov/Regulations-and-Guidance/Guidance/Manuals/Downloads/bp102c07.pdf

Centers for Medicare & Medicaid Services. (2017b). Medicare fee for service recovery audit program. Retrieved from https://www.cms.gov/Research-Statistics-Data-and-Systems/Monitoring-Programs/1/Recovery-Audit-Program/

Improving Medicare Post-Acute Care Transformation (IMPACT) Act of 2014, Pub. L. No. 113-18 (2014).

Review Questions

1. What are the Home Health Conditions of Participation, and why are they important?
2. What is the purpose of the initial assessment?
3. How does the initial assessment differ from the comprehensive assessment?
4. How is homebound status determined?
5. Define medical necessity.
6. What is OASIS? Why is it important?
7. Which disciplines can establish eligibility for the home health benefit?
8. What must be included in the home health POC?
9. Who may review home health documentation?
10. What should be included in the documentation of each visit?

Activity A

Mr. Adams has been referred for home health speech-language pathology services following a recent cerebrovascular accident. Describe the assessments that would be needed to establish his eligibility for home care, and create the POC.

Activity B

Review each of the following statements. Determine whether the statement meets the criteria for homebound status. If not, indicate what is missing.

1. Patient has no one to transport him to outpatient therapy.
   Yes_____ No_____ The missing aspects are:
2. Patient requires 24-hour supervision due to confusion and combative episodes following his recent closed head injury.
   Yes_____ No_____ The missing aspects are:
3. Patient is extremely weak due to ongoing chemotherapy. She is unable to ambulate more than 10 feet within her home before needing to sit and rest.
   Yes_____ No_____ The missing aspects are:
4. The patient refuses to leave home because someone will kidnap her and kill her.
   Yes_____ No_____ The missing aspects are:
5. The patient exhibits impaired mobility due to recent bilateral knee replacements.
   Yes_____ No_____ The missing aspects are:

Appendix 13-A
Sample Template to Address the Components Required to Establish the Plan of Care

Speech-Language/Swallowing Evaluation

Background Information

- Reason for referral
- Primary diagnosis
- Secondary diagnosis
- Pertinent history
- Prior videofluoroscopic swallowing study or fiberoptic endoscopic evaluation of swallowing
- Prior level of function

Medical Information

- Vital signs
- Blood pressure
- Temperature
- Pulse
- Respirations
- Oxygen saturation
- Oxygen use
- Compliance with O_2 safety
- Respiratory status
- Pain/location/controlled with
- Edema
- Wound/skin condition
- Mental status

Swallowing Evaluation/Oral Motor Assessment

- Current diet
- Structure/dentures
- Oral motor function
- Velar function
- Laryngeal function
- Oral phase
- Pharyngeal phase
- Swallowing assessment summary

Cognitive-Communication Evaluation

- Objective tests/measures used
- Hearing
- Vision
- Handedness
- Orientation
- Spoken language comprehension
- Spoken language expression
- Motor speech production
- Attention
- Memory
- Problem solving
- Reading comprehension
- Pragmatics
- Writing
- Voice
- Voice following tracheostomy
- Augmentative and alternative communication
- Alaryngeal communication
- Fluency

Assessment Summary, Including Problems and Awareness of Deficits

- Supplies and equipment needed
- Safety measures
- Medications
- Functional status/objective findings
- Statement of medical necessity
- Rehabilitation potential
- Patient's goal for this episode of care
- Homebound status
- Home social environment
- Communication/care coordination

Appendix 13-B
Case Example

Now let's follow a patient through the course of his home health episode. In this example, the speech-language pathologist is not involved in the initial assessment, and her role in the comprehensive assessment is to complete her discipline-specific assessment.

1. Patient is referred to the agency for skilled nursing and physical and speech therapy following a recent motor vehicle accident that resulted in a traumatic brain injury
2. Required assessments are completed.
   a. Initial assessment establishing eligibility was completed by the nurse, and the patient meets eligibility requirements for home health.
   b. Comprehensive assessment was also completed by the nurse.
   c. OASIS Start of Care Assessment (as required) was completed by the nurse. (Only one discipline is allowed to complete OASIS, which is different from the other post-acute settings, so the speech-language pathologist does not have to do anything on the OASIS.)
   d. From the results of the assessments, the patient requires nursing, physical therapy, and speech-language pathology services. The speech-language pathologist completes the discipline-specific assessment and develops an appropriate treatment plan, including long- and short-term goals, specific interventions, rehab potential, the patient's goal for the episode of care, any special equipment and/or supplies needed, statement of medical necessity, statement of homebound status, and the frequency and duration of home visits planned for the 60-day episode. This is documented in the patient record according to the agency policies and practices. The plan is discussed with the physician overseeing the patient's care and, if agreed upon, is incorporated into the overall POC, which includes treatment to be provided by all disciplines.
3. The speech pathologist then performs and documents each visit according to CMS guidance and agency policies. The speech-language pathologist must document the content of each visit, including the treatment provided, the response to such treatment, the progress or lack of progress toward goals, the medical necessity for that particular visit and future visits as appropriate, the homebound status of the patient, any patient or caregiver education and the response to such education, communication with other disciplines and/or the physician, and any additional pertinent information.
4. If the frequency of visits in a week is not met and is unable to be rescheduled due to unusual circumstances, such as patient illness or conflicting appointments, a missed visit note is completed according to agency policies and submitted to the physician. Documentation of submission, such as a fax cover sheet or e-fax documentation, is required. Whenever possible, missed visits should be rescheduled within the agency's workweek to meet the ordered frequency of visits.
5. Near the end of the episode, during the last 5 days of the episode of care, each discipline, including speech-language pathology, will assess the patient's progress and determine whether any home care services continue to be medically necessary. If so, the recertification OASIS assessment is completed during the last 5 days of the episode. This assessment requires a home visit. The recertification OASIS assessment can be completed by a skilled nurse, physical or occupational therapist or speech-language pathologist. Only one discipline can complete the recertification assessment, but each discipline continuing services is required to reassess the patient and establish new goals and interventions for the next 60-day episode. The overall POC for the upcoming 60-day episode is based on the reassessment findings and submitted to the physician for approval and signature.

14

Outpatient Settings
Adult

Nancy B. Swigert, MA, CCC-SLP, BCS-S

Medicare Providers

If the speech-language pathologist works at a facility that sees adult outpatients, it is almost certain the facility is billing Medicare, Medicaid, and most private insurance plans. If a speech-language pathologist in private practice wants to see outpatients who have Medicare, he or she must enroll to become a Medicare provider and agree to the rates set in the Medicare Physician Fee Schedule. The speech-language pathologist cannot bill the Medicare beneficiary directly. The enrollment process is not complicated, and there are many resources from the American Speech-Language-Hearing Association (ASHA) to provide guidance. In particular, *Medicare Survival Guide for Audiologists and Speech-Language Pathologists* provides thorough information about enrolling as a Medicare provider, along with other detailed information about all aspects of Medicare (Satterfield & Swanson, 2016).

Determining Whether Services Will Be Covered Under Medicare Part B

As with any payer, the speech-language pathologist should determine prior to evaluating the client whether the services will be covered by the insurer, in this case Medicare Part B or C. There are some national guidelines that apply to speech-language pathology and dysphagia services, but more detailed information about coverage is found in local coverage determinations (LCDs).

National Coverage Determinations

There are four national coverage determinations (NCDs) related to speech-language pathology and dysphagia services. Some of these are more detailed than others in the

Swigert, N. B.
Documentation and Reimbursement for Speech-Language Pathologists: Principles and Practice (pp. 213-247).

guidance they provide about the services. For example, the NCD on speech-generating devices is very detailed (Satterfield & Swanson, 2016). To ensure that the speech-language pathologist is consulting the most recent version of an NCD, they should visit the website of the Centers for Medicare & Medicaid Services (CMS). Depending on the population served, the speech-language pathologist should read the following:

- NCD 50.1: Speech-Generating Devices
- NCD 50.2: Electronic Speech Aids
- NCD 160.2: Treatment of Motor Function with Electric Nerve Stimulation
- NCD 170.3: Speech-Language Pathology Services for the Treatment of Dysphagia (CMS, n.d.-b)

Local Coverage Determinations for Medicare

CMS contracts with private insurance companies to administer the Medicare program. These insurance companies are called Medicare Administrative Contractors (MACs). Each covers a different section of the country. The MACs develop documents called LCDs, which further define what will and will not be covered. Most MACs have an LCD for speech-language pathology services and one for dysphagia services. The speech-language pathologist should know which MAC administers the program in his state and should read the LCDs for specific guidance about covered services. The LCDs focus on defining what is "reasonable and necessary" (CMS, 2017c; Satterfield & Swanson, 2016).

Advance Beneficiary Notice

An advance beneficiary notice (ABN) is a document the provider must give to the beneficiary before furnishing services that are usually covered by Medicare but are not expected to be paid in a specific instance for certain reasons, such as lack of medical necessity (CMS, 2015).

Level of Supervision for Certain Current Procedural Terminology Codes With Medicare Part B

CMS determines the level of supervision needed for each Current Procedural Terminology (CPT) code. The levels range from not being subject to supervision if performed by a qualified practitioner to being performed under personal supervision, meaning the physician must be in the room during the procedure. In practical terms, these levels of supervision determine settings in which it is not realistic for a speech-language pathologist to perform and bill for a certain procedure. For example, the use of manometry for assessment of pharyngeal dysphagia is growing, but the code for manometry requires personal supervision. Therefore, it is likely that a speech-language pathologist would be performing that procedure only in a physician's office (Satterfield & Swanson, 2016).

CMS also requires that only the professional can bill for Medicare Part B. Graduate students and clinical fellows in states that don't license the clinical fellows require 100% supervision by the speech-language pathologist. The student can provide the treatment and document, but the professional must be in the room for the full session, making skilled determination and taking full responsibility (Satterfield & Swanson, 2016).

Determining What Will Be Covered With Private Insurance and Medicaid

It is sometimes said that if you have seen one private insurance plan, you have seen one private insurance plan. Each client presents with a different plan with different coverage limitations. Do not assume that all plans for a particular insurance company have the same coverage. For example, one client may have a Blue Cross–Blue Shield plan that covers some communication disorders under certain very specific circumstances. Another client, also with a Blue Cross–Blue Shield plan, may have entirely different coverage restrictions. It is the client's responsibility to determine what his or her insurance covers, although he or she will often ask the speech-language pathologist to look at the policy or provide information about what services (i.e., CPT codes) will be used. The speech-language pathologist can easily share information about the likely CPT evaluation and treatment codes that will be used but should encourage the client to discuss that information directly with the insurance company. The client might want to obtain in writing what the insurance company says they will cover. There are often limitations based on medical necessity, similar to Medicare, and even when services are covered for a particular disorder, there are often limitations on the number of visits that will be covered during a calendar year.

Each state has its own Medicaid program. The coverage may be structured like a fee-for-service insurance plan, but more and more Medicaid programs are utilizing a managed care approach. Some will require preapproval be obtained before the evaluation, and most require authorization after the evaluation before treatment is rendered.

Case History and Interview Forms

In outpatient settings, it is customary to have the client/caregiver complete a case history form before he or she arrives for evaluation. A case history form collects demographic information as well as information about the presenting problem. The form can be basic and generic, used for any type of client. See Appendix 6-A for an example of a generic adult case history form.

However, case history forms designed for specific disorders can gather more detailed information. The more information that can be obtained before the evaluation begins, the more efficient the speech-language pathologist can be during the evaluation session. The case history form can then also serve as the format for the clinician to interview the client to fill in any gaps in the information provided. See Appendices 14-A and 14-B for example case history forms for mild cognitive impairment/memory and voice.

Regardless of the form or format used to gather the information, the speech-language pathologist should be certain to learn the client's or caregiver's perspective on why the evaluation is needed. His perspective may be very different than that of the person who made the referral.

Gathering Information From the Client/Caregiver Interview

Sometimes a detailed interview form can be used to guide the clinician through that part of the evaluation. Such interview forms are especially helpful to a clinician with less experience or who beginning to see a new type of client. As the clinician gains experience and expertise with a particular patient population, the flow of the interview and types of questions to ask become second nature. The case history form would be worded with full sentences and questions for the client to read, whereas the interview form can include just terms or words to trigger the speech-language pathologist about what to ask. See Appendix 14-C for a voice interview questionnaire.

EVALUATIONS

Evaluations in outpatient settings may be completed in an electronic health record (EHR), typed in a Microsoft Word document, or, less likely, handwritten. Regardless of the format, the speech-language pathologist should find ways to be as efficient as possible in the documentation of the evaluation.

Templates, Standard Paragraphs, and Appendices

If the outpatient setting is not using an EHR, the evaluation reports are likely in the form of a Word document. Templates should be developed to help organize the information and to streamline the documentation process. The header for the template can likely be the same regardless of the age of the client or type of evaluation being completed. The header typically contains the following:

- Demographic information on the client
  - Name
  - Date of birth
  - Age
  - Address
  - Phone
- Facility-specific identifying information, such as case number
- Referral source
- Date of evaluation
- Time of evaluation
  - Time in
  - Time out required if using a timed evaluation code
  - Any additional report-writing time if required with that code
- CPT/procedure code(s)

A generic template can be used that includes the main areas that should be included in each report. See Appendices 7-B and 7-C for template examples.

A way to further streamline the report-writing process is to develop slightly different templates, based on the disorder or type of client being evaluated. These templates also make it easier for the reader to follow. The basics of each template will be the same, with slight changes based on the disorder. See Appendices 14-D and 14-E for examples of templates for voice and mild cognitive impairment/memory.

When standardized tests are used, it is helpful to the reader if a description of the test and any specific information about how to interpret scores is included in the report. The speech-language pathologist should not have to create that standard paragraph each time a report is written. The clinic or practice can develop a standard paragraph for each of the tests used in the setting. Appropriate citations should be included. Then, these paragraphs, saved electronically, can be inserted into the report (Figure 14-1).

If a number of standardized tests are used, it is more efficient for the speech-language pathologist, and easier for the reader of the report, if these standard paragraphs are attached as appendices. When this format is used, the report can often be condensed to a one-page summary, with attached appendices the reader can peruse if more detail is desired. Sometimes it is more efficient to include an appendix if only one standardized assessment was utilized. See Appendix 14-F for a videofluoroscopic evaluation report with an appendix/addendum.

If an EHR is used, the process will be efficient only if it was built correctly. Too often, EHRs end up requiring just as much typing as a Word document, but in a less efficient way. EHRs are meant to be mostly point and click, with some annotation. However, they must also be complete enough to meet all documentation requirements and

The Repeatable Battery for the Assessment of Neuropsychological Status Update (RBANS® Update)

This tool is a widely used neuropsychological test for clients (Ages 12.00–89.11) with neurological injury or disease such as dementia, head injury, and stroke. The RBANS includes 12 subtests that assess the following cognitive domains: Attention, Visuospatial Function, Verbal Learning, Verbal Recall, and Psychomotor Speed. Standard scores (Index Scores) are highly correlated with full-scale IQ measures (Mean 100, Standard Deviation 15). Individual subtest scores are also obtained.

Subtest	Index Score	Percentile	Qualitative Description
Immediate memory			
Visuospatial constructional			
Language			
Attention			
Delayed memory			

Figure 14-1. Example of standard paragraph. (Adapted from Randolph, C. (2012). *The Repeatable Battery for the Assessment of Neuropsychological Status Update (RBANS® Update)*. San Antonio, TX: Pearson Education Inc.)

produce a document/report format that can be easily read, either within the EHR by professionals who have access or in paper format sent to other professionals. See Chapter 3 for more information on EHRs.

Documenting Medical Necessity

Regardless of the payer source, the evaluation should document medical necessity because Medicare, Medicaid, and private insurance all require that the services be medically necessary. Templates can include a list of choices of phrases that are used to support medical necessity. Examples of such statements are as follows:

- At risk to aspirate when eating/drinking
- Dysphagia resulting in weight loss
- Dysphagia prevents adequate intake
- Needs to learn compensatory strategies in order to eat/drink safely
- Unable to communicate well enough to participate in own care
- Unsafe to stay at home alone
- Unable to communicate emergency needs
- Difficulty communicating wants and needs
- Impaired breathing interferes with physical activity
- Patient's cognitive ability indicates need for therapy to learn compensatory techniques
- Cognitive-communication deficits impacts ability to participate in activities of daily living

Current Procedural Terminology Codes for Evaluations

Most evaluation CPT codes used by speech-language pathologists are not timed (Table 14-1). That is, regardless of the amount of time spent with the client, only one CPT code will be billed, and it will be reimbursed at the level that payer has agreed to pay for that service. In situations of private pay, the clinic or practice may establish different rates for different types of evaluations, and the individual will be billed different rates. However, when billing a third-party payer, most contracts are set with one fee per CPT code.

However, there are some evaluation codes that are time based (Table 14-2). To bill a timed code, the time spent must exceed the halfway point dictated by the code. This is often referred to as the *8-minute rule* because to use a 15-minute code, you have to spend at least 8 minutes with the client, or more than half of the time. In other words:

- 1-hour unit ≥ 31 minutes
- ½-hour unit ≥ 16 minutes
- 15-minute unit ≥ 8 minutes

Some of these timed evaluation codes, prescription of speech-generating device (92607) and auditory rehabilitation (92626), have a base code for the first hour and a different code for the subsequent period of time, either a 15-minute or 30-minute subsequent period of time. The subsequent units billed may not be counted until the full value of the first unit of time plus half of the value of the second unit of time is exceeded (Figure 14-2).

Two of the timed assessment codes, aphasia (96105) and standardized cognitive performance testing (96125), are per-hour codes. That is, there is not a separate code for the additional time, but rather the speech-language pathologist might bill more than one of that base code. These two codes also allow the inclusion of time spent on interpretation and reporting for billing Medicare (Figure 14-3).

The speech-language pathologist's documentation must break down the time spent on those activities. The evaluation report should include time in and time out, and this amount of time should match the amount of time billed for the evaluation. The time documented in the report must correspond to the number of units billed on the claim (Figure 14-4).

Table 14-1

Speech-Language Pathology Current Procedural Terminology Evaluation Codes: Untimed

CPT Code	Descriptor
31579	Laryngoscopy, flexible or rigid fiberoptic, with stroboscopy
92511	Nasopharyngoscopy with endoscope (separate procedure)
92512	Nasal function studies (e.g., rhinomanometry)
92520	Laryngeal function studies (i.e., aerodynamic testing and acoustic testing)
92521	Evaluation of speech fluency (e.g., stuttering, cluttering)
92522	Evaluation of speech sound production (e.g., articulation, phonological process, apraxia, dysarthria)
92523	Evaluation of speech sound production (e.g., articulation, phonological process, apraxia, dysarthria); with evaluation of language comprehension and expression (e.g., receptive and expressive language)
92524	Behavioral and qualitative analysis of voice and resonance
92551	Screening test pure tone, air only (*Note*: Not paid by Medicare)
92597	Evaluation for use and/or fitting of voice prosthetic device to supplement oral speech
92610	Evaluation of oral and pharyngeal swallowing function
92611	Motion fluoroscopic evaluation of swallowing function by cine or video recording
92612	Flexible fiberoptic endoscopic evaluation of swallowing by cine or video recording
92613	FEES: Interpretation and report only
92614	Flexible fiberoptic endoscopic evaluation, laryngeal sensory testing by cine or video recording
92615	Interpretation and report only
92616	Flexible fiberoptic endoscopic evaluation of swallowing and laryngeal sensory testing by cine or video recording
92617	FEESST: Interpretation and report only

Abbreviations: FEES = fiberoptic endoscopic evaluation of swallowing; FEESST = flexible endoscopic evaluation of swallowing with sensory testing.

Adapted from American Speech-Language-Hearing Association. (n.d.-a). Current Procedural Terminology (CPT) codes. Retrieved from http://www.asha.org/Practice/reimbursement/coding/SLPCPT/

Medicare Functional Outcomes Reporting

One of the challenges in documenting for adult clients with Medicare Part B is reporting the required functional outcomes. Sometimes Congress legislates changes as a trial to see if the change will be effective in lowering the costs of Medicare. In 2012, effective beginning January 2013, Congress mandated that therapy services report the functional outcomes of those services. The stated purpose was to capture information about the outcomes of rehabilitation services. There are significant questions as to whether the system developed will actually yield meaningful information about the outcomes of rehabilitation services, but the reporting is nevertheless required. One of the limitations, for example, is that the speech-language pathologist can only report on one functional area at a time, even though typically the therapy will focus on all deficit areas that have been identified. The reporting of functional outcomes, commonly called *G-codes*, is only required for Medicare Part B services. The most detail is included in this chapter for outpatient adult services, but these requirements also apply to some Medicare patients in acute care hospitals and skilled nursing facilities and those receiving services through home health if the services are paid by Part B. See Chapters 11, 14, and 15 for more detail about G-codes in those settings (CMS, 2016).

TABLE 14-2

SPEECH-LANGUAGE PATHOLOGY CURRENT PROCEDURAL TERMINOLOGY EVALUATION CODES: TIMED

CPT CODE	DESCRIPTION	TIME
92607	Evaluation for prescription of speech-generating device	First hour
92608	Evaluation for prescription of speech-generating device	Each additional 30 minutes
92626	Evaluation of auditory rehabilitation	First hour
92627	Evaluation of auditory rehabilitation	Each additional 15 minutes
96105	Assessment of aphasia, with interpretation and report	Per hour
96125	Standardized cognitive performance testing (e.g., Ross Information Processing Assessment) per hour of a qualified health care professional's time, both face-to-face time administering tests to the patient and time interpreting these test results and preparing the report	Per hour

Adapted from American Speech-Language-Hearing Association. (n.d.-a). Current Procedural Terminology (CPT) codes. Retrieved from http://www.asha.org/Practice/reimbursement/coding/SLPCPT/

Determining Number of Evaluation Units

Speech-Generating Device Evaluation: The evaluation time with the client for prescription of a speech-generating device totaled 2 hours, 50 minutes:

92607: Evaluation for prescription of speech-generating device; first hour = 1 hour
92608: Each additional 30 minutes

Bill 2 units of 92607 and 2 units of 92608. The two additional units of 92608 are allowed because the full 30 minutes were spent and then least 16 minutes were spent on the second 30 minute code (in fact, 20 minutes were spent).

Aural Rehab Evaluation: The evaluation for aural rehabilitation totaled 1 hour, 10 minutes with the client:

92626: Evaluation of auditory rehabilitation; first hour = 1 hour
92627: Each additional 15 minutes

In this case, the speech-language pathologist should bill 1 unit of 92626. Because more than 8 minutes were spent in the next unit, then one unit of 92627 can also be billed. 8 minutes are required in order to bill a 15 minute unit.

Figure 14-2. Determining evaluation units on timed codes with base and added code.

Aphasia Evaluation: The evaluation of aphasia took 50 minutes with the patient. Interpretation and report writing was documented in the record to take an additional 45 minutes. The total billable time for the code is 95 minutes.

96105 = 1 hour for each unit billed.

To bill a second unit of 96105, 91 minutes (first hour + minimum of 31 minutes for second unit) must be documented on evaluation, interpretation, and report.

In this case, 95 minutes are documented in the record. It is appropriate to bill 2 units of 96125.

Figure 14-3. Timed units for aphasia evaluation.

SPEECH-LANGUAGE PATHOLOGY
OUTPATIENT EVALUATION

Patient Name: Keith Emory
Address: 26 Gap Court
Friendly, KY

Birthdate: 09/25/53 **Age:** 63

Referral: V. Supportive, MD

Date of Evaluation: 02/14/17
Start Time Patient Contact: 10:40
Stop Time Patient Contact: 11:30 (50 mins)
Analysis/ report writing: 45 mins
Patient#: 2222222222

Procedure Codes: 96105X2

Medical history related to referral: Mr. Emory was an inpatient at Happy Valley Hospital from January 20, 2017 through February 2, 2017, secondary to a CVA in the distribution of the left MCA resulting in aphasia. He received intervention during that stay and has now been referred for continued outpatient services.

Figure 14-4. Documenting time spent in evaluation for aphasia. (CVA = cerebrovascular accident; MCA = middle cerebral artery)

G-Codes and Severity Modifiers

The G-codes are not discipline specific, but there are seven functional areas in communication and swallowing most typically used by speech-language pathologists. There is one *Other* category that can be used for other communication disorders treated. For each functional area, there are three G-codes: Current status, goal status, and discharge status (Table 14-3) (CMS, 2017a). A seven-point severity rating is used to describe the status of each by applying a modifier of two letters, C+ another letter. The speech-language pathologist must specify how the severity level was determined. For speech-language pathologists who participate in National Outcomes Measurement System (NOMS) data collection, specifying how the determination was made is easy because NOMS Functional Communication Measures (FCMs) are also seven-point scales that map to the seven-point modifier scale (Table 14-4) (ASHA, n.d.; CMS, 2017a).

The G-code and the modifier are reported on the claim, but they must also be documented in the client's record at appropriate times. These might be reported in an evaluation report, treatment plan/certification, treatment note, progress report, or discharge summary. Examples of an evaluation template and treatment plan with G-codes are included in Appendices 14-G and 14-H. These rules for when to report which G-codes are described throughout the rest of the chapter and summarized in Table 14-5.

Reporting Functional Outcomes in the Evaluation Report

When evaluating a client with Medicare Part B, each area that was assessed needs to be rated in severity with a G-code and severity modifier. However, because only one area can be reported as primary during treatment, the clinician must decide which of those areas will be primary. Typically, the area on which the most time will be spent in treatment, or the area on which treatment will have the biggest impact, is selected as primary. Only the current status and projected goal will be reported on the area that will be the primary focus of treatment. For all other areas assessed, the speech-language pathologist will report a current status, projected goal, and discharge status (CMS, n.d.-a).

Reporting Functional Outcomes When It Is Evaluation Only

There are several reasons the client might be seen for an evaluation only. Perhaps the evaluation did not reveal deficits that needed treatment, or there was not a prognosis for any improvement with treatment. Perhaps the client declined to pursue treatment or is going to receive treatment elsewhere. In any of these cases, the evaluating speech-language pathologist would report all three G-codes for each area assessed.

Preauthorization for Treatment

Some third-party payers, such as private insurance payers, some state Medicaid plans, and Medicare Part C plans, may require the speech-language pathologist to obtain a preauthorization for treatment. Each company may have a slightly different process and different forms that need to be completed. If the facility fails to obtain the preauthorization, the third-party payer is not obligated to reimburse for the services. In order to ensure minimum delay between the evaluation and the beginning of treatment, the speech-language pathologist will need to complete the evaluation

Table 14-3

G-Code Functional Reporting Areas

G-Code	Functional Area
G8996	Swallowing current
G8997	Swallowing projected
G8998	Swallowing discharge
G8999	Motor speech current
G9186	Motor speech projected
G9158	Motor speech discharge
G9159	Spoken lang comp current
G9160	Spoken lang comp projected
G9161	Spoken lang comp discharge
G9162	Spoken lang express current
G9163	Spoken lang express projected
G9164	Spoken lang express discharge
G9165	Attention current
G9166	Attention projected
G9167	Attention discharge
G9168	Memory current
G9169	Memory projected
G9170	Memory discharge
G9171	Voice current
G9172	Voice projected
G9173	Voice discharge
G9174	Other funct limit current
G9175	Other funct limit projected
G9176	Other funct limit discharge

Reprinted with permission from Centers for Medicare & Medicaid Services. (2017a). Descriptors of G-codes and modifiers for therapy functional reporting. Retrieved from https://www.cms.gov/Outreach-and-Education/Medicare-Learning-Network-MLN/MLNProducts/Downloads/G-Codes-Chart-908924.pdf

report and treatment plan in a timely way because these documents are sometimes requested along with the other required forms.

Treatment Plans, Certifications, and Recertifications

Chapter 7 provided information about the development of treatment plans. Treatment plans should be established in collaboration with the client and any caregivers, with a focus on function. The treatment plan outlines the long- and short-term goals of the planned intervention.

For Medicare patients, these treatment plans are called *certifications* and require the signature of the provider who ordered the services. At the time of the evaluation, the speech-language pathologist estimates the length of treatment that will be needed. This is the *certification period*, which can be established for a period of up to 90 days. At the end of that time, the clinician prepares an update on the goals, adds new goals as needed, and sends this document, then called a *recertification*, back to the physician for approval and signature for up to another 90 days.

Medicare is not the only payer that requires a recertification of services. Some private insurers and state Medicaid agencies require periodic reports and requests for more therapy visits.

Treatment Notes

Chapter 8 discussed treatment notes that can be completed for each session or perhaps once per week. In outpatient settings, it is typical for a treatment note to be written each time the client is seen. The note should conform to the requirements described in that chapter. The treatment note also typically lists the CPT code(s) that were billed for that session. The treatment codes typically used by speech-language pathologists are listed in Table 14-6. Most of these treatment codes are untimed, and most third-party payers reimburse a flat rate regardless of how long the session was. There are a few timed treatment codes, although certain payers may restrict their use. For example, some MACs do not reimburse for cognitive therapy. When using a timed treatment code, keep in mind the 8-minute rule to determine how many units of the code can be billed.

TABLE 14-4

SEVERITY MODIFIERS FOR G-CODES

MODIFIER	% SEVERITY LEVEL	SEVERITY LEVEL DESCRIPTOR	NOMS
CH	0%	Impaired, limited, or restricted	7
CI	1% to 19% impaired	At least 1% but < 20% impaired, limited, or restricted	6
CJ	20% to 39% impaired	At least 20% but < 40% impaired, limited, or restricted	5
CK	40% to 59% impaired	At least 40% but < 60% impaired, limited, or restricted	4
CL	60% to 79% impaired	At least 60% but < 80% impaired, limited, or restricted	3
CM	80% to 99% impaired	At least 80% but < 100% impaired, limited, or restricted	2
CN	100% impaired	100% impaired, limited, or restricted	1

Adapted from American Speech-Language-Hearing Association. (n.d.). National Outcomes Measurement System (NOMS). Retrieved from http://www.asha.org/NOMS/; Centers for Medicare & Medicaid Services. (2017a). Descriptors of G-codes and modifiers for therapy functional reporting. Retrieved from https://www.cms.gov/Outreach-and-Education/Medicare-Learning-Network-MLN/MLNProducts/Downloads/G-Codes-Chart-908924.pdf

Medicare 10th Visit Progress Report

Progress reports are required by the Medicare program at a minimum every 10th treatment. These reports and the plan of care will be used by medical reviewers and auditors to determine whether the services were medically necessary and skilled. The progress note and the daily visit/treatment note can be one and the same, but, if so, the note needs to clearly distinguish which information is the daily treatment note and which is the 10th visit. See Appendix 14-I for an example that combines a treatment note and 10th visit note.

The progress reports must contain the following:

- Who performed the treatment
- Assessment of improvement or the extent of progress made toward therapy goals, including objective measurements (e.g., standardized patient assessment tools, outcome measurement tools, measurable data that capture function)
- Information about need for continuing treatment and any revisions to the treatment plan
  - Changes to the long- or short-term goals
- Functional outcomes reporting
  - Current status
  - Goal status
  - Corresponding G-codes and severity modifier for the primary area (CMS, 2016)

These progress reports are the most logical place to report on the closure of one G-code (functional area) and the opening of another G-code (functional area). The progress report does not have to be done on the 10th visit. It can be done before that. For example, if you have treated the client for eight sessions with a focus on swallowing and want to begin reporting on motor speech, you could complete the progress note after the eighth visit and report projected goal and discharge status for the swallowing. Then, on the next treatment visit, you could report current status and projected goal for motor speech. You cannot report the closing of one functional area and the opening of another on the same date of service.

REHABILITATION VERSUS MAINTENANCE THERAPY NOTES

Most clients are receiving therapy services because improvement is expected. This would be described as *rehabilitative therapy* and suggests the client has the potential to improve with therapy. However, for some clients with a progressive or degenerative disorder, intermittent periods of therapy may be indicated to maintain skills or slow the deterioration. Different third-party payers may or may not reimburse such maintenance therapy, but Medicare will reimburse for these services if they are necessary to maintain, prevent, or slow deterioration of functional status and can only be provided safely and effectively with a skilled professional. Maintenance therapy that can be accomplished by the patient, caregiver, or unskilled professional should not be billed to the Medicare program. During each of the periods of maintenance therapy, a maintenance, or home, program should be established and then revised and updated so that the patient and caregiver can work to ensure optimal performance of the skills or generalize the skills (CMS, 2017b).

If the client being seen for maintenance therapy is covered by Medicare Part B, G-codes need to be reported. It is likely that the severity modifier for the current status and for the projected goal will be the same because no improvement is expected.

Table 14-5

When to Report G-Codes and Where to Document

Situation	Report Current Status	Report Projected Goal	Report Discharge Status	In What Documentation You Could Report the Functional Status With G-Codes
You evaluate the client in one area (e.g., receptive language) and plan to treat.	X	X		Evaluation report and/or the treatment plan (certification)
You evaluate the client in multiple areas (e.g., receptive language, expressive language, motor speech).	X	X	Report discharge on the areas that you will not primarily be reporting (you can be working on all of them)	Evaluation report and/or the treatment plan (certification)
You evaluate the client in one area or more areas but will not be treating at your facility.	X	X	X	Evaluation report
You evaluate the client in one or more areas, but you are not sure he or she will return to receive services at your facility.	X	X	X	Evaluation report
Client comes for first treatment visit at your facility	Report on the primary area you will work on	Report on the primary area you will work on		Treatment note or treatment plan (certification)
Client has been seen for 10 visits (can be fewer), and you plan to keep working on the same primary area	X	X		10th Visit Progress Note
Client has been seen for 10 visits (can be fewer) and you want to close this functional area and start reporting on another.		X	X	10th Visit Progress Note
Client's next visit when you start reporting the new area (even though you may have been working on it all along with the other area). The current status is as of this date, not the status when you first evaluated that area. *Note*: You cannot start reporting a new area on the same date of service you close the other area.	X	X		Treatment note
Client's treatment at your facility is completed.		X	X	Discharge summary or treatment note

Adapted from Satterfield, L.. & Swanson, N. (2016). *Medicare survival guide for audiologists and speech-language pathologists*. Rockville, MD: ASHA Press.

Table 14-6

Speech-Language Pathology Treatment Current Procedural Terminology Codes

CPT Code	Description	Notes
92507	Treatment of speech, language, voice, communication, and/or auditory processing disorder; individual	Not timed
92508	Group, two or more individuals	Not timed
92526	Treatment of swallowing dysfunction and/or oral function for feeding	Not timed
92606	Therapeutic service(s) for the use of non–speech-generating device, including programming and modification	Not timed; not reimbursed by Medicare
92609	Therapeutic services for the use of speech-generating device, including programming and modification	Not timed
92630	Auditory rehabilitation; prelingual hearing loss	Not timed; not reimbursed by Medicare
92633	Postlingual hearing loss	Not timed; not reimbursed by Medicare
97532	Development of cognitive skills to improve attention, memory, problem solving (includes compensatory training), direct (one-on-one) patient contact by the provider	Each 15 minutes
97533	Sensory integrative techniques to enhance sensory processing and promote adaptive responses to environmental demands, direct (one-on-one) patient contact by the provider	Each 15 minutes
97535	Self-care/home management training (e.g., activities of daily living and compensatory training, meal preparation, safety procedures, and instructions in use of assistive technology devices/adaptive equipment), direct one-on-one contact by provider	Each 15 minutes

Adapted from American Speech-Language-Hearing Association. (n.d.) Medicare CPT coding rules for speech-language pathology services. Retrieved from https://www.asha.org/practice/reimbursement/medicare/SLP_coding_rules/

Discharge Summaries

Chapter 9 addressed discharge summaries. Completing a discharge summary for any outpatient seen should be standard practice. The document provides a snapshot of the intervention provided and the client's response to the treatment.

Reporting Functional Outcomes at Discharge

For clients with Medicare Part B, the functional area that was last being reported needs to be closed. The clinician would report the projected goal and the discharge status on that functional area. Sometimes clients drop out of therapy, and it is not possible for the speech-language pathologist to accurately rate the discharge status. Also, there is not a visit to which those discharge ratings can be attached. Therefore, reporting of G-codes at discharge is not required but should be completed whenever possible.

Follow-Up After Discharge

Many outpatient settings establish a process for scheduled follow-up for certain patients. For example, for patients with a degenerative condition like Alzheimer's disease or amyotrophic lateral sclerosis, scheduling the follow-up visits can be done at the time of discharge. The client or caregiver can always be encouraged to contact the clinic sooner if communication or swallowing skills change more rapidly than anticipated. The follow-up plan can be reported in the discharge summary. Perhaps routine calls, for example every 2 to 3 months, will be scheduled. Those calls should be documented and included in the client's record. Appendix 14-J provides an outpatient case example of Medicare Part B with functional outcomes reporting.

References

American Speech-Language-Hearing Association. (n.d.). National Outcomes Measurement System (NOMS). Retrieved from http://www.asha.org/NOMS/

Centers for Medicare & Medicaid Services. (n.d.-a). Functional reporting: PT, OT, and SLP frequently asked questions (FAQs).Retrieved from https://www.cms.gov/medicare/billing/therapyservices/downloads/functional-reporting-pt-ot-slp-services-faq.pdf

Centers for Medicare & Medicaid Services. (n.d.-b). National Coverage Determinations (NCDs) alphabetical index. Retrieved from https://www.cms.gov/medicare-coverage-database/indexes/ncd-alphabetical-index.aspx?bc=BAAAAAAAAAAA

Centers for Medicare & Medicaid Services. (2015). Medicare advance written notices off noncoverage. Retrieved from https://www.cms.gov/Outreach-and-Education/Medicare-Learning-Network-MLN/MLNProducts/downloads/abn_booklet_icn006266.pdf

Centers for Medicare & Medicaid Services. (2016). IMPACT Act: Connecting post-acute care across the care continuum [Training presentation]. Retrieved from https://www.cms.gov/Medicare/Quality-Initiatives-Patient-Assessment-Instruments/HomeHealthQualityInits/HHQIQualityMeasures.html

Centers for Medicare & Medicaid Services. (2017a). Descriptors of G-codes and modifiers for therapy functional reporting. Retrieved from https://www.cms.gov/Outreach-and-Education/Medicare-Learning-Network-MLN/MLNProducts/Downloads/G-Codes-Chart-908924.pdf

Centers for Medicare & Medicaid Services. (2017b). Medicare Benefit Policy Manual: Chapter 15—Covered medical and other health services. Retrieved from https://www.cms.gov/Regulations-and-Guidance/Guidance/Manuals/downloads/bp102c15.pdf

Centers for Medicare & Medicaid Services. (2017c). Medicare home health benefit. Retrieved from https://www.cms.gov/Outreach-and-Education/Medicare-Learning-Network-MLN/MLNProducts/Downloads/Home-Health-Benefit-Fact-Sheet-ICN908143.pdf

Martin-Harris, B. (2010). *Modified Barium Swallow Impairment Profile* [Assessment tool]. Gaylord, MI: Northern Speech Services.

Satterfield, L., & Swanson, N. (2016). *Medicare survival guide for audiologists and speech-language pathologists.* Rockville, MD: ASHA Press.

Suggested Reading

Centers for Medicare & Medicaid Services. (2016). Medicare quality initiatives: Patient assessment instruments. Retrieved from https://www.cms.gov/Medicare/Quality-initiatives-patient-assessment-instruments/hospital-value-based-purchasing/index.html

Review Questions

1. What is the difference between a Medicare NCD and LCD?
2. What are two strategies for streamlining documentation if an EHR is not being used?
3. Explain Medicare functional outcomes reporting. What is the stated purpose? Give an example of what you would report after an evaluation in which client will not be seen for treatment.
4. What is the difference in a treatment note and a 10th visit progress report? For what payer is the 10th visit progress report required?
5. Explain the 8-minute rule and give an example of a speech-language pathologist evaluation code where this would apply.

Activity A

Using Appendices 14-A through 14-C as examples, select one of the disorders listed here and develop a case history/intake form or an interview form with questions specific to that disorder:

- Acquired motor speech disorder: Apraxia
- Dysphagia secondary to head and neck cancer
- Motor speech/voice: Parkinson's disease
- Fluency
- Aphasia following CVA

Activity B

For each of the following assessments, determine which CPT evaluation code would be most accurate. If it is a timed code, indicate how many units would be charged.

What Was Done	Payer	Which Code(s) to Use
22-year-old with moderate fluency disorder. Seen for 75 minutes for evaluation of fluency. Hearing screening performed.	Private insurance has authorized the evaluation	
65-year-old with early cognitive impairment. 70 minutes spent administering standardized cognitive tests. Additional 35 minutes scoring and writing report.	Medicare Part B	
45-year-old new-onset voice disorder. Evaluated voice with in-depth interview and clinical tasks. Then completed acoustic and aerodynamic measures and screened hearing.	Private insurance	
72-year-old with confusion and declining memory and word retrieval deficits. In denial about deficits, so used informal methods of evaluation and interview with patient's daughter. Spent 75 minutes with patient and daughter and additional 25 minutes in writing report. Screened hearing.	Medicare Part B	
81-year-old status post-CVA. Evaluated motor speech as has moderate apraxia. This took 20 minutes. Then spent 40 minutes more with patient assessing aphasia and additional 20 analyzing and writing report. Declined hearing screening as has hearing aids.	Medicare Part B	

APPENDIX 14-A

Mild Cognitive Impairment Case History Form

Caregiver Case History Form

Memory Clinic

Contact Information:

Patient name: ______________________ Name of caregiver completing form: ______________________

Birth date: ______________________ Relationship to patient: ______________________

Address: ______________________ Address: ______________________

Phone: ______________________ Phone: ______________________

Current Living Situation:

Where does the patient currently live? ______________________

____

____

Who lives with the patient? ______________________

____

____

How long has the patient been in this current living situation? ______________________

____

____

If the patient lives alone, what kind of support is provided (e.g., stopping by to check in, preparing meals)? ______________________

____

____

Medical History:

Current medical diagnoses: ______________________

____

____

Current medications (if it is easier, you can attach a copy of the medication list): ______________________

____

____

Any history of surgeries in the head or neck region? Please provide years: ______________________

____

____

Can the patient independently manage medications? ______________________

____

____

Does the patient have any swallowing difficulty? If yes, please describe: ______________________

Does the patient have any hearing or vision difficulties? If yes, are hearing aids and/or glasses used? ______

When did you first notice changes in the patient's thinking, memory, or behavior? Please describe: ______

Has the patient ever gotten lost? Please describe: ______________________

Is the patient easily distracted or having difficulty paying attention? ______________________

Does the patient have trouble remembering new information? Please describe: ______________________

Daily Life:

If the patient cooked, grocery shopped, or completed household chores in the past, can he or she now? ______

If the patient read in the past, is he or she able to now? ______________________

Can the patient keep finances in order? Is this a change? ______________________

What is the patient's current activity level? Exercise? Please describe: ______________________

Is the patient involved in any social or community activities? How many days per week? ______________________

Doe the patient drive? If no, how long has it been since he or she stopped? ______________________

Does the patient ever block on a word and is unable come up with it? ____________________

____

____

Does the patient initiate conversation or just respond to questions? Is the patient becoming quieter? ____________________

____

____

Is the patient more passive now, letting other people make decisions and initiate activities? ____________________

____

____

Is the patient aware of the changes in his or her memory? ____________________

____

____

Have you noticed any significant mood changes lately? If so, please describe. ____________________

____

____

What are the patient's sleep patterns like? About many hours of sleep per night? Napping during the day? ____________________

____

____

Is there anything else you want to tell us about the patient? ____________________

____

____

Please list any question you hope we will answer during the visit: ____________________

____

____

APPENDIX 14-B
Voice Case History Form

Adult Client Voice Case History

Name: ______________________ Birthdate: ______________________

Address: ______________________

____

Home phone: ______________________ Work/cell phone: ______________________

Emergency contact (name, relationship, phone number): ______________________

____

Place of employment: ______________________

Occupation: ______________________

Education completed: ______________________

Evaluation by referring MD: ______________________

Date(s) of evaluation(s): ______________________

Results (what did the doctor say about your throat and larynx?): ______________________

____

____

Why did the doctor send you to see us? ______________________

____

____

Current medications (especially for reflux, allergies/drainage): ______________________

____

____

Significant medical diagnoses/conditions: ______________________

____

____

Significant operative/invasive procedures: ______________________

____

____

Have you had any therapy for your voice in the past? ______________________

____

____

Please answer these questions to provide more information about your voice:

What changes have you noticed in your voice? ______________________________

When did you first notice these changes? ______________________________

Was it a sudden change or did it happen gradually? ______________________________

Is there anything you can think of that caused these changes? ______________________________

Has your voice gotten worse, better, or stayed the same since you first noticed these changes? ______________________________

Is your voice better in the morning or later in the day? ______________________________

Does your vocal quality get worse the more you use the voice or stay the same? ______________________________

Is there anything you do that makes your voice better? ______________________________

Is your voice affected by stress? ______________________________

If you rest your voice, does it then sound better for a while? ______________________________

How do you use your voice on a typical day?

- Recreational/church/semiprofessional singing? ______________________________
- Excessive phone talking? ______________________________
- Yelling/shouting at sporting events or with family/children? ______________________________
- Voice use for job/profession? ______________________________

How much water do you drink per day? ______________________________

How much caffeine do you intake per day? ______________________________

Do you smoke or have you smoked in the past? ______________________________

- If you smoked in the past, how long ago did you quit? ______________________________
- If you smoke presently, how much do you smoke per day? ______________________________

Do you consume alcohol? How much per day? ______________________________

Do you experience tightness, tension, soreness, etc. when using your voice? ______________________________

Do you experience shortness of breath or run out of air when using your voice? ______________________________

Do you have difficulties with seasonal allergies, excess mucus, or postnasal drip? ______________________________

Is there anything else you want to tell us about your voice? ______________________________

APPENDIX 14-C

Interview Form for Client Presenting With Voice Symptoms

Patient name: ______________________ Date completed: ______________

Speech-language pathologist: ______________________________

Voice Disorders Interview/Questionnaire

General History Voice (referral/start/sudden/event/better/first time/how long problem in past/treated how?)

____

____

____

____

____

____

____

How do you feel? Excellent, Good, Fair, Poor ______________________________

Medical (hospitalization)/surgical history/current medications/recent changes?

____

____

____

____

____

Chronic problems: Y N

Colds Sinus Allergies Chronic obstructive pulmonary disease Headaches

Thyroid Blood pressure Heart/circulatory Lung Diabetes

Kidney Liver Bladder Arthritis

Neurological? (Tremor, stroke, epilepsy, etc.)

Anxiety/depression: 0 1 2 3 4 5 6 7 8 9 10

1. Dysphonia/Voice/Care of Voice

Increased effort? ______________________ Speaking: Little Moderate Lot

Fatigues? ______________________ Singer? Y N

Range: ______________________

Voice loss? ______________________

Abuses/talk over noise: ______________________

Variability? ______________________ Cough: Dry/productive; throat clearing

What makes voice worse/better? ______________________________

Fluid consumption:

Water ____________ Coffee ____________ Tea ____________ Soda ____________ Alcohol ____________

Juice ____________ Milk ____________

Situations in which voice used:

Throat pain/discomfort: 0 1 2 3 4 5 6 7 8 9 10

Location: ______________________________

Other sensations: Dryness, tickle, phlegm, lump, tightness, scratchy, raw, post nasal drip.

Examiner rating voice quality: Mild Moderate Severe

Quality: ______________________________

Pitch: ______________________________

Loudness: ______________________________

2. Dysphagia

How long?: ______________________________

Worse with: liquids solids Swallow study? Modified Barium Swallow (MBS)/FEES

Food sticking? Y N When/where? ____________________

Coughing? Y N After meals/generally? ____________________

Choking? Y N After meals/only occasionally? ____________________

Regurge? Y N Whole? Y N

Pneumonia? ____________ Weight loss? ____________________

Reflux diagnosis? Y N

Meds? Y N How long? ______________________________

Probe questions: Heartburn, sour taste, lump in throat, regurgitation? Certain types of foods?

3. Airway

Shortness of air: Y N

Asthma? Y N Had a Pulmonary Function Test? Y N When? ____________________

Results: ______________________________

Inhalers? Y N Do they help? ____________________ Last use? ____________________

Sleep apnea? (Continuous Positive Airway Pressure or Bilevel Positive Airway Pressure) Y N ____________

COPD? Y N

Allergies? Y N Testing? ______________________________

When? ______________________________

Sinus? Y N Tests? CT? ______________________________

Bronchitis? ______________________________

Current Smoker? Y N How much? ____________________

If quit, when and how much and how long as past smoker? ____________________

Chronic cough: barking, honking, brassy, self-propagating, loose, productive, non-productive

How often? ______________________________________

spells per day? ____________________ Triggers? ____________________

Time of day/night? ____________________ What makes better/worse? ____________________

If responses indicate possible paradoxical vocal fold motion, continue:

4. Paradoxical Vocal Fold Movement

When? ____________________ Wheezing? Inhale/Exhale ____________________

Activities? ____________________ Stridor? Inhale/Exhale ____________________

Chemicals/perfumes/grass? ____________________ Tightness? Chest/Throat ____________________

How long episodes last? ____________________ Harder to get air in/out ____________________

What makes it better/worse? ____________________ Wake up at night? Cough/Choke ____________________

APPENDIX 14-D
Template for Voice Report

Speech-Language Pathology Outpatient Evaluation
Voice Disorder

Patient name: ______________________ Date of Evaluation: ______________

Address: ______________________ Start time patient contact: ______________

______________________ Stop Time patient contact: ______________

______________________ Analysis/report writing: ______________

Birthdate: __________ Age: __________ Patient#: ______________

Referral: ______________________ Procedure codes: ______________

Medical history related to referral: ______________________

Medications: ______________________

Reason for referral: ______________________

Patient-reported symptoms:

Vocal effort: ______________________

Fatigue: ______________________

Variability: ______________________

Throat clearing/cough: ______________________

Pain level (0 mild–10 severe): ______________________

Throat sensations: ______________________

Reflux: ______________________

Dysphagia: ______________________

Dyspnea: ______________________

Smoking history: ______________________

Liquid intake: ______________________

Chronic health problems reported: ______________________

The patient completed the **Voice Handicap Index (VHI)**, which provides information about how the voice problem affects daily activities. A VHI score of 0 to 30 represents a low score and indicates minimal handicap associated with the voice disorder. A score of 31 to 60 indicates a moderate amount of handicap. These scores are often observed in people with injuries to the vocal folds. A VHI score of 60 to 120 indicates a significant and serious amount of handicap due to the voice problem. These scores are often seen in patients with new-onset vocal fold paralysis or severe vocal fold dysfunction.

Functional ( ); Physical ( ); Emotional ( ) Total =

This patient demonstrates the most effect in the ______________ aspect of the VHI.

The patient completed the **Reflux Symptom Index (RSI)**, which provides information about how various symptoms of reflux may be affecting the patient's daily life. An RSI greater than 10 is considered to be abnormal. The patient's RSI was a total of __________. The patient especially noted the following:

The clinician completed the **Consensus Auditory-Perceptual Evaluation of Voice** during spontaneous speech. The Consensus Auditory-Perceptual Evaluation of Voice aids the clinician in rating the quality of a patient's voice based on how the patient's voice sounds. The patient's voice quality is rated on several different parameters.

Severity rating: Consistent or inconsistent:

Overall severity: ______________________________

Roughness: ______________________________

Breathiness: ______________________________

Strain: ______________________________

Pitch: ______________________________

Loudness: ______________________________

Voice was characterized as: ______________________________

____

____

Laryngeal function studies (acoustic and aerodynamic):

The Visi-Pitch was used to record acoustic information about the voice that could be analyzed for planning voice treatment. Aerodynamic measures were also obtained.

TASK	FUNDAMENTAL FREQUENCY	RANGE	NORMATIVE DATA	INTERPRETATION

Acoustic and aerodynamic measures indicate: ______________________________

Hearing acuity: ______________________________

Screening for other communication deficits: ______________________________

Diagnosis/ICD-10 code: ______________________________

Summary: ______________________________

Recommendations: ______________________________

Medical necessity: ______________________________

Frequency/duration of treatment: ______________________________

Prognosis: ______________________________

Discussed probable outcomes of treatment with: ______________________________

____

____

Speech-Language Pathologist: ______________________________

CC:

Date sent:

Appendix 14-E
Template for Mild Cognitive Impairment/Memory

Speech-Language Pathology Outpatient Evaluation

Mild Cognitive Impairment/Memory

Patient name: ______________________ Date of evaluation: ______________

Address: ______________________ Start time patient contact: ______________

______________________ Stop time patient contact: ______________

______________________ Analysis/report writing: ______________

Birthdate: ____________ Age: ____________ Patient #: ______________

Referral: ______________________ Procedure codes: ______________

Medical history related to referral: ______________________

Reason for referral: ______________________

Patient's stated concerns regarding memory: ______________________

Family's stated concerns regarding memory: ______________________

The following tests were administered: ______________________

______ Repeatable Battery for Neurocognitive Status Update

______ Function, Reason, Orientation, Memory, Arithmetic, Judgment, and Emotional

Mental Status Guide ______ Geriatric Depression Scale Short Form______

Other: ______________________

Behavioral observations: ______________________

Clinical findings: ______________________

Hearing acuity: Patient denies difficulty with hearing. Hearing was within functional limits for conversation.

Summary: ______________________

Screening for other communication/swallowing disorders:

Diagnosis/ICD-10 code: ______________________

Recommendations: ______________________

Medical necessity: ______________________

Frequency/duration of treatment: ______________________

Prognosis: ______________________

Discussed probable outcomes of treatment with: ______________________

____

Speech-Language Pathologist: ______________________

CC:

Date sent:

Appendix 14-F

Report Template Using Appendix/Addendum

Modified Barium Swallow

Patient name: ______________________ Patient #: ______________________

Birth date: ______________________ Age: ______________________

Address: ______________________ Referring physician: ______________________

____

____

______________________ CPT: ______________________

Phone: ______________________

ICD-10: ______________________

Date of study: ______________________ Start: ______________________

Diagnosis/history pertinent to dysphagia:

Reason study needed: The patient has dysphagia (R13.10), with the following complaints indicating possible pharyngeal involvement.

Summary: The patient was administered a standardized MBS following the Modified Barium Swallowing Impairment Profile (MBSImP) protocol and scoring. The patient was given thin liquid, nectar, pudding, and cookie coated with pudding in lateral and anterior-posterior (A-P) views. Specific MBSImP scores can be found in the addendum. The patient was seen by the speech-language pathologist and radiology physician's assistant for the study.

Oropharyngeal swallowing skills noted during this exam. Initiation of swallow response for all consistencies for patient's age and gender penetration or aspiration was noted during this evaluation. There was residue in the hypopharynx.

Radiology physician's assistant screened esophageal phase in upright position and noted *Please see radiology report for further details.*

Diagnosis:

Patient/significant other teaching: The results of the evaluation were discussed with the patient, who understood/did not understand.

Medicare outcomes reporting

G 8996 Current status	
G 8997 Goal status	
G 8998 Discharge status	

Positive expectation to begin treatment:

Recommendations:

Speech-language pathologist: ______________________

CC:

Date sent:

Modified Barium Swallow Impairment Profile:

The following table reflects the standardized MBS following the MBSImP (Martin-Harris, 2010) protocol and scoring developed by Bonnie Martin-Harris, PhD, CCC-SLP, BRS-S. The MBSImP provides a reliable way to score 17 individual physiologic components of the oral, pharyngeal, and esophageal phases of swallowing. An overall impression score is given for each component, rated on the worst performance on the component. That is, the patient may have done better with a specific texture on a component, but the score assigned reflects the highest level of impairment with any texture. Components that were significantly impaired and contributed to the functional deficits are described here.

MBSImP Impaired Physiology	OI
Lip closure (0–4) *thin*	
Tongue control during bolus hold (0–3) *thin; cued to hold*	
Bolus prep/mastication (0–3) *pudding/solid*	
Bolus transport/lingual motion (0–4) *pudding/solid*	
Oral residue (0–4) *pudding/solid*	
Initiation of pharyngeal swallow (0–4) *thin*	
Soft palate elevation (0–4) *thin*	
Laryngeal elevation (0–3) *thin*	
Anterior hyoid movement (0–2) *thin*	
Epiglottic movement (0–2) *thin*	
Laryngeal vestibular closure (0–2) *thin*	
Pharyngeal stripping wave (0–2) *thin*	
Pharyngeal contraction (0–3) *nectar A-P*	
Pharyngoesophageal segment opening (0–3) *thin*	
Tongue base retraction (0–4) *pudding/solid*	
Pharyngeal residue (0–4) *pudding/solid*	
Esophageal clearance upright (0–4) *nectar A-P or oblique*	
0 indicates skills are within normal limits	
Adapted from Martin-Harris, B. (2010). Modified Barium Swallow Impairment Profile [Assessment tool]. Gaylord, MI: Northern Speech Services.	

Appendix 14-G

Outpatient Evaluation Template With International Classification of Functioning, Disability and Health *Categories and G-Code Reporting*

Speech-Language Pathology

Name: ____________ Gender: ____________ Patient ID number: ____________

Date of birth: ____________ Referral source: ____________

Age: ____________ Physician(s): ____________

Spouse: ____________ Date of evaluation: ____________

Time in/out: ____________

Address: ____________

Telephone: ____________

Background information related to referral (including health condition): ____________

Reason for referral: ____________

Tests given/sources/measures used (see scores and comments attached):

____ Behavioral checklist:

____ Standardized tests:

____ Client/caregiver interview:

____ Observation:

Clinical findings (including body structure and function): ____________

Impact on activities and participation: ____________

Hearing screening: ____________

Diagnosis/ICD-10 code(s): ____________

Impressions: ____________

Functional Outcomes Reporting Primary Area (ASHA NOMS FCMs used to determine modifier)

G-Code for Functional Area		Modifier
G	Current status	
G	Goal status	

Functional Outcomes Reporting Other Area(s) Assessed (ASHA NOMS FCMs used to determine modifier)

ASHA NOMS FCM:

G-Code for Functional Area		Modifier
G	Current status	
G	Goal status	
G	Discharge status	

Prognosis: ____

Personal and environmental factors impacting prognosis: ____________________

Recommendations: ____

Frequency/duration of treatment: ________________________________

Speech-language pathologist signature, title, degree(s), credentials: ________________

CC: Referral source

Physician(s)

Appendix 14-H
Treatment Plan With G-Codes

Speech-Language Pathology
Treatment Plan (Certification)/Recertification/Discharge Summary

Patient name: ____________________

Patient #: ____________________

Medical diagnosis/ICD-10: ____________________

Problem areas to be addressed: ____________________

Date treatment initiated: ____________

Estimated amount, frequency, and duration of treatment: ____________________

Reasonable expectation to meet treatment goals: Good

Date of report: ____________

Medicare outcomes reporting by ASHA NOMS FCM:

G-Code for Functional Area		Modifier
G	Current status	
G	Goal status	

Long-term functional goal(s):

Date Established	Speech Therapy/Swallowing Therapy for Short-Term Goals in Functional/Measurable Terms	Progress/Date

Speech-language pathologist: ____________________

Date:

Outpatient Certification

1. The speech-language pathology services are, or were, furnished while the patient was under a physician's care.
2. A plan for furnishing such services is, or was, established by the speech-language pathologist and periodically reviewed by a physician.
3. The speech-language pathology services are, or were, reasonable and necessary for the treatment of the patient.

Referring physician signature ____________________ Date: ________ Time: ______

CC:

Date sent:

Appendix 14-I

Combined Treatment Note and 10th Visit Progress Note

Speech-Language Pathology
Treatment Note

Patient: D'Ron Summer   Patient #: XXXX

Date: 7/14/16   Time: 1330-1410

CPT: 92507

S: Patient reported that his voice use was typical over the past week. Patient also stated that his wife thinks it's easier to understand him/voice is louder.

O: Vocal function exercises: The CD of vocal function exercises was used as a model. The exercises were completed at the following levels.

E/F: 9 sec/10 sec: Patient was able to sustain the sound "eee" on musical note F with a nasal/front focus for 9 seconds on trial 1 and 10 seconds on trial 2. Correct placement achieved with moderate cues. Patient encouraged to perform this exercise as loudly as possible.

Stretching (low to high): Correct placement achieved with moderate cues. Patient encouraged to perform this exercise as loudly as possible. Patient utilized the word "whoop."

Contracting (high to low): Correct placement achieved with min-mod cues. Patient encouraged to perform this exercise as loudly as possible. Patient utilized the word "boom."

The patient sustained the following musical notes on the word "knoll" with a lip buzz. Two trials were elicited. Speech-language pathologist modified cues and then patient achieved correct placement.

C: Not timed; focused on "think loud" and "front focus"

D: Not timed; focused on "think loud" and "front focus"

E: Not timed; focused on "think loud" and "front focus"

F: 8 sec/9 sec

G: 9 sec/10 sec

A: Patient was responsive to feedback and the clinician answered questions regarding home therapy program. Clinician provided instruction re: pairing adequate diaphragmatic breath with front focus for longer production of sounds.

P: Next therapy session is scheduled for next Thursday. Clinician will continue to instruct in vocal function exercises and will provide further instruction re: diaphragmatic breathing as needed.

10th Visit Progress Report

Patient has received nine therapy visits since the initial voice evaluation. Progress on goals:

Date Established	Goals and Treatment Objectives	Progress/Date 07-14-16
06-02-16	1. Patient will institute vocal hygiene techniques:	1. Achieved with consistent adequate fluid intake and very infrequent cough.
	a. Increase current water intake	
	b. Substitute hard swallow or silent cough for throat clear	
	2. Patient will reduce hyperfunctional use of the vocal mechanism via:	
	a. Improved use of diaphragmatic breathing in conjunction with home exercise program	a. States he is practicing daily
	b. Improved use of diaphragmatic breathing in conjunction with connected speech	b. Uses diaphragmatic breathing consistently with cues when standing
	c. Reducing tension in oropharyngeal area	c. Needs more practice when seated
	d. Increased glottal closure in conjunction with voice use	d./e. Use of vocal function exercises has been very successful, with patient demonstrating significantly decreased tension and clearly engaged vocal fold closure with exercises
	e. Improved tone focus for easy phonation	
	f. Patient will be able to project voice over noise using appropriate breath support	f. 80% successful in structured situations
	3. Patient will monitor symptoms of gastroesophageal reflux disease (GERD)/laryngopharyngeal reflux (LPR) and will consult physician re: medical management of GERD/LPR if RSI does not decrease in 4 to 6 weeks	3./4. Patient reported significant reduction in symptoms with behavioral management and thus did not discuss with physician.
	4. Patient will utilize behavioral management of GERD/LPR symptoms	

Medicare Outcomes Reporting:

G 9171 Current status	CI
G 9172 Goal status	CH
G 9173 Discharge status	

Recommendations:

1. Patient needs to continue treatment on voice therapy goals. Focus will be on extending use of techniques to conversational speech and to different situations with varied background noise.

Speech-language pathologist: Luis Larynx, MS, CCC-SLP

CC: E. Nose, MD

Appendix 14-J
Adult Outpatient With Medicare Part B Case Example

Date	Actions	Billed and Coded	Documented
March 25	74-year-old with Parkinson's disease with recent-onset memory impairment and reduced reasoning skills referred. Physician has also requested an assessment of vocal quality. Has Medicare Part B. No preauthorization required, so evaluation is scheduled.		Case history form specific to Parkinson's and additional form for memory sent to patient.
April 5 Visit #1	Evaluation of cognitive skills completed. Spent 55 minutes assessing cognition with standardized testing instruments. Another 40 minutes in interpreting and writing the report. Voice evaluation completed after the cognitive testing was finished. These codes are untimed, but the total time on the report should reflect that two areas were assessed. The voice evaluation included both the behavioral and qualitative analysis through obtaining case history and detailed information on voice use and also laryngeal function studies utilizing the Visi-Pitch. Data entered into NOMS national database for voice and memory (unlike G-codes/functional outcomes reporting, in NOMS, any area being addressed is scored with FCM). *Note*: If a hearing screening had been done, cannot bill for the hearing screening because Medicare does not reimburse for screening.	CPT codes for evaluation: 92520 Laryngeal function studies 92524 Behavioral and qualitative analysis of voice and resonance 96125 Standardized cognitive performance assessment (2 of this code billed: 60 minutes spent = billing 1 code; additional 35 minutes justifies the second code). Note: These G-codes and modifiers are listed on the bill with either \$0.00 or \$0.01 (but no reimbursement is given; the \$ amount is needed to show on the bill).	Decision made to focus first on memory, so G-code for that functional area reported only in current and projected. Facility participates in NOMS, so FCMs used to rate severity. Current G 9168 CJ Projected G 9169 CI As voice was also assessed but will not be first focus in treatment; report all three G-codes: Current G 9171 CJ Projected G 9172 CI Discharge G 9173 CJ Current and discharge are rated the same severity. The evaluation counts as #1 session of the first 10 visits. The evaluation report showed time in as 1000 and time out as 1245 and noted that 35 minutes was spent after the session in interpretation and report writing for the cognitive codes. Report included clear headers to indicate the different areas evaluated. Treatment plan/certification developed to reflect goals for both memory and voice and period of 90 days listed as certification period. April 5 to July 5. Document sent to ordering provider for signature.

Date	Actions	Billed and Coded	Documented
April 8 Visit #2	Treatment with client and partner for memory. Session lasted 35 minutes.	97532 Development of cognitive skills x2	Treatment note in SOAP (subjective, objective, assessment, plan) format
April 14 Visit #3	Treatment with client and partner for memory. Session lasted 50 minutes.	97532 Development of cognitive skills x3	Treatment note in SOAP format
April 19 Visit #4	Treatment with client and partner for memory. Session lasted 50 minutes. Client and partner are utilizing strategies taught. Speech-language pathologist, client, and partner agree to change focus to working on voice/volume. The memory strategies will continue to be reinforced, and perhaps new ones taught, but for functional outcomes reporting the work will be considered closed. *Note*: The speech-language pathologist could do a 10th visit progress note now or can report the G-codes in the treatment note, which is what she decided to do. Cannot open the G-code for voice functional area in the same visit.	97532 Development of cognitive skills x3	Treatment note in SOAP format G-codes need to be reported to close the work on memory. Current G 9168 CJ Projected G 9169 CI Discharge CI
April 25 Visit #5	Lee Silverman Voice Technique (LSVT) treatment initiated. 50-minute session.	92507 Individual therapy (untimed code)	Treatment note G-codes for voice Current G 9171 CJ Projected G 9172 CI
April 26 Visit #6	LSVT treatment session. 50 minutes.	92507	Treatment note
April 27 Visit #7	LSVT treatment session. 50 minutes.	92507	Treatment note
April 28 Visit #8	LSVT treatment session. 50 minutes. Reinforced memory strategies.	92507	Treatment note
May 2 Visit #9	LSVT treatment session. 50 minutes.	92507	Treatment note

DATE	ACTIONS	BILLED AND CODED	DOCUMENTED
May 3 Visit #10	LSVT treatment session. 50 minutes.	92507	Treatment note Because this is the 10th visit, a Progress Report needs to be completed as well. The progress report should summarize the improvement with memory and the work done on voice. The voice G-codes are reported. The current status has not changed since reported on April 25, and goal remains the same. Current G 9171 CJ Projected G 9172 CI
May 4 Visit #1	LSVT treatment session. 50 minutes.	92507	Treatment note
May 5 Visit #2	LSVT treatment session. 50 minutes. Added a new memory strategy	92507	Treatment note
May 9 Visit #3	LSVT treatment session. 50 minutes.	92507	Treatment note
May 10 Visit #4	LSVT treatment session. 50 minutes.	92507	Treatment note
May 11 Visit #5	LSVT treatment session. 75 minutes. However, client reports that the distance traveled to treatment is more than they can handle and indicates that he will have to discontinue treatment. Additional time spent with client and partner outlining home program they can follow to maintain gains and hopefully see more improvement. NOMS discharge information entered into national data base.	92507 (just because the session is longer, you can't bill anymore because this is an untimed code). 97535 Home Management might seem an appropriate code to use, but the MAC does not allow that code to be used by speech-language pathologists.	Treatment note Copy of home program Discharge summary Information needs to be provided on both the memory goals and the work on voice with LSVT. G-code for voice needs to be reported to close it. Even though client has not completed the recommended course of treatment, he has improved on severity level. Projected G 9172 CI Discharge G 9173 CI

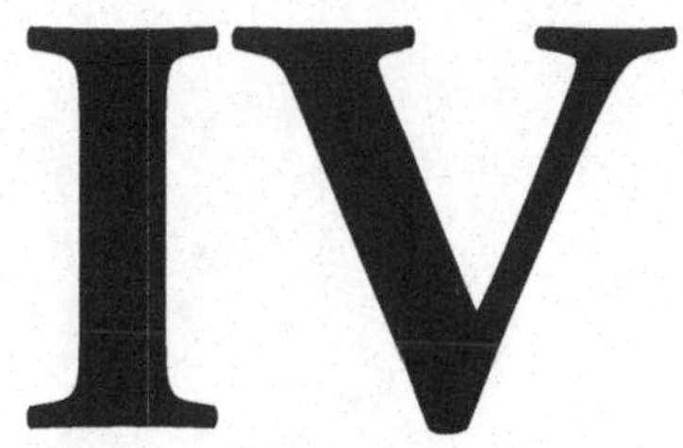

Documentation and Reimbursement in Pediatric Settings

The chapters in Section I of this book provided the basics of documentation. Section II described documenting the different types of services, with the focus mostly on health care. Sections III and IV delve into the specifics of documentation and reimbursement in specific settings. Section III addressed five different settings in adult health care: Acute care, inpatient rehabilitation, skilled nursing facilities, home health, and outpatient settings (e.g., hospital outpatient departments, clinics, private practices).

Section IV focuses on documentation and reimbursement in pediatric settings:

- Early intervention (birth to 3 years)
- Schools
- Outpatient settings

The majority of this book focuses on documentation in health care settings (i.e., any setting except schools). Chapter 16 is focused entirely on documentation in the school setting. The rules, forms, and processes in schools are very different than in any health care setting.

Each chapter in this section is authored by speech-language pathologists who have extensive experience practicing in those settings. The chapters will reinforce the basics from Section I and the types of services covered in Section II but will go into more depth about the particular requirements in that setting. You will find information on the following:

- Documentation requirements in that setting (from evaluation to discharge)
- Tips on how to document efficiently
- Basics of reimbursement for clients/patients in that setting and how reimbursement rules impact documentation in that setting
- Any tips on coding (diagnostic and/or procedural)
- Examples of evaluation, treatment plans (including examples of long- and short-term goals for some typical disorders), progress notes, discharge summaries, and any specific outcomes tools or other forms that must be filled out
- A case history example from each setting to help you understand the coding, reimbursement, and documentation rules

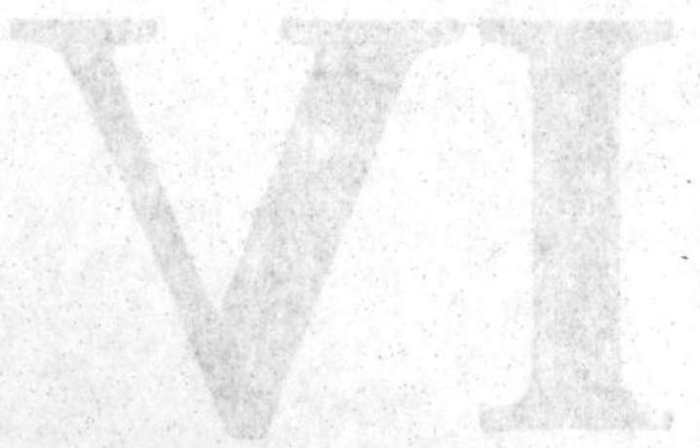

15

Early Intervention (0 to 3 Years)

Karyn Lewis Searcy, MA, CCC-SLP

Individuals with Disabilities Education Act Part C

History

Early intervention for children with communication deficits is currently available through many facilities throughout the United States, but few resources were available prior to 1950. In the 1960s, civil rights advocates worked beside parents to promote federal legislation for early intervention. Research emerged in the late 60s and early 70s that revealed better long-term success related to earlier access to treatment. Further, evidence emerged indicating that families who were directly involved in the intervention process learned to become stronger advocates for their children (Derrington, Kelly, Shapiro, & Smith, 2003). Although specific treatment techniques are critical skills for speech-language pathologists to establish, families also benefit from working with therapists who can efficiently direct them to funding sources and empower them in their lifetime journey of supporting their children.

Early intervention was designed to minimize delays and maximize development for children who are considered at risk for disabilities. It was intended to begin at birth or upon diagnosis, and continue until age 3, at which time the child either ages out of early intervention and into an educational program or has developed skills to a level commensurate with chronological age. It was also meant to support family patterns of interaction that facilitate a child's development (Guralnick, 1997). Frequently overlooked by clinicians working in early intervention is an understanding that caregivers outside our system do not know how to navigate through it and may not even know there is anything to navigate.

The Early Intervention Program for Infants and Toddlers with Disabilities is a federally supported program through the Individuals with Disabilities Education Act (IDEA), known as Part C (Part B covers children from 3 to 22 years). IDEA Part C helps each state implement comprehensive programs of early intervention services for babies with disabilities ages birth through 3 years, and their families (National Dissemination Center for Children with Disabilities, 2005; Palmaffy, 2001). In some states, children stay with the same programs from birth to 5 years (shifting from Part C to Part B funding), whereas others transition from early start individual treatment with parent involvement to public school district special education programs at age 3. The federal program provides state funding for early intervention services to address the physical, cognitive, communication, social-emotional, and adaptive developmental needs of infants and toddlers (feeding and swallowing could be considered physical or adaptive developmental needs). Services are delivered by providers, such as

Swigert, N. B.
Documentation and Reimbursement for Speech-Language Pathologists: Principles and Practice (pp. 251-291).

speech-language pathologists, who are contracted or vendored with early start funding agencies to meet the needs of the family. These needs are determined through a screening and evaluation process and defined on an Individualized Family Service Plan (IFSP) by service coordinators (i.e., social workers who work with families to coordinate Part C services) and caregivers, most often meaning the parents.

IDEA Part C has been amended since its inception. The current version (P.L. 108-446) stipulates many state requirements, including minimum components that must be provided to children. Individual states, however, can set their own criteria for eligibility. As a result, definitions of eligibility differ from state to state. This causes confusion not only for parents, but also for service providers who struggle to keep up with changes and variations in access to programs within their own communities. Information regarding Part C criteria and implementation regulations and recommendations can be found at the following sites:

- Office of the Federal Register: https://www.federalregister.gov/documents/2011/09/28/2011-22783/early-intervention-program-for-infants-and-toddlers-with-disabilities
- U.S. Department of Education, Office of Special Education Programs: https://www.osepideasthatwork.org/
- Building the Legacy of Our Youngest Children With Disabilities: http://www.parentcenterhub.org/repository/legacy-partc/
- Wrightslaw Early Intervention (Part C of IDEA): http://www.wrightslaw.com/info/ei.index.htm

After eligibility has been established, execution of Part C funding and services is determined by each state. Each governor can select a lead agency to implement funding and administration of the IDEA Part C program, in collaboration with an Interagency Coordinating Council (ICC), composed of service providers (e.g., therapists, agency administrators) and parents of young children with disabilities who become advisors to the lead agencies. Currently, all states and eligible territories are participating in the Part C program, with annual funding based upon census figures of the number of children under the age of 3 in their general population. This allows each state to design its own federally supported program relative to the specific needs of their community. Federal guidelines are provided, but, as noted, implementation varies from state to state, which makes it complicated for families and therapists to follow (Andrews Mackey & Taylor, 2007). Definitions of criteria for IDEA Part C eligibility for each state were updated in March 2015 and can be viewed through online at http://ectacenter.org/~pdfs/topics/earlyid/partc_elig_table.pdf.

Speech-Language Eligibility Through Individuals with Disabilities Education Act Part C

As previously noted, each state varies in its implementation of their early intervention program, so speech-language pathologists must learn the policies of their particular state in order to provide comprehensive and holistic services to children under 3 and their families. Even within each state, delivery of services can vary from county to county. For example, in California, some counties allow speech-language pathology assistants to provide direct early intervention services, whereas others do not.

Another variation in implementation of Part C from state to state is eligibility criteria. For example, some states require 33% delay in two areas of communication development (e.g., comprehension and expression) or 50% delay in one area, whereas others require a 25% delay in two areas. Eligibility criteria within an individual state is fluid and can change, so speech-language pathologists need to stay informed about their state's current requirements. Clinicians can check their state's regulation at http://ectacenter.org/partc/statepolicies.asp.

Early Intervention Reimbursement

Under Part C of IDEA, the following services are provided at no cost to families:

- Child find services
- Evaluations and assessments
- Development and review of the IFSP
- Service coordination (typically social workers who coordinate a service plan)

Subpart F of IDEA Part C, however, stipulates that funding cannot be used to pay for additional services (e.g., speech-language therapy) if a child can be covered through public or private sources. This means that Part C is the payer of last resort, requiring families to exhaust efforts to obtain funding through private insurance or Medicaid. This process can be overwhelming to parents, particularly those in states where service coordinators, whose caseloads are extraordinarily high, cannot help them navigate the insurance system quickly. Speech-language pathologists who are knowledgeable about this process can provide an additional level of support. Service coordinators (i.e., Part C social workers) may be able to provide funding for families while they are in the process of securing private insurance reimbursement, but attempts must be documented, which is another area where speech-language pathologist can be of help. Although services may be covered by private health insurance or Medicaid, funding sources cannot be contacted without explicit permission from the insured. If permission is not provided, child services through Part C still cannot be denied.

The Early and Periodic Screening, Diagnostic, and Treatment (EPSDT) program requires states to cover a comprehensive set of benefits and services for all individuals enrolled in Medicaid who are under the age of 21 (McCarty & Romanow, 2009). Each state administers its own program and establishes eligibility requirements. In California, for example, children diagnosed with developmental disabilities are eligible for MediCal (California's Medicaid program) through a medical waiver, and it is not contingent on family income. Unfortunately, Medicaid reimbursement rates are often substantially lower than other funding sources and may be financially realistic only to non-profit agencies who are eligible for subsidies, grants and donations, and do not rely solely on third-party payments, such as a private practice might.

Although some states will fund insurance copayments, others may require a share of cost to families, called Family Cost Participation (FCP), for specific services, including speech and language. This aspect of Part C is executed differently depending on each state's early intervention policy. In October 2002, a Part C National Survey (Andrews Mackey, 2003) identified the position of states and territories related the use of family cost participation for individual services. Information gathered from 34 states and 1 territory revealed the following:

- 11 states used FCP in the form of both insurance and direct family fees
- At least 14 states had some policy regarding use of family private insurance
- 6 states used FCP in the form of family fees
- 4 states report no policies for FCP

These funding variables further complicate the navigation through the early intervention process for both clinicians and families. Speech-language pathologists can clarify funding information by directly contacting service coordinators through their early intervention Part C agency. Updated information is also available through individual state organizations who fund local Part C agencies. Specific details about each state's lead agency for their early intervention program can be obtained through the Early Childhood Technical Assistance Center website (www.ectacenter.org). Clinicians can also help parents learn more about the Part C system by directing them to the Center for Parent Information and Resources (http://www.parentcenterhub.org/repository/ei-overview).

Early Intervention Level of Service

The amount of treatment hours allotted through Part C is also variable from state to state, with some limiting speech and language services to 1 hour/week. Thirty-minute sessions, although valuable to most children under 3 and their parents, can be difficult to schedule, particularly for in-home rather than clinic-based sessions. If 1-hour sessions are provided, the child and family will only be seen once per week, which can minimize or delay progress. Speech-language pathologists can advocate for more sessions if they are able to document multiple areas of need.

Summarizing Part C Screening, Evaluation, and Eligibility

Any child who demonstrates potential communication delays or atypical development can be evaluated to determine eligibility for specific testing. The developmental evaluation is completed through Part C funding by trained assessors at no cost to families upon request. In San Diego, for example, trained assessors meet with families, typically in their homes, and complete the Infant-Toddler Development Assessment (Provence, Erikson, Vater, & Palmeri, 1995), which assesses all areas of development. If results reveal developmental delays, children are referred for formal testing to professionals licensed in identified areas of need. An IFSP is then developed by the team, which generally includes parents, service coordinators, and initial assessors, although families can invite others to attend. The goals of the plan and related service referrals are based on the needs and concerns expressed by the family if they fall within 16 domains (Table 15-1) (California Department of Developmental Services, 2005).

After the goals are developed by the IFSP team, formal assessments are scheduled through specific specialists, such as speech-language pathologists for children with communication delays, developmental disabilities, feeding disorders, and swallowing dysfunctions (Steedman, 2005; Wrightslaw, 2017).

Final Word on Navigating the IDEA Part C System

Speech-language pathologists working in the early intervention system need to know how to maximize funding for needed services and what resources are best used to garner support. Clinicians who chose to work in this field have learned how to incorporate funding issues with evidence-based clinical practices to support children with special needs. Parents who have unrelated experiences, careers, jobs, and responsibilities are often unaware of how to navigate through early intervention funding. Complicating matters even more is that families may learn how to access early intervention in one state but then move to another where they are confronted with an entirely new set of rules. Although that might not seem a substantial adjustment to make, parents who are racing to meet that important window of early treatment for their child with a disability fear that minor deviations represent critical lost time. As

Table 15-1

The 16 Domains of the Individual Family Service Plan

1. Assistive technology devices	9. Family training and counseling
2. Medical services	10. Nursing services
3. Physical therapy	11. Service coordination
4. Special instruction	12. Transportation and related costs
5. Health services	13. Nutrition services
6. Occupational therapy	14. Psychological services
7. Social work service	15. Speech-language therapy
8. Vision services	16. Audiology

Adapted from *Here's How to Do Early Intervention for Speech and Language: Empowering Parents* (p. 7) by Karyn Lewis Searcy, Copyright © 2012. Plural Publishing, Inc. All rights reserved. Used with permission.

treating speech-language pathologists working with these families, it is our responsibility to help them navigate the system. First, however, we have to identify the families who need our help.

Current Trends

Pediatrician Referrals

Civil rights activists in the 1960s worked with caregivers to establish federal legislation, enabling early childhood programs to expand exponentially. Unfortunately, many parents are still unaware that they exist. Of significant concern is the inconsistency recorded in referrals for treatment by pediatricians when young children present with communication delays or feeding aversions. This inconsistency, although explicitly addressed by the American Academy of Pediatrics (AAP), continues to exist and often delays adequate and efficient guidance for parents. In 2006, the AAP acknowledged that early identification of developmental disorders should be considered a primary responsibility of pediatric health care professionals because of its impact on the well-being of children and their families. The AAP noted that delays may increase the risk of behavior disorders that require specialized evaluation, diagnosis, and treatment, but their investigation discovered inconsistent referral outcomes. Results of their study suggested that physicians were not seeing delays in very young babies as significant and, therefore, were not directing families to federally supported early intervention programs (Council on Children with Disabilities et al., 2006). They also discovered that detection of developmental disorders was reportedly lower than actual prevalence. Despite organizational and national efforts to improve developmental screenings, few pediatricians were implementing effective screenings. In an effort to remediate this tendency, the AAP developed a list of recommended screening tools for pediatricians.

They also established guidelines for doctors to integrate into routine visits, including the following:

- Informal developmental evaluation of children younger than 3 months during well-child visits
- Standard developmental screenings of children at 9, 18, and 24 to 30 months
- Referrals for more testing and to early intervention programs for children not passing screenings (Council on Children with Disabilities et al., 2006)

A 2010 study of 17 pediatric practices revealed that many pediatricians were still not following the AAP guidelines, even if they had concerns about a child's development (King et al., 2010). Although 53% of the practices studied reportedly conducted developmental screenings, none of them followed AAP screening guidelines. On an almost monthly basis, speech-language pathologists meet families of children older than 2 years who report their pediatricians told them not to worry about their child's delayed communication skills. That is a source of frustration to many parents, who often feel unheard and discounted and later shaken by guilt that they had not advocated more rigorously. According to Nathan (2011), this disconnect between pediatricians and parents may be related to several factors (Table 15-2).

A family's experience with pediatricians regarding developmental delays or disabilities often varies depending on the etiology of a child's disorder or delay. Congenital disorders, such as Down syndrome, are often identified before the child's birth. As a result, parents can take an active role in researching options and establish early relationships with support groups, funding sources, and specialists who can direct them to services even prior to the birth of their children (National Early Intervention Longitudinal Study, 2007). For others, however, a developmental delay or

Table 15-2

Doctor Versus Parent Perspective

Pediatrician	Parents
• Keeping your child alive and healthy • Getting all of the vaccinations in on time • Making sure your child is safe • Making sure that he or she is growing well enough and does not have diseases • Getting done on time and charting everything	• Is my child okay? • Is my child healthy? Eating enough? • How can we sleep better, behave, poop and pee right? • Is it safe to talk about worries I have about my child? • Our parents, friends, and teachers are worried about my child.

From *Here's How to Do Early Intervention for Speech and Language: Empowering Parents* (p. 30) by Karyn Lewis Searcy, Copyright © 2012. Plural Publishing, Inc.

disorder may take longer to identify. That delay can create a sense of intermittent reinforcement, characterized by seemingly typical development, followed by blips of atypical patterns, then a return to typical stages. Parents have reported that just when they were about to talk to their pediatrician or call a resource group about developmental concerns, their babies suddenly appeared to be okay. Despite substantial empirical evidence supporting the importance of early intervention on the developing brain and on the healthy progression of the parent-child relationship (Daro, 2009), there still are professionals, well-meaning strangers, and relatives who minimize a parent's fear, stating, "Don't worry! He's just a late talker; he'll catch up." This creates a need for objective direction from unbiased, compassionate, and knowledgeable developmental specialists. Pediatricians need to be familiar with early intervention services, particularly for families of children aged 0 to 5 years, because they are often the only professionals seeing children at that stage of development during healthy baby visits (Lipkin, 2008). Speech-language pathologists can help families struggling to be heard by their pediatricians by sharing general information regarding simple screening procedures recommended by the AAP for physicians.

Early Intervention Screenings

Speech-language pathologists in private practice can offer free preschool screenings, which serve to build community awareness about the importance of early intervention, in addition to identifying young children who may need treatment. Day care centers and private preschool facilities welcome clinicians who offer this service to their families. The screenings can be completed quickly (approximately 10 minutes per child) and may be executed by trained volunteers (including speech-language pathology undergraduate students) in order to identify which children should be referred to funding agencies for comprehensive assessments. Children cannot be screened without signed parent permission, and no diagnoses can be formed from screening results.

After the screenings are complete, the volunteer or student can review outcomes with a speech language pathologist, who will share the official screening outcome and recommendations with the day care center or preschool and with the family. Appendix 15-A can be used as a template to report this information. It is important to provide specific referral sources that will allow families to easily follow through with recommended suggestions.

Determining and Securing Eligibility for Funding

The process of determining eligibility, particularly from private third-party agencies such as insurance companies, is, at best, a daunting task. The insured parent can review the insurance plan summary (typically a 150-page document), which breaks down plan exclusions and limitations in detail, but most find that task overwhelming. Families can also call their insurance company and wait on hold, or meet with their human resource department at work if the insurance is provided by their employer, to determine if their child's therapy will be covered. Parents have reported becoming so frustrated by the inaccurate information they have been given that they either abandoned the reimbursement process and paid out of pocket or removed their child from much-needed treatment. Based on IDEA requirements, however, they must determine what their private insurance will fund because, again, Part C is the payer of last resort, and their child will age out by age 3.

Prior to meeting new families, even if they are initially funded through Part C, clinicians can obtain initial intake information to prepare for their first meeting and begin the funding navigation process. Without a system to assist new families who are unfamiliar with the early intervention process, many flounder without clear focus. One example of the complexity of the process relates to military families who are funded through Tricare, the health care program of the U.S. Department of Defense Military Health System. Families covered through this system often bypass Part C completely, meaning they may forfeit coordination of services. Tricare is divided by region with different restrictions and funded by an insurance company, which can change. Up through 2016, United Healthcare Military & Veterans was the funding source for the Western Tricare region, with a shift to Healthnet proposed in 2017. A speech-language pathologist should refer all early intervention families to their Part C program, even if they have adequate funding through private insurance, such as what typically happens with Tricare. They may enter a clinic with authorization for treatment but no Part C support, which can help coordinate all services, including transition out of the early intervention program. Similarly, service coordinators may refer a child for early intervention services following the completion of an Infant-Toddler Development Assessment, without knowing what their private insurance will cover, if anything. A speech-language pathologist who understands the funding maze can guide most families through the process during a time when they often feel the most vulnerable.

Clinicians can obtain insurance information either during the intake process or at the time of the first visit, after it has been determined that an evaluation will be funded by Part C. To alleviate familial frustration, speech-language pathologists can, with permission from the insured, contact insurance companies directly, armed with specific questions requiring explicit responses regarding treatment. A clinician or agency can ask the insurance representative whether a particular plan has exclusions or limitations for a specific diagnosis when calling to determine benefits. Insurance policies and plans are highly variable, and many details that need clarification prior to starting an evaluation or treatment must be confirmed. Although the back-up plan allows for Part C funds if necessary in early intervention, alternative funding options must be explored and documented.

Parents and speech-language pathologists often obtain information indicating that an insurance policy will fund a service, which is later denied when the claim is submitted. Acquiring all necessary information in advance can alleviate some, but never all, of these conflicts. Some insurance companies, but not all, require prior authorization or a physician's prescription to verify therapeutic need. If an insurance company will fund treatment only with a prescription, it must be obtained prior to the first appointment to ensure payment. There are less risks involved for children who are eligible for Part C because, as the payer of last resort, denied funding will be covered, but procuring all relevant documents in advance clarifies the process for everyone. Additionally, when a child ages out of early intervention at age 3 in some states, families will know what funding they may be able to access through their private insurance if they elect to continue private speech and language services. Appendix 15-B is a sample letter to physicians used to request a prescription for ongoing services to be submitted to insurance.

Insurance Appeal Process

Children younger than 3 years old receiving speech-language therapy are covered through Part C, but because the governing agency is the payer of last resort, private insurance can become the funding source if the service is covered by the insurer's policy. It should be noted, however, that even when clinicians or agencies confirm insurance eligibility prior to the onset of treatment, it is not uncommon for billing claims to be denied. This is both frightening and frustrating for parents who are anxious to provide their children with much-needed services. It is important to remind families that Part C will fund necessary services that are not covered by private insurance. Even when insurance does cover therapy, coinsurance, copayment, or deductible is reimbursed through Part C in some states.

If an insurance claim is denied, clinicians or their agencies must file an appeal, not only in an effort to exhaust attempts to procure funding, but also to advocate for the relevance of medical necessity for speech-language therapy services. The appeal process used to be a three-tiered system, but now varies depending on the specific insurance company, with most now allowing only one or two appeals. Regardless of the individual plan, the process can be overwhelming for families to navigate. Therefore, it becomes the responsibility of the clinician or administrative agency to create a viable and familiar system to clarify the medical need for treatment. This system can include the following:

1. First appeal letter
2. Second appeal letter with research information regarding the disorder
3. Internal medical review

Step 3 used to involve a third appeal that would allow a clinician to speak directly with a medical reviewer, but recently most companies have been sending subsequent appeals straight to internal medical review. Increasingly, clinicians are less able to have a conversation with the medical reviewer, instead receiving a letter stating that all supporting documents submitted have been "taken into account and it has determined that…and the denial is upheld." On some occasions, the medical reviewer actually addresses the specific issues included in the appeal letter, but more commonly a standard form letter is used in response. Speech-language pathologists are encouraged to seek a telephone consult with a medical reviewer if possible to help promote awareness of the substantial issues supporting the appeal and need for funding.

If the final appeal is also denied, a decision must be made regarding whether this particular case simply will not be funded under this particular insurance plan or policy. If it is decided that the denial is not fair, however, it may be reviewed by the state's insurance commissioner, who can make an unbiased decision and overturn the denial if the appeal is deemed viable. In many cases, however, the denial is returned back to the insurance company, or the state may recommend ombudsman assistance. Not all policies qualify for state review, and insurance companies can uphold their final denial of a claim. Self-funded or employer funded plans, for example, are not subject to review from the state commissioner's office. Families should be informed about the process before embarking on that journey.

Another issue that might impact insurers in addition to medical necessity is the end of lifetime or annual coverage caps. Families and their Part C service coordinators should be notified in advance that if a child receives ongoing weekly therapy funded by a capped insurance policy, they are likely to reach their annual or lifetime cap before completion of needed services. Under the Affordable Care Act, insurance companies could no longer impose lifetime or annual benefit caps, but with changes proposed in 2017, it is unclear whether that policy will be preserved. In some states, such as California, insurers cannot cap individual benefits, meaning an insurance company cannot limit the number of speech-language or physical therapy sessions if the treatment is approved for an autism spectrum disorder. Some states have issued parity acts, which stipulate that limits set for a specific treatment, such as mental health services, cannot be imposed if they were not also imposed on at least two-thirds of all other treatments for other related conditions (unless the plan is grandfathered). Speech-language pathologists who are billing insurance companies need to be knowledgeable about their state's insurance regulations. Although this does not specifically impact children in the early intervention program because they will be covered by Part C if not through private insurance, clinicians can empower and help advocate for all their patients by understanding local laws. Appendix 15-C is an example of a letter parents can use to request continued coverage for speech-language therapy services for a child with autism spectrum disorder under California insurance law.

Another reason for an early intervention claims denial sometimes offered by funding agencies (including private insurance and Part C funders) is *cognitive* or *developmental readiness*, which is not a valid factor in considering eligibility for speech-language therapy. According to a 2002 American Speech-Language-Hearing Association (ASHA) technical statement, children with disabilities whose language skills are commensurate with their cognitive skills can still benefit from language intervention (National Joint Committee for the Communication Needs of Persons With Severe Disabilities, 2003). ASHA's Joint Committee in 2002 concluded that decisions about eligibility for communication services and supports for individuals with severe disabilities must be based on communication abilities and needs, not on a presumed cognitive or developmental readiness. Unfortunately, some clinicians use this readiness argument to deny direct treatment. In fact, some agencies encourage their clinicians to offer families of children with Down syndrome multiple sessions per week with an early intervention teacher and only 4 hours per year of consult with speech-language pathologists. Increasing numbers of parents, however, are rejecting these offers, knowing that communication, speech production, eating, and swallowing difficulties often associated with a diagnosis of Down syndrome require the unique skills and expertise of speech-language pathologists.

Clinicians can empower families by knowing how to file appeals to claims denied for any reason. Supportive documentation is vital to any appeal and can include the following:

- Assessments inside and outside the agency, especially medical supportive assessments and referrals
- Correspondence and dates of communications with insurance representatives and reference numbers documenting those communications
- Documented dates of service

Families should be involved in funding appeals process. According to the Centers for Disease Control and Prevention (Boyle et al., 2011) the prevalence of developmental disabilities increased 17.1% from 1997 to 2008, with approximately 1.8 million more children diagnosed from 2006 to 2008. This increase, clearly impacting more families, may be influencing the improved support noted in the human resources (HR) departments of employers who offer employer-funded insurance. Clinicians and agencies can provide insured families with their appeal documentation and arguments. Then parents can contact their HR department, who directly contacts the insurance company. In many cases, claims get paid with little more discussion and less direct participation by the clinician. Many families do not know to contact their HR department, however, without being directed there by their speech-language pathologist.

Timeliness of Claims Submissions

Timely filing is critical when an insurance company puts a limit on claims submission. For example, if a payer has a 90-day timely filing requirement, that means the claim must be submitted within 90 days of the date of service. With increased accessibility of electronic billing, this aspect of the system has become easier. It makes the most sense for agencies to submit billing at the time of service or at least within the same week. The challenging element of timely submissions is knowing what each funder's time frame is because there is no set standard among all payers. That means that while a speech-language pathologist is treating patients, determining diagnosis codes, and submitting claims, someone has to keep track of all contracted requirements. If a claim is submitted late, reimbursement denials will arrive, and they typically cannot be appealed.

Early Intervention Speech-Language Evaluation

After a child has been found eligible for an evaluation through the early intervention process, it is time to get started. Evaluations are reimbursed at a flat rate through Part C. Insurance Current Procedural Terminology codes for communication and feeding/swallowing disorders are untimed, which is different from other therapies, such as occupational and physical therapy. That means that a 1-hour evaluation will be funded at the same reimbursement rate as a 2-hour evaluation, neither of which typically covers the cost of the speech-language pathologist's time. This does not factor in the amount of time needed to complete writing the report. Further, a 45- to 60-minute interaction with a young child can hardly provide a clear assessment of skills, and reliable impressions cannot be based on initial meetings. In part, that is why eligibility determination through the evaluation process is different from a comprehensive assessment, particularly in early intervention. Clinicians initially need to determine whether a child should receive treatment (i.e., are they eligible for services), and later probe specific areas of need and response to strategies during therapy sessions. After eligibility has been determined and funding secured (i.e., a child is not functioning at a specific developmental level or not at a stage commensurate with same-aged peers, whatever measure is stipulated by the funding source), diagnostic treatment can be initiated. Standardized and criteria-based testing provide eligibility information, but goals will be determined by establishing baseline measures (i.e., percentage of accuracy or incidence of occurrence at the onset of treatment) in each discrete communication skill area. Most states determine early intervention service recommendations based on percentage of delay, but standardized assessments do not always reliably quantify specific areas of need. Therefore, eligibility requirements are not always neatly aligned with clinical judgment or recommendations, which is often difficult for both parents and therapists to reconcile.

ASHA (2008) recommends informal techniques be incorporated into the early intervention communication evaluation and described in the evaluation report, including a blend of standardized with non-standardized assessments, such as the following:

- Observation of the child with familiar communication partners and family members
- Interaction with the child
- Dynamic assessment
- Caregiver-supplied information

In addition to the valuable information families provide, the process of dialoguing with them about their observations serves to strengthen their belief that they are active and valued partners in the early intervention process at the onset of our relationship with them.

Standardized and Non-Standardized Early Intervention Tests

Standardized testing provides information under a standard set of conditions, which may distort our ability to observe communication performance within authentic contexts that reflect daily interactions, because not all children can effectively participate within those conditions. Further, few standardized assessments measure all aspects of communication. Identifying the role each family member plays in that interaction is often limited by the restrictions inherent in the standardization process (ASHA, 2008). If a 24-month-old can participate in formal testing, such as the Preschool Language Scales, Fifth Edition (PLS-5; Zimmerman, Steiner, & Pond, 2011), a speech-language pathologist can collect hard data. Most of the time, however, the clinician relies on parent report, clinical observation, and/or non-standardized assessment tools in addition to clinical intuition.

ASHA reviewed categories of evaluation tools in their 2008 report of the role and responsibilities of speech-language therapists in the early intervention process (ASHA, 2008). In order to identify very young children at risk for communication delays and disorders, non-standardized tests, criterion-referenced assessments (which measure a fixed set of predetermined developmental standards such as what a child should be doing at a specific age), and developmental scales are typically used. Scores on criterion-referenced tests indicate what children *can* do and not how they have scored in relation to their peers (Linn & Gronlund, 2000). Other forms of non-standardized tests include parent and other familiar adult descriptions (sensitive to cultural diversity), play-based or routine-based observations by a therapist, and informal probes for stimulability. The following are examples of different assessment tools often used to determine eligibility in early intervention.

- Standardized tests
  - PLS-5 (Zimmerman, Steiner, & Pond, 2011): Direct test and interview
  - Clinical Evaluation of Language Fundamentals Preschool, Second Edition (Semel, Wiig, & Secord, 2004): Direct test and interview
- Non-standardized tests
  - MacArthur-Bates Communicative Development Inventories (Fenson et al., 2007): Parent report
  - Rossetti Infant-Toddler Language Scale (Rossetti, 1990): Direct test, interview, parent report

Decisions regarding which diagnostic tool to use are often based on reimbursement requirements rather than on a clinician's professional choice. For example, some funding sources, such as Easter Seals or Kaiser insurance, require specific tests to be used, and then readministered for reauthorizations. That means if a child became eligible based on results of the Rossetti Scale (Rossetti, 1990) but improved enough to now be assessed using the PLS-5, the speech-language pathologist may need to readminister the Rossetti anyway, which may not be sensitive enough to capture the child's improved skills or current areas of need. Unfortunately, it is necessary to identify the funding source, know what their eligibility requirements are, report results accordingly, and maintain your integrity as an early intervention speech-language pathologist. After a child is identified as eligible, therapists can initiate diagnostic therapy, allowing for the collection of information while jump-starting the child's learning. Regardless of what measures are used, speech-language pathologists must produce replicable data to determine whether a child is eligible for funding through IDEA and insurance companies in most states.

Informal Probes

Informal probes can also provide clinicians with valuable baselines measures from which to design therapy targets and track response to treatment. Particularly with young children who are exhibiting little to no communication skills, functional abilities are often difficult to tease out. Is it motor planning, a cognitive deficit, language processing disorder, lack of stimulation? Structured, informal probes can provide anecdotal data and baselines that can be used to document progress over time and be measured in terms of percentage of accuracy. Appendix 15-D is an informal probe inventory sheet that can be adapted as a tool to establish baseline measures of functional communication skills.

Early Intervention Report Writing

As previously discussed, early intervention evaluations are typically reimbursed at a relatively low rate that rarely covers the clinician's preparation time, actual assessment, and report writing. Further, most speech-language pathologists note that report writing tends to monopolize time that might be better used treating other children or expanding their knowledge base. Nonetheless, there are no options: An evaluation or treatment performed without written documentation cannot be reimbursed because there is no proof of implementation. Additionally, written documentation ultimately helps clinicians identify and focus on important targets. Designing templates that can be adapted to include all pertinent information for families, physicians, social workers, allied therapists (e.g., occupational and physical therapists, applied behavioral analysis therapists), and preschool teachers can streamline the report writing process. The following are some tips to consider in report writing:

- Describe what you see, but do not label it (e.g., "The child flapped his hands when watching a top spin" is better than "The child exhibited self-stimulating behaviors").
- Always use "speech-language" in your writing and never only "speech therapy," which diminishes the extent of our clinical focus.
- Instead of the term "eating," use "feeding/swallowing" because this better describes the intent behind recommended services.
- Minimize use of speech-language pathology jargon, which not all readers will recognize.
- Be concise and explicit.
- Always include measurable data related to all areas of communication (baselines as well as any standardized measures).
- Carefully review your final edits to be sure name and birthdate are correct, even in footers (therapists often cut and paste general information and may forget to customize details).

Concise and efficient documentation is critical to all funding sources and may be reviewed by agency personnel who might not have a working knowledge of the specifics involved in speech-language therapy. It is not uncommon, for example, for an insurance medical reviewer to make a decision regarding the medical necessity of speech-language services. That can mean that a geriatric renal specialist representing an insurance company may be placed in a position to authorize speech-language services for a young child diagnosed with autism.

Some funding agencies may require clinicians to use their prescribed template, but most allow them to create their own. Appendix 15-E is an example of a simplified Early Intervention evaluation report template that covers areas to address in an early intervention assessment in one Part C region (San Diego County). This can be adjusted to include more detailed information for a child's private insurance if they become the primary funding source. Speech-language pathologists need to confirm what details and measures are required to receive funding from their Part C lead agency. Additional information might be needed for private insurance funding, which can vary depending on the company, so clinicians need to know specific requirements of each funding agency.

From Early Intervention Evaluation Through Treatment

Immediately following an early intervention evaluation and finding that a child is eligible for speech-language treatment, therapy should be scheduled with direct parent or caregiver participation whenever possible. This is not feasible for children treated in day care or preschool facilities, but it is an important element of treatment to include families, based on the importance of creating a treatment

Table 15-3

Goal Writing

Element	Description	Example
When	By annual review	By January 22, 2018,
Who	Child's name	Joe Doe
What	Target	will identify object verbally labeled from field of 3
Prompt	Type and number of prompting	when provided no more than 1 gestural prompt
Accuracy	Percentage of accuracy	with 80% accuracy
Stability	Ability to recreate mastery over time	over 3 consecutive sessions
Staff responsible	Who will be tracking data	as measured by speech-language pathologist.

program that incorporates familial culture, preferences, and dynamics.

Although Part C funders do not require Current Procedural Terminology or *International Classification of Diseases, Tenth Revision, Clinical Modification* (ICD-10-CM) codes, insurance companies do. Because the payer of last resort will transition families to their private insurance companies whenever possible, clinicians need to identify both diagnostic and treatment codes. Unfortunately, there are few evaluation and procedure codes for speech-language and feeding/swallowing services provided in early intervention, requiring clinicians to learn which codes best capture each child's current needs. Clinicians can check the ASHA website for the most up-to-date coding information relevant to their clients.

Where applicable, it is important to remind parents that IDEA Part C stipulates that services should be available to all eligible families at no personal cost beyond the FCP, required by some, but not all, states. If there is a coinsurance or copay fee associated with their insurance plan, families may be reimbursed through their Part C funding agency, depending on individual state regulations.

Setting Early Intervention Goals

Some early intervention funding agencies require specific long- and short-term goals, whereas others rely on treating speech-language pathologists to address specific needs and do not require explicitly detailed targets. When they are required, goals should include only one measurable variable that concisely and explicitly defines targets based on initial baseline information and include level and type of prompting (e.g., "when provided no more than three gestural or phonemic cue prompts"). Table 15-3 is an example of a goal commonly used for children in early intervention.

Terminology used for goals should be clear to anyone reading them, with measurements easily understood. They are typically written to either report percentage of accuracy regarding set number of trials, (e.g., verbally labeling to request objects with 80% accuracy) or counting the number of targeted occurrences during a prescribed period of time (e.g., number of times a child visually references an adult during a 30-minute session).

Daily Notes

Speech-language pathologists are moving toward electronic daily notes for record keeping, although many find it cumbersome to use when dynamically engaging very young children and their families, stating it interrupts the interactive flow. Regardless of how notes are collected, data has to be recorded for every therapy session in order to receive reimbursement from any funding source. Dates, including the year (which is often omitted), need to be included on every entry, along with the clinician's initials or signature. Funding sources periodically request daily notes when they are questioning whether a billing claim is valid or medically necessary, and treating speech-language pathologists must submit them within a timely manner.

Collecting data in early intervention can be challenging because most children can be either in constant movement or challenging to engage. Further complicating data collection in early intervention is that children may have few foundational communication skills when initially beginning treatment, and goals may include non-verbal subtle elements, such as attention to an object, visual referencing, joint attention, and even parent response to therapist coaching. Speech-language pathologists must turn these targets into objective and measurable elements of treatment. Data collection should include specific types of prompting used (i.e., gestural, tactile, or verbal) and the number of prompts needed per task. Appendix 15-F is an example of SOAP (subjective, objective, assessment, plan) notes that can be used to track during daily sessions.

Progress Notes/Reports

Periodic reports on which progress on treatment targets is summarized are required by all funding sources and should be completed even in the rare case of self-funding, when no third-party payer will request them for review. Progress report requirements, in terms of content, vary according to the funding source. Some funders, such as Easter Seals, supply a specific progress template that must be used and do not allow for therapist customization. Most other funding sources allow for customized reports but stipulate information that must be included.

Frequency of progress report submission to funding sources is variable as well. Some funding agencies will authorize therapy for 3 months, whereas others will authorize 20 sessions. Either will require reauthorization by the time those sessions are completed. Speech-language pathologists must prepare progress reports prior to the completion of authorized sessions in order to avoid a gap in ongoing services. Progress reports should include the number of sessions completed to date, measure of movement from initial baseline results to current performance in each target area, need for continuing treatment, possible revised targets or goals, and approach to those targets. Appendix 15-G is a sample progress report that has been successfully used for early intervention families, multiple insurance companies, and Part C funders.

A graphic that helps visualize progress is a chart that illustrates movement from baseline measures to current status, which can easily be added to reports using Microsoft Excel or similar software (Table 15-4). These graphs not only document progress achieved in therapy for funding sources and for families, but they help speech-language pathologists identify a child's response to treatment and next steps. It is not uncommon for new early intervention therapists to wonder whether they are making a difference. Data collection and review with visual representation often helps everyone—families, clinicians, and funding sources—identify the progress the children and their parents have achieved.

Discharge Summary

Discharge reports should be completed whenever a child transitions out of treatment, regardless of the reason. This is critically important for children who are aging out of the Part C early intervention program. Most will transition into a public school special education system, and the information provided by the early intervention speech-language pathologist will help the school therapist and the entire preschool team.

The discharge summary should include information regarding the child's performance in all communication, feeding, and swallowing areas measured since the last progress note until discharge. It should include current measures in target areas, reason for discharge, and recommendations for further treatment or monitoring. Appendix 15-H provides an example of an early intervention discharge summary report.

Implementation of Services

Where Early Intervention Services Are Provided

In addition to variable eligibility issues, another area of inconsistency in early intervention is where services are delivered. The 2011 IDEA Part C stipulates that treatment must be provided within a child's "natural environment," which is defined as "settings that are natural or typical for a same-aged infant or toddler without a disability, may include the home or community settings, and must be consistent with the provisions of §303.126." This is a relatively subjective determination with logistic as well as ethical and emotional overlays.

Most providers agree that an infant's natural environment is the home, but from there, opinions and realities diverge. In some states, funding sources can only provide services if a family's private insurance denies treatment. The irony is that many clinicians who accept insurance do not provide home-based treatment, primarily because of costs involved that are not reimbursable (e.g., travel time and mileage) and challenging schedules (e.g., 30-minute sessions in each home). Collaboration with allied professionals, although feasible in-home, can be challenging to schedule. Further, inner-city therapists have reported that they do not feel safe traveling alone into unstable neighborhoods or areas, which results in creating an underserved community of young children with special needs. Table 15-5 is an informal comparison of service delivery site options for speech-language therapy.

In some states, treatment in the natural environment involves weekly sessions with tutors, early interventionists, or infant educators, with periodic consultation by the speech-language pathologist who can provide support to the family's efforts to communicate with their child during everyday activities or help them with feeding issues. ASHA (2008) notes that the natural environment implies more than just location of services. Clinicians are encouraged to equally consider the context of treatment, which should be the shared and preferred activities of the family. Based on the number of single parents and two-career parents,

Table 15-4

Graphing Progress

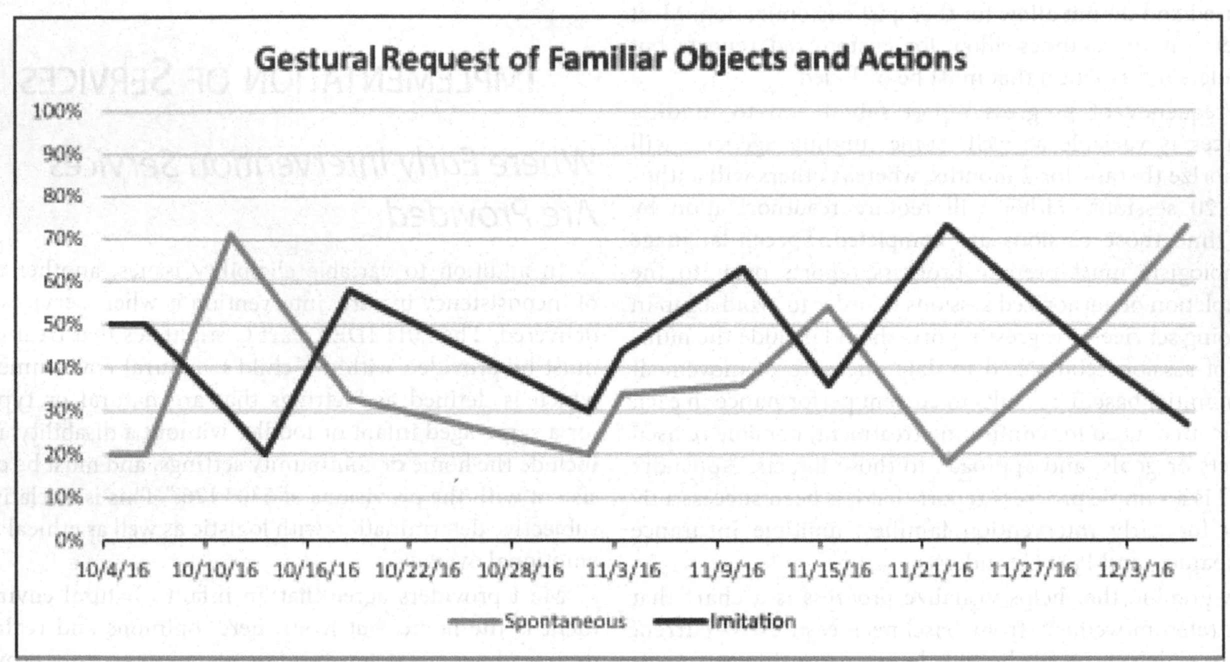

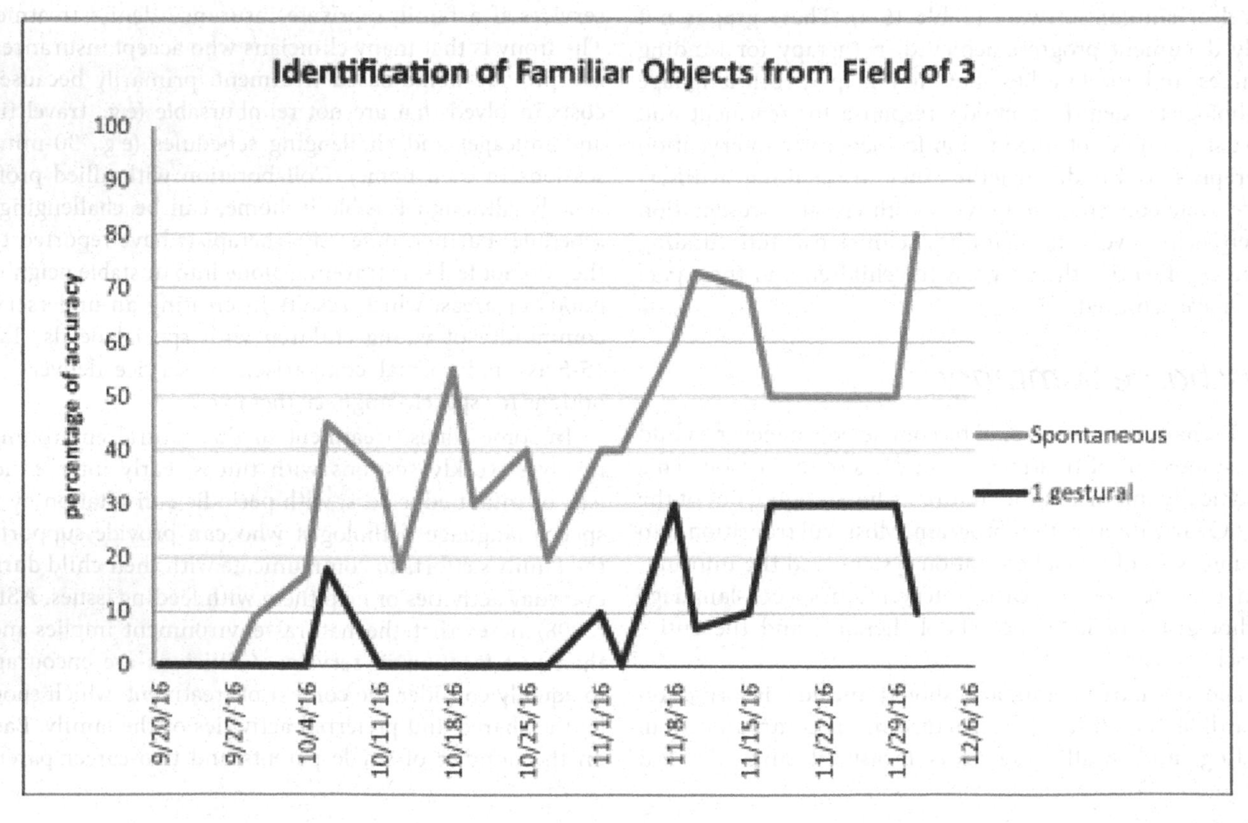

Table 15-5

Comparing Service Delivery Sites for Speech-Language

Home-Based	Center-Based
• Provided in natural environment; often 50-minute sessions 1 time/week. • Parents are often more relaxed and not frazzled by carting all their children out of the home. • Provides use of everyday objects and everyday routines. • Demonstrates strategies in natural, non-artificial environment how parent can stimulate and motivate child. • Multiple family members (e.g., grandparents and siblings) can be directly involved in treatment.	• Can provide multiple 30-minute sessions per week for increased carryover. • Therapist can reduce wait list by providing services to many children per day. • Therapist can collaborate with other clinicians and receive direct supervision. • May allow for collaboration with other therapy disciplines, including occupational and behavioral therapy. • Some parents are not ready to be that intimately involved and do not want strangers in their homes.

From *Here's How to Do Early Intervention for Speech and Language: Empowering Parents* (p. 17) by Karyn Lewis Searcy, Copyright © 2012.

the geographical spread of families, and the number of children in need of multiple services, early intervention delivery must be available in a variety of settings, all of which are focused on preserving the values of the individuals involved. Good therapy is not about where the service is provided, but rather about the fit for the family. If daily routines and values specific to the family are incorporated into treatment, location issues become less pressing. Remembering that children learn through participating in everyday, natural activities and meaningful experiences with their caregivers is more critical than place of service (Woods, 2008). Interactions that are fun for parents and children yield better engagement, with long-term positive outcomes for the child and family. When parents are given the tools to embed learning opportunities into the child's daily routines, maximum and lasting developmental gains can be achieved. Speech-language pathologists can simulate the home environment in any setting within which they can control the variables (e.g., no pets, not too many toys, no personal phone calls) and model an appropriate backdrop for stimulating a child's interaction, as long as the caregiver is directly involved in the treatment. The how is more important than the where. Finally, it should be noted that many insurance company will only reimburse clinic-based facilities and will not pay for services provided in-home, which creates a conflict between what Part C requires and what some funders will reimburse.

Transitioning From Early Intervention

IDEA ensures a free and appropriate education (FAPE) to children, but implementation is inconsistent not only between states, but even within the same school districts in the same county. Early intervention speech-language pathologists can help parents understand the process and know what to request before the transition. As stipulated by IDEA, children transition from individual early intervention services between the ages of 3 and 5, as determined by each state, with most entering a school district–funded program (U.S. Department of Education, n.d.). Whether a child initially received therapy at home, an outpatient hospital, or a private clinic, the transition from the known to the unknown can be overwhelming for the entire family. In many cases, children have completed 6 to 12 months of individual therapy, which results in a relatively intimate connection between child, parent, and clinicians. Speech-language pathologists working in early intervention are familiar with the transition routine, but for families who only recently entered the early intervention world, the shift from one-on-one attention with parent involvement to a group program without direct observation is not always a welcomed change. Early intervention clinicians are often the ones with whom families began this journey, and they can help build awareness about the transition system, buffering their exit from early intervention. By providing families with concrete references and describing the process, speech-language pathologists can demystify some of this shift.

In some states, this transition is relatively seamless, with children remaining in the same programs with the same therapists and teachers. In other states, therapists, teachers, and place of service seemingly change abruptly when children turn 3. Service coordinators, social workers, or case managers try to prepare families for the transition, but clinicians often have had more consistent contact because they worked directly with families on a weekly basis, allowing them to establish a strong alliance. Speech-language pathologists should remember that a child's limited ability to effectively communicate can be the greatest source of stress for families (Bristol & Schopler, 1984) and may continue to be a primary area of concern during the transition process. Our role should not stop until the transition process has a clear end and the family is firmly acclimated into this next phase.

Regardless of who parents turn to for support, the change is often disruptive. It can force to the surface the realization that the child continues to demonstrate delays, and the very need to enroll in a special education program is another of many blows sustained by parents. Although clinicians may be familiar with the system, it is new to most families, who are often caught off guard by the terminology used. One parent reported that she was looking for the classroom where her 3-year-old's Individualized Education Plan (IEP) was being held and was stunned when she was told to follow signs to the special education department. Another recounted the jolt she felt when informed that her son's meeting was being held in the department of developmental disabilities. These terms frequently roll off clinicians' and administrators' tongues with little thought and certainly no malice, but it becomes our responsibility to be aware of the impact they may have on new families. As one mother said, "These strangers didn't even know how those words sounded to me." Knowledge of procedural basics, in addition to regional specifics, help clinicians guide parents. Unless children achieve substantial gains prior to testing at age 3, they will continue to qualify for services. If this occurs in a state where the early intervention service is a separate funding agency, eligibility testing is usually completed by the new funding team (i.e., the school district), with input accepted from the early intervention therapists.

Speech-language pathologists can be instrumental in the often-awkward transition process, by discussing it with families throughout the early intervention program. At least 7 months prior to the transition, parents should have an idea of what this will look like. No matter how many times they may have been told by clinicians or service coordinators, this is new territory where repeated review of the procedural changes will strengthen a family's understanding. This new system treating their children has its own set of terms, acronyms, and abbreviations. Providing them with a cheat sheet similar to that in Table 15-6 can help familiarize them with the process.

Families may also benefit from a checklist to reference during their first meeting with the school district to help them remember to discuss all areas of concern after entering this new arena. Table 15-7 helps simplify this process.

Finally, providing a brief description of the process from IFSP to IEP can preload families with information that may ease some their angst over shifting from individual treatment with an early intervention speech-language pathologist to the school district. Appendix 15-I provides an explanation of the process for families who will need to move from an IFSP to an IEP developed by the school district for children over 3 years. This can be adapted by adding specific details relevant to a speech-language pathologist's state or local educational district.

In a perfect world, early intervention providers and service coordinators would work together directly with the school transition team, but unfortunately, coordinating everyone's schedules in most regions is challenging, and follow-through with all participants tends to be inconsistent. Helping parents organize their professional relationships with the school district can promote a preliminary sense of knowing who will play an integral role in the treatment of their child. Children enrolled in early intervention typically will be assessed by an IEP team through their public school district by age 2, with goals and placement discussed prior to age 3, at which time they can begin attending the district program. Table 15-8 illustrates the transition process from early intervention to public school special education placement.

Additional Issues in Early Intervention

Most early intervention speech-language goals target communication disorders or delays in children. Related issues that may also require attention include feeding and swallowing disorders, and introduction of augmentative and alternative communication (AAC) options. Not all treatment facilities or in-home programs can efficiently target these related areas of need.

Feeding and Swallowing

Early intervention clinicians working with children who exhibit swallowing disorders may need access to medical support teams and assessment tools, such as videofluoroscopic studies. According to ASHA's Scope of Practice in Speech-Language Pathology (ASHA, 2016), speech-language pathologists are important in the assessment, diagnosis, and treatment of infants and children with swallowing and feeding disorders. The professional

Table 15-6

School District Terminology and Abbreviations

Term	Definition
SPED	Special education
LRE	Least restrictive environment: Student should have the opportunity to be educated with non-disabled peers, to the greatest extent appropriate
DHH	Deaf/hard of hearing
AUT	Autism spectrum
MD	Multiply disabled
OHI	Other health impaired
RSP	Resource Specialist Program
SDC	Special Day Class
SLP	Speech-language pathologist
IDEA	Individuals with Disabilities Education Act
SAI	Specialized Academic Instruction
IEP	Individualized Education Program
FAPE	Free appropriate public education
DIS	Designated instruction and services, which are available when they are necessary for the pupil to benefit educationally from his or her instructional program; child must qualify for an IEP before qualification for DIS is determined (includes speech-language)
IEE	Independent Educational Evaluation is a private assessment at public expense if parents disagree with a school district assessment; request should be dated and in writing
SLI	Speech-language impaired

From *Here's How to Do Early Intervention for Speech and Language: Empowering Parents* (p. 238) by Karyn Lewis Searcy, Copyright

roles and activities in speech-language pathology include clinical/educational services (i.e., diagnosis, assessment, planning, and treatment), prevention and advocacy, education, administration, and research. Clinicians need to know when to refer families out to dysphagia specialists for assessments and when a feeding disorder reflects behavioral patterns, sensory reactions, and food aversions rather than physiological differences. Appendix 15-J is a sample feeding and swallowing consultation note that can be completed through observation and caregiver report.

Play-based techniques can be introduced to families and children with eating disorders if physiological limitations are ruled out. Speech-language pathologists often collaborate with occupational therapists or behavioral specialists to help families introduce new textures and tastes and progressively expand a child's repertoire of food experiences. The advantage of having a feeding team assembled is that each clinician plays a different but equally critical role, including physical positioning, behavioral reinforcement, and oral motor manipulation of a variety of textures. Caregivers should be directly involved so they understand the behavioral, sensory, and physiological components to feeding babies who have aversive reaction to food. Oftentimes, parents become highly anxious when their children will not eat items that typically developing children will. Adult tension can be transmitted to the child, which exacerbates the problem and does not promote a pleasant interchange between parent and child. Caregivers and clinicians can work collaboratively to establish feeding goals and objectives.

Home-based pediatric dysphagia intervention is a mandated service, but according to Sheckman Alper and Bell (2010), there are challenges to providing services to children and their families in a home or community setting. They note that an educational model of intervention, not a medical model, must be used, suggesting clinicians coach the family and other team members rather than directly intervening with the child. A growing number of high-risk infants are entering early intervention programs (ASHA, 2001), but attempts to classify pediatric feeding problems are complicated because of the multiple characteristics associated with them (Burklow, Phelps, Schultz, McConnell, & Rudolph, 1998). The most frequently coded

Table 15-7

Checklist of Concerns During Transition to Preschool

_______ Comprehension	_______ Sensory issues
_______ Conversation	_______ Self-help skills
_______ Sound production	_______ Pre-academic skills
_______ Social skills	_______ Dietary/feeding
_______ Play skills	_______ Toileting
_______ Gross motor skills	_______ Fine motor skills

Other: ____

____

____

____

____

____

____

____

____

____

____

From *Here's How to Do Early Intervention for Speech and Language: Empowering Parents* (p. 236) by Karyn Lewis Searcy, Copyright

Table 15-8

Transitioning from Early Intervention to Special Education Preschool

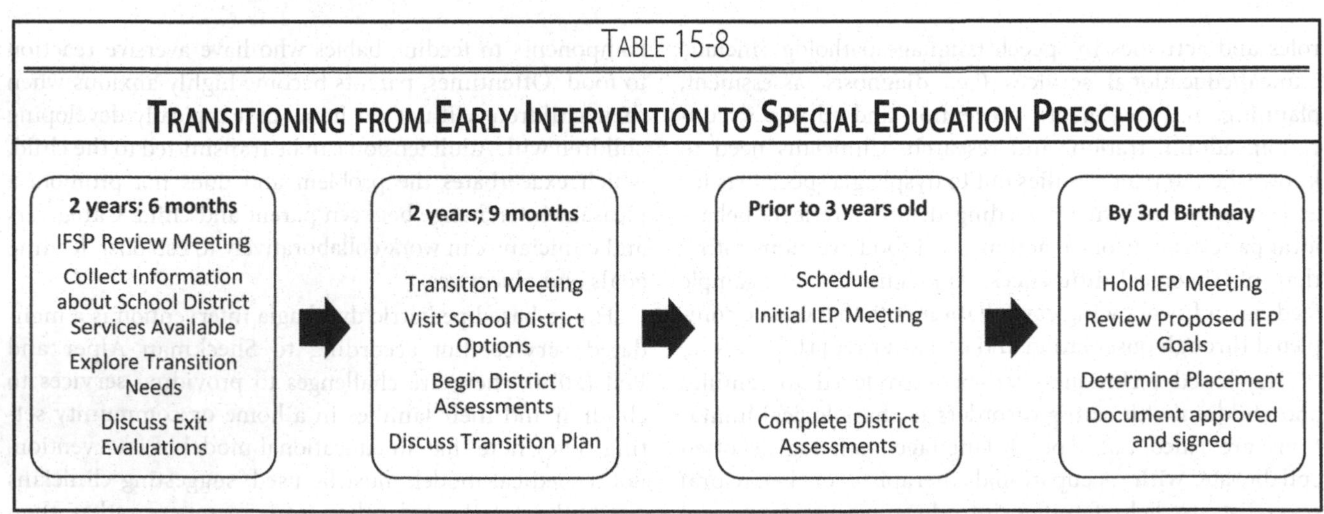

Table 15-9

Identifying Communicative Opportunities

Instruction to parent: Identify five activities or objects your child enjoys. Briefly describe how you know each is a preference and together we will identify how we can use it to develop a communicative exchange.

My Child Likes	My Child Gets It By	Turn It Into Communicative Act

Core Vocabulary Throughout the Day: Progressive Expansion

Instruction to parent: Based on preferences identified, what one-word and two- to three-word combinations can we target?

Object or Activity	One Word	Two Words	Three Words

Adapted from *Here's How to Do Early Intervention for Speech and Language: Empowering Parents* (pp. 169, 170) by Karyn Lewis Searcy,

categories identified by Burklow et al. (1998) were the following:

- Structural-neurological-behavioral (30%)
- Neurological-behavioral (27%)
- Behavioral (12%)
- Structural-behavioral (9%)
- Structural-neurological (8%)

They concluded that complex pediatric feeding problems are bio-behavioral conditions. This means biological and behavioral aspects mutually interact, and both need to be addressed to achieve normal feeding.

Augmentative and Alternative Communication

IDEA Part C also mandates that children under 3 with a disability can use assistive technology devices and services, as needed. AAC can help them communicate basic and functional needs to their caregivers, which can alleviate some frustration and help reset parent-child interaction.

AAC used with babies generally falls into the following three major categories:

1. Simple and naturalistic, such as gestures and modified signs
2. Symbolic but low- or no-tech, such as photos, pictures and graphic symbols, and communication
3. High-tech electronic systems with speech-generation capability, such as computers, tablets, and other mobile devices

Multiple modalities can be combined to maximize communicative opportunities and to allow clinicians to determine which device or technique is most effective for each parent and child.

The AAP (Council on Communications and Media, 2016) issued a policy statement addressing the use of media for children under 24 months, advising restricting use only when paired with parent interaction. The danger is considered when use is isolating rather than when used to promote relationships between child and adult. This is a separate issue than whether the use of technology meets the needs of children with developmental disabilities. Many parents express concern that using any form of communication other than verbal speech will inhibit the development of oral language. These caregivers will need guidance to understand how AAC actually promotes communication development and can jump-start that system. Unfortunately, there is often a tendency to use AAC with the child but inconsistently confirm that families understand the modality used and how to do so efficiently and functionally. Clinicians need to directly assist families in the choice of the type of AAC used and how to implement consistent use of it in the home. One effective method of including families in the use of any form of AAC is to get their buy-in through establishing a functional core vocabulary based on family's preferences and lifestyle. Table 15-9 illustrates how worksheets can be used to identify core vocabulary and adapted to address the specific form of AAC used. Step-by-step guidelines for AAC and early intervention are available at Penn State's Early Intervention: Evidence-based step-by-step guidelines for AAC and early intervention by Janice Light and Kathy Drager (http://aackids.psu.edu/index.php/page/show/id/1/).

Conclusion

Speech-language pathologists working with any early intervention population must be prepared to treat more than a communication, feeding, or swallowing disorder. All patients interact and engage with their families, who play a critical role in their habilitation or rehabilitation. Generalization of skills cannot be promoted without the support of parents, spouses, and other integral family members.

Parents and caregivers of very young children who struggle to communicate, interact, or participate in traditional feeding activities most often feel incompetent because they do not know how to help their children. While speech-language pathologists work with families to facilitate overall development, they can also ease the additional frustration many experience as they scramble to find financial resources. Although IDEA guarantees funding for children from 0 to 3 years old, families must try to obtain personal funding because Part C is the payer of last resort, as is Medicaid. Clinicians who understand how to effectively and efficiently navigate through the funding maze can empower parents by leading them toward funding supports in addition to coaching them in their efforts to interact with their children.

References

American Speech-Language-Hearing Association. (2001). Roles of speech-language pathologists in swallowing and feeding disorders: technical report [Technical Report]. Retrieved from www.asha.org/policy./

American Speech-Language-Hearing Association. (2008). Roles and responsibilities of speech-language pathologists in early intervention: Guidelines. Retrieved from http://www.asha.org/policy/GL2008-00293.htm

American Speech-Language-Hearing Association. (2016). Scope of practice in speech-language pathology. Retrieved from https://www.asha.org/policy/SP2016-00343/

Andrews Mackey, S. (2003). Part C system of payments: Family cost participation. *IDEA Infant and Toddler Coordinators Association.* Retrieved from http://www.ideainfanttoddler.org/pdf/ITCAFCPSurveySum_A.pdf

Andrews Mackey, S. D. & Taylor, A. (2007). *To fee or not to fee: That is the question!* (NECTAC Notes No.22). Chapel Hill: The University of North Carolina, FPG Child Development Institute, National Early Childhood Technical Assistance Center.

Bristol, M. M., & Schopler, E. (1984). A developmental perspective on stress and coping in families of autistic children. In J. Blacher (Ed.), *Severely handicapped young children and their families* (pp. 91-141). New York, NY: Academic Press, Inc.

Burklow, K. A., Phelps, A. N., Schultz, J. R., McConnell, K., & Rudolph, C. (1998). Classifying complex pediatric feeding disorders. *Journal of Pediatric Gastroenterology and Nutrition, 27,* 143–147.

California Department of Developmental Services. (2005). *Compilation of Early Start statutes and regulations,* (8th Ed.). Sacramento, CA: California Department of Developmental Services.

Council on Children with Disabilities, Section on Developmental Behavioral Pediatrics, Bright Futures Steering Committee and Medical Home Initiatives for Children with Special Needs Project Advisory Committee. (2006). Identifying infants and young children with developmental disorders in the medical home: An algorithm for developmental surveillance and screening. *Pediatrics, 118*(1), 405–420. doi:10.1542/peds.2006-1231

Council on Communications and Media. (2016). Media and young minds. *Pediatrics, 138*(5). doi:10.1542/peds.2016-2591

Daro, D. (2009). Embedding home visitation programs within a system of early childhood services. *Chapin Hall Issue Brief.* Retrieved from http://www.chapinhall.org/sites/default/files/publications/Issue_Brief_R3_09_09_09_0.pdf

Derrington, T., Kelly, G., Shapiro, B., & Smith, B. (2003). Earlier is better! Predictiveness of early delays. *University of Hawai'i Center on Disability Studies.* Retrieved from http://www.seek.hawaii.edu/Products/4-Info-Binder/LR-Predictors.pdf

Fenson L., Marchman V. A., Thal D. J., Dale P. S., Reznick S., Bates E. (2007). *MacArthur-Bates communicative development inventories* (2nd ed). Baltimore, MD: Brookes Publishing.

Guralnick, M. (1997). *The effectiveness of early intervention.* Baltimore, MD: Paul H. Brookes.

King, T. M., Tandon, S. D., Macias, M. M., Healy, J. A., Duncan, P. M., Swigonski, N. L., . . . Lipkin, P. H. (2010). Implementing developmental screening and referrals: Lessons learned from a national project. *Pediatrics, 125*(2), 350–360.

Linn, R. L., & Gronlund, N. E. (2000). *Measurement and assessment in teaching* (8th ed.). Upper Saddle River, NJ: Prentice Hall.

Lipkin, P. (2008). Accessing early intervention and education. *Pediatric News,* 32. Retrieved from https://www.kennedykrieger.org/sites/default/files/overview_related_files/11-08.pdf

McCarty, J., & Romanow, K. (2009). Navigating the early intervention system: A guide to scope and funding of programs. *The ASHA Leader, 14,* 1–45. doi:10.1044/leader.PA1.14042009.1

Nathan, G. (2011). *How to talk to your doctor about your child.* Presented at San Diego Regional Centers. San Diego, CA.

National Dissemination Center for Children with Disabilities. (2005). A parent's guide: Finding help for young children with disabilities (birth–5). Retrieved from http://www.fmptic.org/sites/default/files/Finding%20Help%20for%20Young%20Children%20with%20Disabilities%20Birth%20-%205.pdf

National Joint Committee for the Communication Needs of Persons With Severe Disabilities. (2003). Position statement on access to communication services and supports: Concerns regarding the application of restrictive "eligibility" policies [Position Statement]. *American Speech-Language-Hearing Association.* Retrieved from https://www.asha.org/policy/PS2003-00227/.

National Early Intervention Longitudinal Study. (2007). SRI International. Retrieved from https://www.sri.com/work/projects/national-early-intervention-longitudinal-study-neils

Palmaffy, T. (2001). The evolution of the federal role. In C. Finn, A. Rotherham, & C. Hokanson (Eds.), *Rethinking special education for a new century.* Thomas B. Fordham Foundation and Progressive Policy Institute. Retrieved from http://www.cesa7.org/sped/Parents/ASMT%20Advocacy/wl/spedfinl.pdf

Provence, S., Erikson, J., Vater, S., & Palmeri, S. (1995). *Infant-toddler developmental assessment.* Chicago, IL: Riverside.

Rosetti, L. (1990). *Rosetti infant-toddler language scale.* East Moline, IL; Lingui Systems

Semel, E., Wiig, E. H., & Secord, W. A. (2004). Clinical evaluation of language fundamentals®-preschool-2 (celf®-preschool-2). Retrieved from https://www.pearsonclinical.com/language/products/100000316/celf-preschool-2-celf-preschool-2.html

Sheckman Alper, B., &. Bell, H. R. (2010). Pediatric dysphagia early intervention: Home & community practices & precautions. Poster presented at American Speech-Language-Hearing Association Convention, Philadelphia, PA.

Steedman, W. (2005). 10 tips: How to use IDEA 2004 to improve your child's special education. Retrieved from http://www.wrightslaw.com/idea/art/10.tips.steedman.htm

U.S. Department of Education. (n.d.). Ed. Gov. Part C: Infants and Toddlers with Disabilities. Retrieved from http://idea.ed.gov/explore/view/p/%2Croot%2Cstatute%2CI%2CC%2C

Woods, J. (2008). Providing early intervention services in natural environments. *The ASHA Leader, 13,* 14–23. doi:10.1044/leader.FTR2.13042008.14

Wrightslaw. (2017). Early intervention (Part C of IDEA). Retrieved from http://www.wrightslaw.com/info/ei.index.htm

Zimmerman, I., Steiner, V., & Pond, R. (2011). Preschool language scale (5th ed.). San Antonio, TX: Pearson Education Inc.

Suggested Readings

American Speech-Language-Hearing Association. (n.d.). IDEA milestones: 1975-2005. Retrieved from http://www.asha.org/advocacy/federal/idea/IDEAmilestones.htm

American Speech-Language-Hearing Association. (2008a). Core knowledge and skills in early intervention speech-language pathology practice. Retrieved from https://www.asha.org/policy/KS2008-00292/

American Speech-Language-Hearing Association. (2008b). Roles and responsibilities of speech language pathologists in early intervention: Position statement. Retrieved from https://www.asha.org/policy/PS2008-00291/

American Speech-Language-Hearing Association. (2008c). Roles and responsibilities of speech language pathologists in early intervention: Technical report. Retrieved from https://www.asha.org/policy/TR2008-00290.htm

Bailey, D., Scarborough, A., Hebbeler, K., Spiker, D., & Mallik, S. (2004). Family outcomes at the end of the early intervention. *National Early Intervention Longitudinal Study, Data Report No. 6.* Retrieved from https://www.sri.com/sites/default/files/publications/family_outcomes_report_011405_ls.pdf

Boyle, C. A., Boulet, S., Schieve, L., Cohen, R. A., Blumberg, S. J., Yeargin-Allsopp, M., . . . Kogan, M. D. (2011). Trends in the prevalence of developmental disabilities in US children, 1997–2008. *Pediatrics, 127*(6), 1034–1042.

Bransford, J. D., Brown, A. L., & Cocking, R. R. (1999). *How people learn: Brain, mind, experience, and school.* Washington, DC: National Academies Press.

Case Center for the Advanced Study of Excellence in Early Childhood and Family Support Practices. (n.d.). Retrieved from http://fippcase.learnpointlms.com/

Dunst, C. J., Bruder, M. B., Trivette, C. M., Hamby, D., Raab, M., & McLean, M. (2001). Characteristics and consequences of everyday natural learning opportunities. *Topics in Early Childhood Special Education, 21*(2), 68–92.

Finn, C., Rotherham, A., & Hokanson, C. (2001). Rethinking special education for a new century. *Thomas B. Fordham Foundation and Progressive Policy Institute.* Retrieved from http://www.cesa7.org/sped/Parents/ASMT%20Advocacy/wl/spedfinl.pdf

Foehl, A. (2008). How to win private plan appeals. *The ASHA Leader, 13,* 3–18. doi: 10.1044/leader.BML.13102008.3

Foehl, A. (2009). Making a move away from insurance contracts. *The ASHA Leader, 14,* 26–27. doi:10.1044/leader.IPP.14012009.26

Hebbler, K., Spiker, D., Bailey, D., Scarborough, A., Mallik, S., Simeonsson, R., . . . Nelson, R. (2007). Early intervention for infants and toddlers with disabilities and their families. *National Early Intervention Longitudinal Study, Final Report.* Retrieved from https://www.sri.com/sites/default/files/publications/neils_finalreport_200702.pdf

McWilliam, R. A. (2010). *Routines-based early intervention: Supporting young children and their families.* Baltimore, MD: Paul H. Brookes.

Project TaCTICS. (n.d.). TaCTICS (Therapists as Collaborative Team members for Infant/Toddler Community Services). Retrieved from http://tactics.fsu.edu

Reading, J., & Reading, S. (2006). Standards and practices for determining eligibility in early intervention. Presented at American Speech-Language-Hearing Association Convention, Miami, FL.

Spiker, D., Hebbeler, K., Wagner, M., Cameto, R., & McKenna, P. (2000). A framework for describing variations in state early intervention systems. *Topics in Early Childhood Special Education, 20,* 195–207.

TAcommunities. (n.d.).Part C settings: Services in natural environments. Retrieved from http://www.tacommunities.org/community/view/id/1029/

Wolfendale, S. (1997). *Meeting special needs in the early years: Directions in policy and practice.* London, UK: David Fulton Publisher.

Suggested Websites

The Early Childhood Technical Assistance Center: http://ectacenter.org

Early Intervention for Young Children with Autism, Cerebral Palsy, Down Syndrome, and Other Disabilities: http://aackids.psu.edu/index.php/page/show/id/1/

First Five Years Fund: http://ffyf.org

Thrive Washington: https://thrivewa.org

Zero to Three: Developmental screening: https://www.zerotothree.org/policy-and-advocacy/developmental-screening

Zero to Three: HealthySteps: https://www.zerotothree.org/resources/services/healthysteps

Review Questions

1. When is early intervention for speech-language therapy paid for via Medicare Part C funding instead of by private insurance?
2. Describe the difference between standardized and non-standardized testing.
3. List three elements that must be included in a progress note or discharge summary.
4. List one advantage and one disadvantage associated with natural environment.
5. How often do progress notes need to be written?
6. List three options to pursue if an early intervention billing claim has been rejected.
7. Define cognitive readiness and explain why it is not a valid reason to deny services.

Activity A

Write an insurance appeal letter for a 2-year-old child with Down syndrome whose speech-language treatment was denied based on cognitive readiness.

Activity B

Complete the following tracking form for an 18-month-old who begins individual speech-language therapy at a private clinic until transition into the public school district.

Child's Age	Process	Funding Source Option	Comments
1;6 years	Becomes eligible for early intervention	Part C funding	Must research private insurance eligibility
2 years			
2;6 years			
2;9 years			
3 years			

Appendix 15-A
Speech-Language Preschool Screening Results

Name: ______________________ Sex: M F Date of birth: ______________

Date of screening: ______________ Chronological age: ______________________

Examiner: ______________________ Site: ______________________

	Pass	Recheck	Refer	Comments
Comprehension/understanding language				
Expression/verbal use of language				
Sound production				
Social language/interaction with peers and adults				
Voice				
Fluency				

Based on the results of this screening, your child:

__________ Appears to have adequate speech and language development

__________ Should be reassessed in 3 months

__________ Should receive a comprehensive speech-language evaluation

☐ Your child is under 3 years of age: Please call San Diego Regional Center at (619) XXXXXXX and request an Early Start speech-language assessment

☐ Your child is over 3 years of age: Please call your school district's preschool special education department and request a preschool assessment

__________ Other: ____

Comments: ____

____

____

____

____

____

Appendix 15-B

Authorization Form for Speech-Language Pathologist to Send to Doctor

Current Date

John Smith, MD

Xxxx Drive

Xxxx, CA xxxxx

FAX: xxx xxx xxxx

Re: Joe Doe

DOB: xx/xx/xxxx

Dear Dr. Smith,

Attached please find an updated prescription request form for Joe Doe. We are required by his insurance company to have a completed prescription for speech-language therapy on file so we can include it with all authorization requests for treatment. This prescription may also be used in our appeals process when seeking payment for services provided to him in the future.

Joe's speech-language pathologist at Crimson Center is recommending a 6- to 12-month treatment period for him, for 1-hour sessions, 2 days per week. We have attached a copy of his latest progress report for your review.

Please complete the updated prescription request form and fax it to the Crimson Center at (555) 555-5555.

Thank you very much for your time and assistance.

Sincerely,

Tina Centar,

Enclosures: Prescription request

Speech-language pathology report

Appendix 15-C
Example Letter Requesting Continued Coverage for Speech-Language Therapy Services

INSURANCE COMPANY NAME

Appeals and Grievances

PO BOX 1234

Cypress, CA 90630-9972

Date:

FAX #: (555) 123-4567

RE:

Member Name: Joe Doe
DOB: 07/22/2015

Member ID: XXXXX-XXXX

Authorization Request Reference #: 000000000000

Dear Appeals and Grievances Unit:

The Crimson Center for Speech & Language Pathology received a copy of a letter sent from your company to the parents of Joe Doe, informing them that authorization for the 48 visits and 6 months of speech language therapy requested by John Smith, MD, were denied due to "*lack of medical necessity.*" The letter indicated that the denial was also based on the fact that Joe is transitioning into a school-based speech-language program.

Joe received a medical diagnosis of autism spectrum disorder (ASD; ICD-10: F84.0). The treatment he receives at the Crimson Center is medically based and addresses the speech and language deficits related to this diagnosis. According to the American Speech-Language-Hearing Association (ASHA), ASD is a neurodevelopmental disorder that impairs an individual's ability to process and integrate information. It is characterized by speech, language, and communication impairments and affects social and cognitive abilities. As the term "spectrum" indicates, there can be a wide range of effects. ASD includes Asperger disorder, pervasive developmental disorder, and Rett disorder (Speech-Language Pathology Medical Review Guidelines, 2015).

The range of deficits related to a medical diagnosis of ASD (ICD-10: F84.0) are outside the therapy scope of school-based programs. Medically based speech-language therapy focuses on communication in all contexts, and medically based therapy functions under the principle of using language to communicate needs, self-advocate, and build relationships in all settings, including at home with family, in the community to build independence, and in social situations. Clinic-based therapy includes direct caregiver involvement to maximize generalization across all environments.

Medically based speech language therapy is "reasonable and necessary" to enable Joe to communicate his basic needs, to communicate when he experiences pain, and to understand whether someone is attempting to help or harm him. These communication skills are "**reasonable and necessary to protect life, to prevent significant illness [and] significant injury [and] to alleviate severe pain," and go far beyond the scope of academic skill building provided by a school system.

School-based speech-language treatment is limited to working on communication skills related to academic skills (e.g., participation in group activities, reading and writing), whereas medically based treatment provides the foundational and functional skills upon which academic, school-based communications skills are built. Without medically based speech-language therapy, academic skill building would remain at a minimum. Further, it rarely generalizes to home or community functioning, which impacts the entire family. In an optimum situation, medically based speech-language therapy and school-based communication programs coexist to provide a complete and well-rounded treatment for communication deficits related to ASD.

The referenced authorization request and the physician's prescription dated January 20, 2017, requested 48 visits and a 6-month period of treatment. The denial letter sent to the family states that the medical reviewer, Ms. Smith, does not see the need for 48 therapy visits and a 6-month treatment period and is therefore granting only 12 visits and 3 months. A copy of her denial letter is enclosed.

Although Joe's condition may not meet your company's policy standards regarding medical necessity for speech-language therapy, his condition does fit into California's definition of medical necessity. California law supersedes contrary provisions in insurance company policies, especially in the case of an insurance company's commercial plans. Any contractual terms that provide a more restrictive definition of medical necessity than that provided by California law are unenforceable (**Samson v. Transamerica (1981) 30 Cal. 3d 220, 231.178. Cal. Rptr. 323, 350).

The California Legislature has defined "medically necessary" as all care which is "reasonable and necessary to protect life, to prevent significant illness or significant disability, or to alleviate severe pain" (Welfare & Institutions Code 14059.5). Further, speech-language treatment provides the same benefits to individuals with language impairments as medication or medical procedures provide to individuals afflicted with other physical or bio-neurological disorders.

The Crimson Center for Speech & Language Pathology has been designated by Joe's family to serve as their authorized representative in this appeal, and thereby requests that your company take the above argument into consideration, review the details of this case, and authorize the requested 48 visits and 6-month treatment period.

Should you decide to uphold the denial, the Crimson Center for Speech & Language Pathology, Joe's family, and Dr. Smith request that you provide, in writing, a detailed explanation specific to this case as to why your company believes that the request for treatment is not medically necessary and the reason your policy is not subject to the requirements of California law.

Thank you for your attention to this very important issue.

Appeals Coordinator

Crimson Center for Speech & Language Pathology

Attachments: Joe Doe's denial, IEP report, Crimson Progress Note, prescription

Appendix 15-D
Informal Communication Probe Inventory

Language Area	Probe	Response	Percentage
Receptive vocabulary	Identify objects		
Field of ______	Identify verbs/actions		
	Identify body parts		
	Identify clothes		
	Identify colors		
Receptive language	Match object with function		
	Follow one-step direction		
	Follow two-step related		
	Follow two-step unrelated		
Expressive vocabulary	Label nouns/objects		
	Label verbs/actions		
	Label body parts		
	Label clothes		
Expressive language	Mean length of utterance		
	Noun + verb combinations		
	Modifier + noun combinations		
Imitation	Gestures		
	Words		
	Vowel imitation		
	Consonant imitation		
	CV imitation		
	CVCV replicated imitation		
Spontaneous production	Sound repertoire		
	Individual words		
	Word combinations		
	Novel phrase		
	Rote phrase		
Pragmatic/social language	Eye gaze		
	Communicative intent		
	Joint attention		
	Referencing adult		
	Requesting		
	Commenting		

Non-Verbal communication	Pointing		
	Gestures		
	Modified signs		
	Picture exchange		

Appendix 15-E
Speech Language Evaluation

Client	
DOB	
Chronological age	
Parents/caregiver	
Telephone	
Address	
Medical diagnosis	*Description of diagnosis (ICD-10:)*
Diagnosis	*Description of diagnosis (ICD-10:)*
Report date	

Referral Information—Brief Description

Joe Doe, a 2-year, 9-month-old male, was seen for an evaluation at the Crimson Center for Speech & Language on January 21, 2017, due to parental concerns regarding expressive language and play skills. He was referred to this facility by his service coordinator, Jane Smith, from San Diego Regional Center.

Pertinent Background Information (per parent report)

Prenatal	
Birth	
Health	
Behavioral	
Familial history of delays	
Siblings	
Residing with	
Languages spoken at home	
Interaction	
Additional concerns	
Caregiver goals	

Developmental Milestones (per parent report)

Domain	Skill Acquisition
Sitting	
Crawling	
Walking	
Speech and language	
Feeding	

Assessment

Informal Observations

Response to unfamiliar adult	
Interaction with familiar adult	
With age-appropriate toys	
Behavioral observation	
Primary mode of spontaneous communication	
Oral motor	
Speech	
Voice, resonance, fluency	
Eating/feeding and swallowing	
Responses to environmental/speech sounds	

Formal Test Results

(Report formal results here; this example is regarding the tool most often used in our early intervention community.)

Portions of The Rossetti Infant-Toddler Language Scale (Rossetti, 2006) were administered to establish baselines for language functioning. This information is not standardized and was used as a guideline for obtaining information regarding speech and language development based on examiner observation and caregiver report. Performance is recorded below:

Age Range	Language Comprehension	Language Expression
12 to 15 months		
15 to 18 months		
18 to 21 months		
21 to 24 months		
24 to 27 months		
27 to 30 months		
30 to 33 months		

Interpretation

Comprehension: __% delayed (C.A.XX months)

- Areas of relative strength
  - ✓ (list areas above age)
- Areas of relative weakness
  - ✓ (list areas below age)

Expression: __% delayed (C.A.)

- Areas of relative strength
  - ✓ (list areas above age)
- Areas of relative weakness
  - ✓ (list areas below age)

Clinical Impressions

(Brief summary highlighting main concerns.)

Joe Doe, a 2-year, 9-month-old male, was seen for an evaluation at the Crimson Center for Speech & Language on January 21, 2017, and presented with more than a 25% delay in receptive language and a 33% delay in expressive language. He presented as a reticent child with an unfamiliar adult in an unfamiliar environment. Joe played with toys in a meaningful way and pulled his mother to areas of interest to him.

Recommendations and Treatment Plan

(What you are recommending based on child's needs.)

Intensive, individual speech-language therapy with direct parent coaching is strongly recommended for a minimum of 60 minutes/week, for at least 6 months. Initial therapy targets should include:

- Bullet point at least three targets for treatment

Electronically signed input date and time

Your Name

Speech-Language Pathologist

Appendix 15-F

Sample SOAP Note Format

Client's name: ______________________________ Date: ________________

Subjective				
Objective	Task	Spontaneous	One Prompt	< One Prompt
Assessment				
Plan				

Client's name: ______________________________ Date: ________________

Subjective				
Objective	Task	Spontaneous	One Prompt	< One Prompt
Assessment				
Plan				

Client's name: ______________________________ Date: ________________

Subjective				
Objective	Task	Spontaneous	One Prompt	< One Prompt
Assessment				
Plan				

Appendix 15-G
Progress Report

Speech-Language Progress Report

Patient	
DOB	
Chronological age	
Caregivers	
Telephone	
Address	
Medical diagnosis	
Speech-language diagnosis	
Physician	
Report Date	

Date of initial enrollment			
Frequency of sessions			
Length of sessions			
Total sessions to date			
Current recommendation	______ D/C	______ Cont. Tx	other:

Present Functional Status

Domain	Within Normal Limits	Deficits	Impressions	
Behavioral				
Receptive language				
Expressive language				
Speech sound production				
Oral motor				
Play skills				
Social pragmatic				
Hearing				

Focus of Treatment

Goal	Date of Goal	Baseline % or #	Current % or #	Goal Met	Goal in Progress

Comments:

Summary and Recommendations

With intensive and individualized speech and language therapy ________________________ is:

	Making consistent, significant progress toward speech and language goals
	Not making progress toward goals
	Targeted goals have been met for all goals

It is highly recommended that ________________________________

	Continue to receive intensive, individualized speech and language therapy for a period of ______ months
	Continue to receive intensive, individualized speech and language therapy with a reduction in services
	Discharge from services at this time

Treatment Plan:

-
-
-

For further information, please contact Crimson Center for Speech & Language at 555-555-5555.

Electronically signed by

Speech-Language Pathologist

12/18/17 7:38pm

Appendix 15-H

Discharge Summary Template

Client	
DOB	
Chronological age	
Parents/ caregiver	
Telephone	
Address	
Diagnosis	
Date of report	

Pertinent History

Johnny Doe, a 2-year, 11-month-old male, has been seen at the Crimson Center for Speech & Language since July 22, 2015, for treatment of an expressive language delay. At the onset of therapy *(include one or two sentences describing behavior and communication status at onset of treatment).*

Present Functional Status

(Three or four narrative sentences describing current status.)

The following improvements have been measured on targeted goals:

Task	Baseline	Current

(Can insert a graph here.)

Clinical Impressions and Recommendations

(Two or three sentences summarizing progress, current status, and what you recommend.)

Disposition

(Two- or three-sentence narrative describing why patient is discharged and plan of action. This can include, but is not limited to, the following:

- Child is transitioning to school district and will receive services there—caregivers can initiate contact with Crimson Center at any time if they would like to discuss progress in school.
- Achieved all goals and needs no further treatment at this time. Caregivers can initiate contact with Crimson Center at any time if they want to reassess skills or discuss overall performance without treatment.
- Family is relocating and will receive services in their new location. Copies of all reports will be forwarded to new therapist upon request OR copies of all reports were given to family at the final session. Release has been signed and new therapist can call Crimson Center at any time to discuss details of the reports.
- Child is transitioning to (NEW AGENCY HERE). Copies of all reports will be forwarded to new therapist upon request OR copies of all reports were given to family at the final session. Release has been signed and new therapist can call Crimson Center at any time to discuss details of the reports.
- Insurance has denied claims, and all appeals have been exhausted. Family has been directed to (LIST RESOURCES YOU HAVE SHARED WITH THE FAMILY).
- Family has been unable to maintain current schedule. They have been placed on a waiting list for a time that might better address their schedule.)

Electronically signed on (date and time):
Speech-Language Pathologist:

APPENDIX 15-I
Transitioning Out of Early Start

Understanding the Transition From Individualized Family Service Plan to Individualized Education Program

Why is this transition happening?

This is because of a federal law called the Individuals with Disabilities Education Act (IDEA). The U.S. Congress has determined that children ages birth to 3 years old receive early intervention services under Part C of IDEA, and that children ages 3 to 22 receive services under Part B of the IDEA. Part B and Part C are both sections of IDEA, but they have very different provisions and services.

When will this transition process occur?

The transition process takes place in a series of meetings when a child is 2 years old. Typically, an Individualized Family Service Plan (IFSP) review takes place when a child is 2 years 6 months old (called the *2-6 meeting*). Another meeting takes place when a child is 2 years 9 months old, specifically to address the transition process (the *2-9*, or *transition meeting*). Between the 2-6 meeting and a child's third birthday, the child's school district should assess the child to determine eligibility for special education services. All initial assessments should be completed and an initial Individualized Education Program (IEP) team meeting must be held prior to a child's third birthday.

What will change?

Many things will change. Your school district of residence will become responsible for providing special education to your child. The types of services will change, and the service providers will be different. Services will be provided at a different location. The process will also change from a family-centered, empathetic approach to a more bureaucratic approach that focuses on the needs of your child in the educational environment.

Who will provide services to my child after the transition?

Your school district of residence will provide special education services to your child after your child's third birthday.

Where can I get more information and help?

Ask questions throughout the transition process and follow up in writing with all of your concerns! Find other parents in your community and support groups.

Questions? Contact: ______________________________

From *Here's How to Do Early Intervention for Speech and Language: Empowering Parents* (p. 230) by Karyn Lewis Searcy,

Appendix 15-J
Feeding and Swallowing Consultation

Feeding Arrangements

Type, texture, temperature and quantity of food(s)/beverage(s): ______________________________

____

Seating:

Feeding implements:

______ **Fed self completely** ______ **Partially assisted** ______ **Fed entirely by other(s)**

Name/position of personnel assisting/fully feeding child: ______________________________

Area	**Concern/Comments**	**No Concern**
Neuromuscular Function		
Posture		
Tone		
Reflexes		
Other		
Behavior		
Appetite		
Food acceptance		
Rate of eating/drinking		
Sociocommunicative interactions with feeder(s)		
Other		
Sensory Function		
Vision		
Hearing		
Taste		
Smell		
Defensiveness		
Pain on swallowing		
Other		
Physical Function		
Level of arousal		
Maintenance of alertness		
Heart rate		
Respiration rate		
Respiration pattern		
Other		
n/a indicates information not available to our team.		

AREA	CONCERN/COMMENTS	NO CONCERN
Feeding/Swallowing Function		
Accessing food		
Self-initiation		
Awareness of food in or near mouth		
Awareness of appropriate quantity		
Response to temperature(s)		
Response to taste		
Response to texture		
Control for sucking, sipping, biting, rotary chewing, bolus formation, and preparation for swallowing		
Drooling of saliva		
Food leakage from mouth		
Clearing food from lips and mouth		
Tongue thrust		
Coordination of suck-swallow and breathing		
Elevation of larynx during swallow		
Elevation of larynx during cough		
Rate of feeding		
Duration of feeding		
Energy used to complete feeding		
Persistence		
Need for cueing or encouragement		
Other		
Aspiration Indicators		
Throat clearing		
Coughing		
Gagging		
Color change		
Voice change		
Other		
n/a indicates information not available to our team.		

Feeding/Swallowing Plan

Emergency hospital preference (name, address, phone): ____________________

____

Medication effects that need to be considered: ____________________

____

____

Precautions/emergency procedures related to feeding/swallowing: ____________________

____

____

Appendix 15-K
Developing Core Vocabulary

Identifying Communicative Opportunities

Instruction to parent: Identify five activities or objects your child enjoys. Briefly describe how you know each is a preference, and together we will identify how we can use it to develop a communicative exchange.

My Child Likes	My Child Gets It By	Turn It Into Communicative Act

Core Vocabulary Throughout the Day: Progressive Expansion

Instruction to parent: Based on preferences identified, what one-word and two- to three-word combinations can we target?

Object or Activity	One Word	Two Words	Three Words

Appendix 15-L
Speech-Language Evaluation

Client	GLD
DOB	03/06/2014
Chronological age	1;11 (23 months)
Parents/ caregiver	CRD
Telephone	(555) 555-5555
Address	5555 Westview Lane San Diego, CA 92126
Diagnosis	Expressive language disorder (ICD-10: F80.1)
Evaluation date	2/8/2016
Report date	2/22/2016

Referral Information

GLD, a bilingual (English and Mandarin) male, aged 1;11 (23 months), was seen for an initial evaluation at the Crimson Center for Speech & Language on February 8, 2016, due to concerns regarding communication development. He was referred to this facility by the San Diego Regional Center (SDRC) through the Early Start program.

Pertinent Background Information (per caregiver report)

Prenatal	• No complications noted
Birth	• No complications noted • 4 weeks premature
Health	• No complications noted
Behavioral	• Will bang head against the floor and become physical with others to gain attention or when upset
Familial history of delays	• None reported
Residing with	• Biological parents, maternal grandparents, and older sister (8 years old diagnosed with autism spectrum disorder [ASD])
Languages spoken at home	• English and Mandarin
Interaction	• Interacts and plays with caregivers • Will seek others for comfort and to gain attention
Caregiver goals	• To be age-appropriate with speech and language skills

Developmental Milestones (per caregiver report)

Domain	Skill Acquisition
Sitting	8 months
Crawling	9 months
Walking	14 months
Speech and language	• First words: 16 months • Combine words: 21 months • Primarily communicates through using single words, pointing, or gesturing

Assessment

Informal Observations

Response to unfamiliar adult	• Arrived to the clinic with his maternal aunt and grandfather • Slightly shy at first but engaged with clinician once toys were introduced
Interaction with familiar adult	• Affectionate • Brought toys to each caregiver and held them up to comment on them
With age-appropriate toys	• Demonstrated functional and relational play skills with presented toys • Established eye contact with caregivers and therapist during play • Preferred cars and balls
Primary mode of spontaneous communication	• Guiding, pointing, and using mostly single words to meet needs • Some two-word utterances reported via imitation • Used single words to comment, protest, and label objects
Oral motor	• Structure, function, and control of oral mechanism appeared to be within normal limits
Speech	• Consonant sounds produced included "p, b, t, d, k, g, f, m, n, w, h, sh, ch, j" • Caregiver reported gestures used more often than words; however, both were equally observed within this session • Consistent single-word imitation noted
Swallowing/feeding	• No concerns reported by caregivers • Minimal drooling noted
Responses to environmental/ speech sounds	• Inconsistently responded to name when called • Reportedly responds to environmental sounds

Portions of The Rossetti Infant-Toddler Language Scale (Rossetti, 2006) were administered to establish baselines for language functioning. This information is not standardized and was used as a guideline for obtaining information regarding speech and language development based on examiner observation and caregiver report. Performance is recorded here:

Age Range	Language Comprehension	Language Expression
9 to 12 months	100%	100%
12 to 15 months	100%	77%
15 to 18 months	100%	71%
18 to 21 months	100%	66%
21 to 24 months	75%	38%
24 to 27 months	75%	0%
27 to 30 months	66%	0%

Speech-Language Functioning

Comprehension: Within Functional Limits (C.A. 23 months)

- Areas of relative strength
  - ✓ Follows novel commands
  - ✓ Follows a two-step related command
  - ✓ Points to four actions words in pictures
  - ✓ Understands the concept of one
- Areas of relative weakness
  - ✓ Chooses one object from a group of five upon verbal request
  - ✓ Understands size concepts

Expression: 50% Delay With Scattered Skills up to 21 to 24 Months (C.A. 23 Months)

- Areas of relative strength
  - ✓ Uses single words frequently
  - ✓ Uses 50 different words
  - ✓ Refers to self by name
  - ✓ Verbalizes two different needs
- Areas of significant weakness
  - ✓ Sings independently
  - ✓ Asks "what's that?"
  - ✓ Talks rather than uses gestures
  - ✓ Uses sentence-like intonational patterns
  - ✓ Uses two-word phrases frequently
  - ✓ Uses three-word phrases occasionally
  - ✓ Uses early pronouns

Clinical Impressions

GLD, a 1;11-year-old male, was seen for a speech and language assessment on 02/8/2016 and presented with a moderate-severe expressive language disorder with scattered skills up to 21–24 months. Receptive language skills appeared intact, and his desire to engage with familiar and unfamiliar adults was noted throughout his interactions in an unfamiliar setting. GLD followed novel two-step commands during play and participated in functional and reciprocal play with the examiner. He visually referenced both familiar and unfamiliar adults and maintained attention to others and toys throughout the evaluation. GLD primarily communicated using single words and gestures. Caregivers reported concerns with "aggressive behavioral swings" to communicate displeasure or to seek attention. Expressive language was characterized by single-word utterances, minimal vocal play, and use of jargon.

Recommendations and Treatment Plan

Based on his current delay and history of a sibling with a significant language disorder (ASD), intensive, individual speech-language therapy with parent coaching is strongly recommended for a minimum of 60 minutes/week, for at least 6 months. Initial therapy targets should include the following:

- Expressive Language
  - Establish ability to use gestures, word approximations, single words, and word combinations to request, protest, and comment
  - Facilitate imitation of functional two- and three-word phrases
  - Develop vocabulary based on identification of strongly preferred objects, food, and activities in functional play-based activities
  - Replace physical protest behaviors (e.g., banging head, hitting) with expressive language (verbal or gestural)
- Receptive Language
  - Monitor receptive language development, including object function skills and understanding of basic concepts
- Speech
  - Monitor speech sound development and overall intelligibility
- Feeding/Swallowing
  - Monitor feeding behavior based on sibling's history of textural avoidance

Electronically signed on 2/22/2016 at 1:32 PM

JKL, MA, CCC

Speech-Language Pathologist

16

School Settings

Barbara J. Moore, EdD, CCC-SLP, BCS-CL

Funding and Reimbursement Systems in Public Schools

Unlike health care systems, private clinics, and universities, which have direct billing for speech-language pathology services, school settings receive funding to provide special education services under the Individuals with Disabilities Education Improvement Act (IDEA, 2004). IDEA and state law establish the criteria used to determine whether a student is eligible and in need of such services through an Individualized Education Program (IEP) or, in recent years, through prereferral programs such as response to intervention (RTI). In school services, the speech-language pathologist does not need to deal with insurance billing and Current Procedural Terminology codes; however, this does not mean that funding and reimbursement is not important to those who work in schools. School funding is very complex, and the work that is conducted in schools by special educators, including speech-language pathologists, is strongly influenced by the connection between funding and service.

Payment systems for speech-language pathology services come under one of two different methods. The first is known as *fee-for-service*. In a fee-for-service arrangement, the client or patient pays directly for the service procured. Such an arrangement may be made in a private practice, where the client is obtaining services not covered by insurance or is seeking specialized services from the speech-language pathologist, including such treatment as accent reduction, vocal coaching, or even high-level language intervention for children or young adults who are not eligible for IDEA services. Public schools cannot accept direct payment for special services, including speech-language pathology services, because the obligation under the special education law is to provide a free appropriate public education (FAPE) to the student. For this purpose, *free* is the operative word. It is also unethical for speech-language pathologists who work in schools to agree to work with students who are receiving IDEA services outside of the school setting and to accept direct payment for providing such services because this is perceived to be a conflict of interest.

The vast majority of speech-language pathology services are provided under what is known as a *third-party payment system*. Under such a system, someone other than the consumer of the service is paying for the service. In these cases, an individual meets specific criteria established by the third party, either an insurance company, the government (as in the case of school services), or even a non-profit or university clinic. In all of these examples, someone other than the recipient of service (i.e., a third party) determines the criteria by which an individual may be provided services that will be paid for by the third party.

Swigert, N. B.
Documentation and Reimbursement for Speech-Language Pathologists: Principles and Practice (pp. 293-317).

In the other chapters in this book, descriptions of the importance of documentation for insurance billing relates to potential denial of payment if coding is not correct or other documentation errors occur. In school settings, speech-language pathologists have a responsibility to their employer and the government to ensure that they appropriately and accurately apply criteria ensuring that only eligible students receive services. This is a fiduciary responsibility in addition to the professional obligations related to their position.

School funding is not based on the identification of individual students receiving services. (This is somewhat different for Medicaid funding, which will be described later in this chapter.) In recent years, funding formulas for special education have been revised to ensure that states and local districts are not incentivized for inappropriately identifying students for special services in an attempt to gain funding. Federal and state funding is different, but the fact remains that it is the responsibility of those employed under these laws to ensure that the resources of the system are provided only to those who are eligible for the entitlement.

Education funding comes from federal, state, local, and private sources. Many people would be surprised to learn that the federal contribution to education is only about 8%. This contribution includes funding for the U.S. Department of Education, in addition to what is distributed to states, ultimately to be passed along to Local Education Agencies (LEAs). Approximately $620 billion was spent on education in the 2012–2013 school year, with the majority coming from state, local, and private sources (Institutes on Education Sciences & National Center on Education Statistics, n.d.). The federal allocation for special education was $11,912,848 in 2016, with the same amount requested for 2017 (U.S. Department of Education, 2016). When the first special education law, the Education for All Handicapped Children Act (P.L. 94-142), was passed in 1975, Congress promised that the federal government would pay 40% of the excess costs of special education services provided under this law. Children are considered general education students first. The base amount of funding that is allocated to LEAs for educational services to children includes children with disabilities. Congress realized that special education would cost local agencies more, but the intention was never to cover the entire cost of the services. However, although Congress promised 40% of the costs in 1975, the federal level of funding has never reached that level, causing stress on the fiscal programs of state and local agencies.

Speech-language pathologists in schools may encounter workplace issues that are actually related to funding, including high caseloads; limitations on funding for materials, equipment, or continuing education; and shortages of qualified personnel to fill open positions. Although solutions related to practice and operations certainly will help resolve some of these workplace issues (e.g., salary supplements improve recruitment and retention challenges; improved prereferral systems and using RTI or multitiered systems of support [MTSS] can reduce high caseloads), ultimately some of the solutions still cost money. Funding for special education services is complex and is mostly the responsibility of state and local school districts because the federal contribution is relatively small. Because the actual funds issued to support special education programs are far less than the actual cost of the programs, the requirements to provide such services is known as an *unfunded mandate*, meaning that school districts are required to provide such services even though the revenue to do so falls far below what is required.

Speech-language pathologists who work with children both within and outside school systems do not necessarily need to be experts on school funding, but they do need to have some knowledge of how the funding systems work and why some of the challenges exist related to funding. The rest of this chapter will focus on documentation in schools. The requirements are all related to the mandated requirements under the law. Although speech-language pathologists in schools may not be completing these documents for receiving direct payment, in fact every time an assessment, IEP, or prereferral process is provided, decisions are being made that ultimately will cost the system something, not the least of which is the salary of staff. The cost of services should never enter the consideration of the IEP team when making decisions and recommendations for a specific student's eligibility and services; however, as professionals, we must understand how funding works and impacts our work in schools.

Federal Laws Governing School Services

Documentation in schools reflects adherence to the laws that authorize such services. Local school districts may provide specific training on the requirements, including local procedures and forms. The federal laws identified here lay the foundation for all procedures.

Individuals with Disabilities Education Improvement Act

IDEA is the federal law that authorizes special education programs and services in the United States. Under this law, students with disabilities are provided an FAPE in the least restrictive environment (LRE) after a determination that they are entitled to receive such services. The determination of entitlement occurs through assessment, the IEP process, and re-evaluation. Parents and students are provided protections through procedural safeguards, which are realized in the form of timelines, parent consent requirements, and due process appeal procedures. Documentation provides the evidence that these procedural protections have been offered and followed. This concept is critical as a central theme to this chapter. IDEA is a civil rights law. Procedural protections rise from this foundation. Appropriate documentation will be the evidence that rights were afforded to parents and children and that the legal mandates were followed (Moore & Montgomery, 2018).

Of special mention in terms of a discussion regarding reimbursement and funding is the mandate for the provision of an FAPE to students with disabilities, with a special emphasis on the *free* part of this concept. This is where processes, procedures, and importance of documentation are truly realized. When children are identified as meeting eligibility criteria and requiring special education and related services under IDEA, these students become members of a protected class in the United States. The IEP process is utilized to determine FAPE in the LRE. Free, of course, means that there is no charge to the parents, but it also means that IEP teams cannot take cost into consideration when determining what is appropriate.

Family Educational Rights and Privacy Act

The Family Educational Rights and Privacy Act (FERPA) of 1974 is the law that governs student records, particularly as it pertains to privacy and access. Confidentiality is a key issue under IDEA. The provisions of FERPA outline who may have access to student records and also provide procedures if parents wish to challenge the contents of student records or have the records amended. LEAs (i.e., school districts and other agencies providing educational services) have policies adopted by the governing board regarding student records access (e.g., school board policies). FERPA regulations and local policies outline not only who has access to student records, but also record retention regulations that describe which types of records need to be maintained, how long records need to be maintained, and how to dispose of records when they are no longer needed by the agency. Notably, special education documents contain personally identifiable information about the student and are only available to individuals with legitimate education interest. Speech-language pathologists in schools should contact their local administrator to address any specific record request or retention questions.

The Rehabilitation Act of 1973/Section 504 and the Americans with Disabilities Act

The Rehabilitation Act of 1973/Section 504 and the Americans with Disabilities Act (ADA) are civil rights laws providing antidiscrimination basis and access for individuals with disabilities. Under Section 504, accommodation plans are developed for eligible individuals. Like IDEA, procedural safeguards are provided. An important difference is that 504 does not have funding, nor does it have the significant regulations imposed under IDEA. Despite this, 504 has gained increased utilization. Speech-language pathologists may find themselves providing services and supports under 504 to students who are 504 eligible but not IDEA eligible.

The ADA was originally passed in 1990 and was subsequently reauthorized, most recently in 2009. The 2009 reauthorization ties the ADA and 504 together. The ADA provides for access for individuals with disabilities. Original considerations for access under the ADA were seen in physical access to buildings through ramps and mandated elevators, restrooms that accommodated wheelchairs, and other building accommodations. Additionally, access was provided for individuals with hearing loss who needed sign language interpreting or other amplification. More recently, the courts have become involved in legal disputes that arise out of IDEA or 504 but also allege discrimination based on disability. Again, documentation is key in addressing such challenges.

School Processes and Procedures

Prereferral Processes

The procedural protections afforded to students and families under IDEA include consent, timelines, and the right to appeal. Since the passage of Public Law 94-142, LEAs are obligated to conduct Child Find activities in order to seek and serve students with disabilities. At the same time, the determination for eligibility under special education requires that the student meets established criteria in addition to a determination that the student's needs cannot be met through modification to the general program and that the student requires special education to address identified needs. How teams determine whether a student's needs can be met in general education has become increasingly systematic with the development of intervention models that address both academic and behavioral needs of students. These systems include MTSS, RTI, and positive behavior intervention and support. The concept of MTSS brings together the efforts of RTI, positive behavior intervention and support, Title I, special education, English learner services, mental health support, community support, and support for at-risk students. In this comprehensive system, all services designed to support students with academic, social-emotional, and behavioral needs are coordinated. Increasingly, states are moving to this model of coordinated supports, connecting systems designed to assist students in a more cohesive manner (Moore & Montgomery, 2018; "New standards," 2014). School districts across the country are moving to coordinate school-wide systems designed to provide interventions to students with a variety of background and learning needs. These efforts are also supported and encouraged under the reauthorization of the Elementary and Secondary Education Act, known as the Every Student Succeeds Act (2015).

As members of the educational community at a school site, speech-language pathologists are expected to participate in school-wide efforts to provide interventions and to be engaged in efforts to address student needs at the school. The American Speech-Language-Hearing Association (ASHA, 2010) identifies participation in prevention activities and school-wide efforts as part of the roles and responsibilities of school-based speech-language pathologists.

Instructional Support Teams and Response to Intervention

Each school should have a team of individuals whose function is to discuss individual student needs and recommendations. In the past, these teams have been called student study teams or child support teams, but more current terms are *instructional support teams* (ISTs) or *problem-solving teams*. The main difference between the old model and ISTs is that the team's primary function is to consider what types of instructional supports are needed and/or should be attempted to address a student's needs, rather than looking for deficits within the child to explain his or her school failure.

The IST will function within the MTSS or RTI model of the school but may also serve as part of the Child Find process prior to a special education referral (Figure 16-1). For this reason, the speech-language pathologist may serve as a member of the IST. This role is strongly recommended for several reasons, most specifically because students who have needs in language or speech development, literacy issues, or behavior and/or social communication may be referred to the IST by a concerned classroom teacher. Utilizing appropriate IST and RTI processes ensures that students have ample opportunity for prereferral interventions. Progress monitoring is an important part of the RTI process. Speech-language pathologists are well trained in data collection during treatment. These skills are valuable for data collection during progress-monitoring activities. After an intervention is provided with fidelity for an identified period of time (generally 30 to 60 hours of intervention), the data collected will be reviewed to evaluate the student's RTI. If a student is presenting with needs that are suggestive of disability, an appropriate referral for assessment will be made, and that the referral will contain documentation about the student's specific needs, including interventions attempted and the response, or lack thereof, which will inform the assessment.

The process and forms for IST meetings will generally involve information prepared by the concerned teacher regarding academics, behavior, and other concerns such as attendance, medical issues, or home concerns (see Appendix 16-A for a sample IST form). The IST meeting will generally follow a process where the team considers the whole child and the strengths, needs, and other supports that can be provided both at school and possibly in the community to support the student and the family. The purpose of the IST is to design and focus on support.

The following are documentation tips for ISTs:

- Consider the student's educational history in terms of consistency of instruction. For example, if the student has moved schools several times, the student's opportunity to learn would have been impacted. The IST must have documentation related to the student's educational history.
- Consider what types of interventions could be provided to give strategic instruction in a Tier II model. Intervention programs must be provided with adequate time for the student to learn and respond. Generally, this is considered to be between 30 and 60 hours. Consistency and fidelity are key to ensuring success being able to adequately judge the student's response. The IST must have documentation related to fidelity of intervention and response in Tier II model. Fidelity refers to ensuring that the intervention is implemented in the manner in which it is designed. For example, if the recommended dosage for the intervention is 1 hour/day, daily, for a total 35 hours of intervention, but only 20 hours are implemented every other day, fidelity has not been met. A similar example is when medications are prescribed but the patient quits taking the medication when he or she starts feeling better. When he or she has a relapse or does not fully recover, the temptation is to say that the medication was not effective. The same is true when treatment fidelity is not followed.
- Apply the same considerations in Tier II for Tier III.
- Examples of forms and processes are widespread and readily available on the internet, in school publications, and through professional publications. Documentation is critical for interventions prior to any referral to special education for assessment.

Rudebusch (2008) suggests that the speech-language pathologist can serve in the following roles as part of an RTI model at school: Team member, technical assistance provider, curriculum and instruction advisor, problem solver, and direct service provider for assessment and intervention activities (Figure 16-2). For each of these roles, documentation of the assistance provided within the execution of the role will be necessary. If the speech-language pathologist or other special educators are providing services within an RTI model, this is known as *early intervening services*. When engaging in RTI as a direct service provider and/or considering information that is necessary to determine whether a student would be referred for special education assessment, various types of assessment documentation will be required (Figure 16-3).

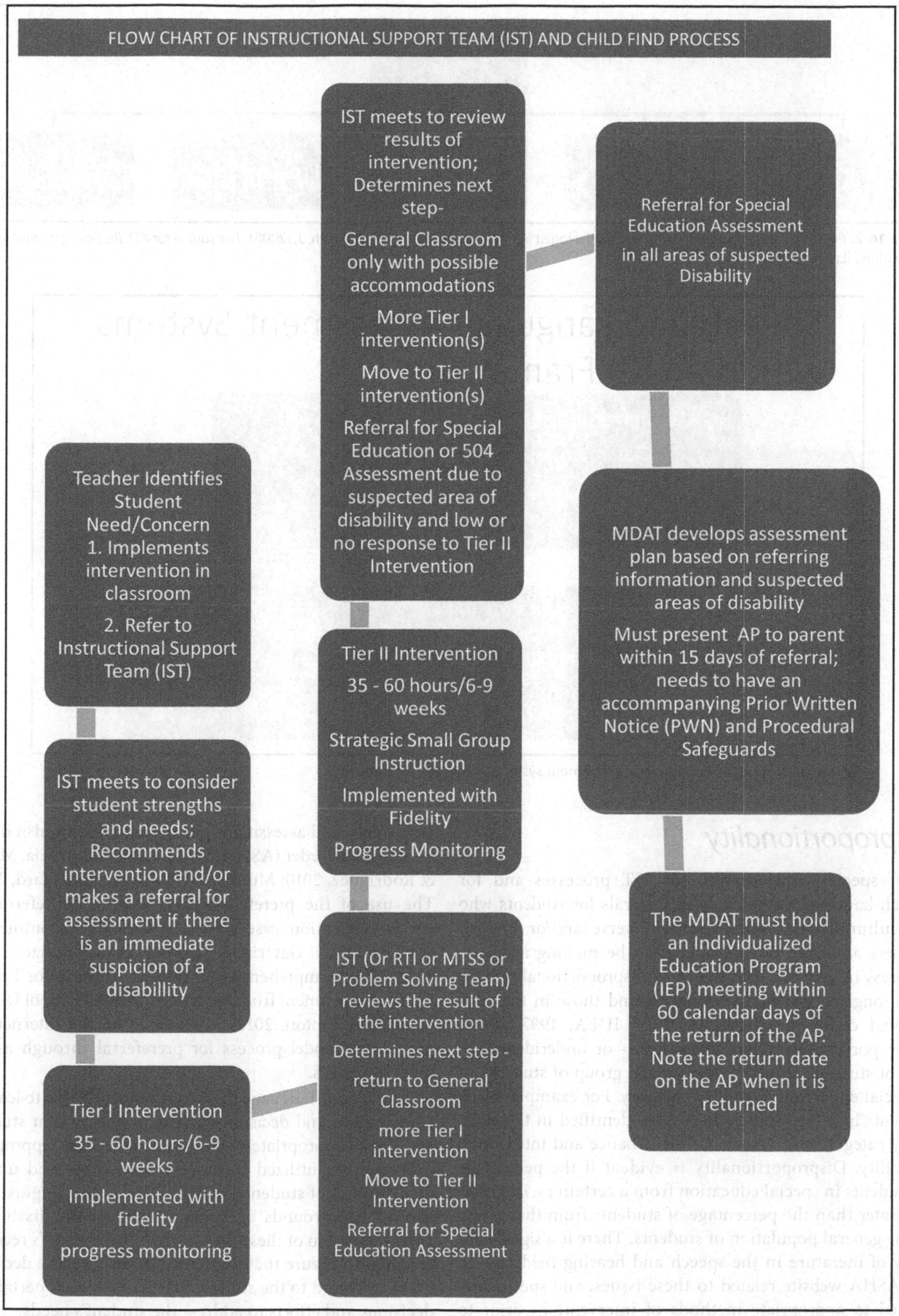

FLOW CHART OF INSTRUCTIONAL SUPPORT TEAM (IST) AND CHILD FIND PROCESS

Teacher Identifies Student Need/Concern
1. Implements intervention in classroom
2. Refer to Instructional Support Team (IST)

IST meets to consider student strengths and needs; Recommends intervention and/or makes a referral for assessment if there is an immediate suspicion of a disabillity

Tier I Intervention
35 - 60 hours/6-9 weeks
Implemented with fidelity
progress monitoring

IST (Or RTI or MTSS or Problem Solving Team) reviews the result of the intervention
Determines next step -
return to General Classroom
more Tier I intervention
Move to Tier II Intervention
Referral for Special Education Assessment

Tier II Intervention
35 - 60 hours/6-9 weeks
Strategic Small Group Instruction
Implemented with Fidelity
Progress Monitoring

IST meets to review results of intervention; Determines next step-
General Classroom only with possible accommodations
More Tier I intervention(s)
Move to Tier II intervention(s)
Referral for Special Education or 504 Assessment due to suspected area of disability and low or no response to Tier II Intervention

Referral for Special Education Assessment in all areas of suspected Disability

MDAT develops assessment plan based on referring information and suspected areas of disability
Must present AP to parent within 15 days of referral; needs to have an accommpanying Prior Written Notice (PWN) and Procedural Safeguards

The MDAT must hold an Individualized Education Program (IEP) meeting within 60 calendar days of the return of the AP. Note the return date on the AP when it is returned

Figure 16-1. Flowchart of IST and Child Find process. (MDAT = multidisciplinary assessment team; AP = assessment plan)

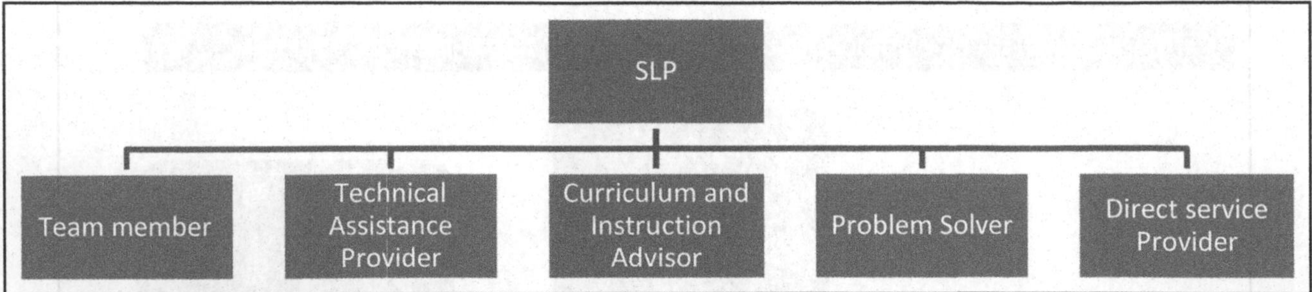

Figure 16-2. Possible roles of speech-language pathologist in RTI. (Adapted from Rudebusch, J. (2008). *The source for RTI: Response to intervention.* East Moline, IL: LinguiSystems.)

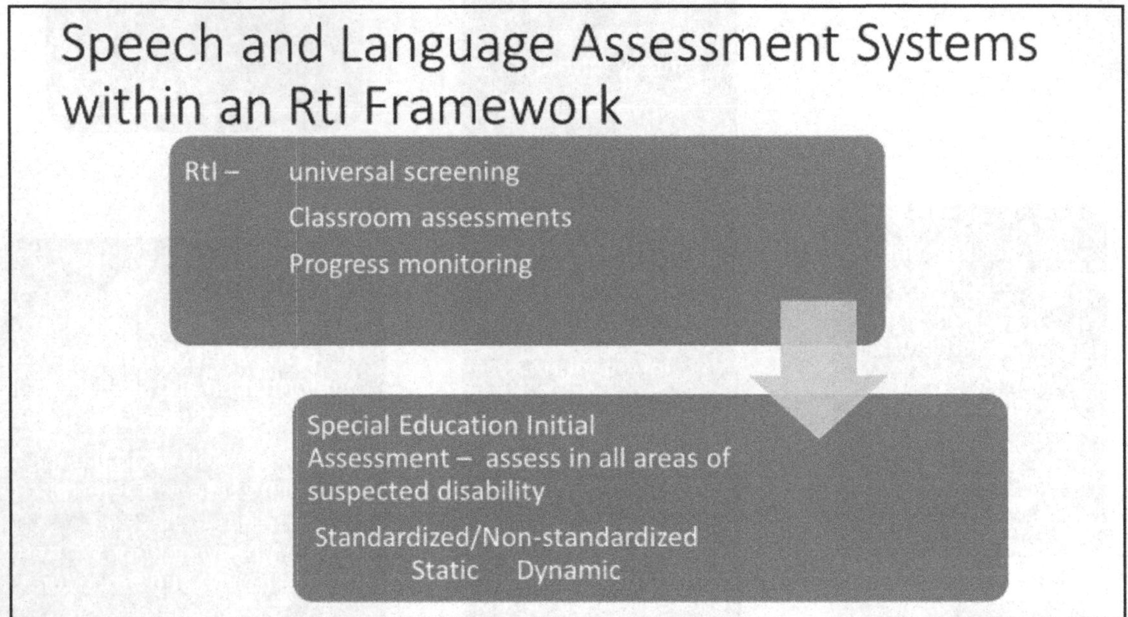

Figure 16-3. Speech and language assessment systems within an RTI framework.

Disproportionality

Of special consideration for IST processes and for speech-language pathologists is referrals for students who are culturally and linguistically diverse and/or English learners and who do not appear to be making adequate progress in schools. The issues of disproportionality have been long recognized by Congress and those in the educational community (Fergus, 2010; IDEA, 1997, 2004). Disproportionality refers to the over- or underidentification of students from a certain racial group of students in a special education eligibility category. For example, Black students have historically been overidentified in the eligibility categories of emotional disturbance and intellectual disability. Disproportionality is evident if the percentage of students in special education from a certain racial group is greater than the percentage of students from that group in the general population of students. There is a significant body of literature in the speech and hearing field and on the ASHA website related to these issues, and specifically related to appropriate methods of interventions prior to assessment and assessment processes to distinguish difference from disorder (ASHA, n.d.-a; Lewis, Castilleja, Moore, & Rodriguez, 2010; Munoz, White, & Horton-Ikard, 2014). The use of the prereferral process prior to referral for special education assessment is strongly recommended (Fergus, 2010; Gaviria & Tipton, 2012; Munzo et al., 2014). The Comprehensive Evaluation Process for English Learners document from San Diego Unified School District (Gaviria & Tipton, 2012) is available on the internet and provides a model process for prereferral through assessment processes.

The speech-language pathologist must be able to lead the conversation and decision making to ensure that students are not inappropriately identified and that appropriate processes are utilized to prevent both over- and underidentification of students from culturally and linguistically diverse backgrounds as being students with disabilities. Documentation of these processes in the student's record is essential to ensure that the record is clear on the decisions made in regard to the student, particularly as it pertains to decisions and efforts to address the student's needs.

Table 16-1

Special Education Timelines

15 days	The number of days that an LEA has to present an assessment plan to the parent from the date of receipt of a referral for special education assessment.
30 days	An IEP meeting must be held within 30 days to review the IEP for a student who has moved into the school district from an outside agency. At this meeting, updates and revisions will be made in consideration of the programs and services in the new district.
60 days	The number of days that an LEA has to hold an IEP meeting from the date of receipt of the signed assessment plan.
1 year	The IEP team must hold an annual meeting to review the student's IEP. This meeting must be held at least annually.
3 years	A triennial evaluation must be conducted every 3 years.
Due process timelines	Due process timelines exist for the agency and district in order to ensure a timely resolution to the filing. Legal and administrative staff are responsible to comply with the timelines.

Assessment for IDEA Eligibility

The standards for documentation in prereferral are focused on student needs and processes that are in place to ensure that students are not inappropriately referred for special education. Once a parent or the IST a recommends that a special education assessment be completed, a series of mandated regulations apply. This process is known as a *referral* and is described here. Educational entities are required to follow legal mandates related to referrals, and if they do not, they are subject to a variety of consequences, including both potential penalties from state and federal agencies and legal challenges from parents and attorneys. Child Find mandates requires LEAs to locate, find, and serve students with disabilities aged 3 to 21, including students who are homeless, attend private schools, are foster youth or wards of the state, and are advancing from grade to grade (IDEA, 2004). Referrals for assessment may come from a variety of places, including from a teacher, IST, parents, physicians, probation officers, or other outside agencies. Ultimately, the parent must give informed consent for the assessment to proceed. Signed assessment plans are an important part of the student record.

Parents and students are afforded procedural safeguards under IDEA. These protections are realized in the form of timelines, informed consent, and the right to appeal.

Timelines

The following timelines apply to IDEA processes. Note that all timelines in special education are calendar days, not school or work days. Timelines toll (i.e., stop) when there are extended breaks, typically over 6 days, such as during the holiday break or summer recess. Documentation of timelines is required in schools. Table 16-1 outlines key timelines in schools.

Assessment Plan

Once a referral for assessment is received by the MDAT, an assessment plan must be prepared and provided to the parent within 15 days of the referral. The assessment is to be conducted in all areas of suspected disability. The referral should indicate the areas of suspected disability. If the referral came from someone other than the parent, it is recommended that an IST meeting be convened with the parent and the referring individual in order to obtain information about why the referring individual or agency is requesting a special education assessment and why the referring individual suspects a disability. Special education assessment is only conducted if there is a suspicion of a disability, so it is important to obtain information about what this suspicion is if the referral comes from the parent or an outside agency. However, the timeline still must be met, so the IST or other parent meeting must occur within the 15 days in order to be able to develop the plan, if that is the determined course of action. If the team determines that an assessment is not warranted, there are procedures for denial, but such action typically requires the involvement and approval of an administrator when a parent requests an assessment. If an agency other than the parent requests assessment, the parent must always be involved because ultimately the parent is the person who needs to give consent to the assessment plan (see Figure 16-1).

Generally, an assessment plan will be developed upon receipt of a request for assessment by the IST or another party. The assessment plan must include consideration of the suspected areas of disability and will reflect the individuals on the MDAT who will complete the assessment. No one individual can conduct an assessment and determine whether a student meets eligibility criteria for special education; therefore, the assessment is conducted by an MDAT. The MDAT will include the team members necessary to ensure that competent assessors are conducting the assessment. These individuals may include the school psychologist, general education classroom teacher, an education specialist (e.g., special education teacher), or other specialists who have expertise in the areas of student needs, such as a speech-language pathologist, behavior specialist, occupational or physical therapist, low incidence specialist for deaf/hard of hearing or visual impairments, audiologist, or other professional with specialized expertise needed to conduct the assessment. The individuals involved must be identified on the assessment plan next to the identified area that will be assessed. Because each assessment is individualized to each child's suspected areas of need, the MDAT's composition will vary depending on the areas that need to be assessed.

Upon an initial assessment, PWN must be provided to the parents to inform them that it is the LEA's intention to conduct an assessment. The PWN must include the following:

- Why the LEA wants to conduct the evaluation (or why it refuses)
- Each evaluation procedure, assessment, record, or report used as a basis for proposing the evaluation (or refusing to conduct the evaluation)
- Where parents can obtain help in understanding IDEA's provisions
- What other options the school considered and why those were rejected
- Any other factors that are relevant to the school's proposal (or refusal) to evaluate the child

PWN forms are generally included with the IEP forms. Be sure to inquire as to when these forms are to be sent and who sends them. Some complicated situations, such as denial of an assessment request, may require involvement of an administrator.

Upon presentation of the assessment plan, the parent must provide informed consent. In order for the parent to provide informed consent, the parent must understand what is included in the assessment plan. This may mean a separate meeting or phone call with the parent, or the parent may be in attendance at the IST or IEP meeting where the referral was made and the plan developed. Such activities should be documented.

The following are documentation tips for assessment plans:

- Develop an assessment plan that includes a plan to assess in all areas of disability, matching the areas of suspected disability from the referring individual(s). Be sure that all areas are included.
- Send parents PWN informing them of the intent to assess, including all required components of PWN. Generally, a form will exist in the district for PWN.
- Issue the plan to the parents within 15 days of the referral. Be sure to document dates sent and received. If the parents do not return the plan within a week, it is recommended that a phone call, email, or other communication with the parent be made. Document the communication. Remember that parents are busy people and may have lost or forgotten to return the document. Do not rely on the student to carry the document back and forth. Send all mail to the parents regular U.S. mail, certified if there is no response. Communicate with administration if parents do not respond to the assessment plan. Follow-up will be necessary.
- Document the date of receipt when the parent returns the assessment plan. Generally, this is done on the assessment plan itself.

Assessment, Eligibility Criteria, and Assessment Report

Each member of the assessment team will perform the testing and other assessment processes and procedures necessary to gather information about the student's performance and needs. Speech-language pathologists and other specialists receive training in assessment methods in their training programs; however, the assessment process in schools is more than testing. Assessment is part of an evaluation where a decision will be reached as to whether a student meets eligibility criteria and requires special education to address goals in the areas of need. Clear documentation of the processes and procedures that lead to addressing this question are key to the decisions made for children. Additionally, the information solicited and entered into the record will guide future professionals who work with the student to know why certain decisions were made about student needs and the decisions that were made regarding eligibility and service.

The assessment completed by the speech-language pathologist will seek to answer a referring question. It is not enough to ask, "Does the student have a speech-language impairment?" The assessment must be structured to address the question of whether the student meets eligibility criteria, what the identified learning needs are within the suspected area(s) of disability, and what recommendations would arise out of identification of those

Table 16-2
IDEA Eligibility Categories
• Autism • Deaf • Deaf-blind • Emotional disturbance • Intellectual disability • Multiple disabilities • Other health impairment • Orthopedic impairment • Speech-language impairment • Specific learning disability • Traumatic brain injury • Visual impairment

needs. Review Appendix 16-B closely for the legal requirements related to assessments. Speech-language pathologists must closely adhere to and document adherence to the requirements.

If the first step in assessment is selection of the instruments, tools, and procedures to determine eligibility and student need, the second step is establishing eligibility. Eligibility determination is the responsibility of the IEP team, but the speech-language pathologist will bring information and make recommendations. There are 13 eligibility categories under IDEA (Table 16-2). The MDAT may be conducting assessment in one or several suspected areas of disability. Following assessment, the team will consider all the information gathered and make an eligibility determination at the IEP meeting. Communication among the members of the team is strongly recommended so that the team can know and understand the needs presented by the student. In some districts, one report may be written to demonstrate that it is a team report and the evaluation is a team effort. In many school districts, it is expected that an eligibility statement be included in the assessment report, with the caveat that the final determination is made by the IEP team. If a student is eligible under any of the disability categories and is determined to be in need of specially designed instruction, then he or she is determined to be eligible for special education. For example, a student may be eligible in the area of autism and be determined to have needs that will require specially designed instruction (e.g., special education services) to address the student's unique learning needs. Based on needs identified in the assessments, the team will establish goals and then determine services.

Speech-language pathologists, special and general educators, and parents are often confused by what it means to qualify. First, there is no such thing as qualifying for services. A student must meet eligibility criteria, and then, based on identified needs and the need for specialized instruction, goals are established and services determined. So, for example, a student who is determined to meet the criteria for autism will have needs in the area of communication, including expressive and/or receptive language and/or social communication, because deficits in this area are part of the eligibility criteria. This student does not also need to meet the eligibility criteria for speech-language impairment because the speech and language needs are a component of the student's autism. Sometimes, the IEP team will choose to find that the student has a secondary eligibility, but in reality, identification of a secondary eligibility is only necessary if the areas of need are not related to the primary disability.

The eligibility category of speech-language impairment is defined as follows:

> Speech or language impairment means a communication disorder, such as stuttering, impaired articulation, a language impairment, or a voice impairment, that adversely affects a child's educational performance. C.F.R.: Part 300/A/300.8/c/11

Assessment for speech-language impairment would include evaluation in the appropriate area as it pertains to the referral and the student's presenting needs. In many states, further regulations exist defining how each of these areas is determined to be deficit. Such regulation gives guidance to how the assessment is to be conducted. Additionally, it is critical to note the criteria that the communication disorder must adversely affect the child's educational performance. This is notable because it closely ties to the observation requirement and the need for the speech-language pathologist to describe the connection between the disability to how the student's academic progress is impacted. (Note: This requirement is also contained in the IEP development discussed later.)

Finally, the information gathered in the assessment and evaluation must be documented in an assessment report. Many school districts have templates or formats for staff to follow. The following information from Moore and Montgomery (2018) provides specific information about what should be included in the assessment report:

> An assessment is not just standardized testing but a comprehensive analysis of the student. Assessments must comply with the education code. An assessment may include review of records, standardized testing, non-standardized testing, classroom observations, observations in other relevant areas, and parent, teacher, and student interviews. Speech-language pathologists must be sure the report includes a pertinent background, a discussion of assessment results, and an explanation of the choice of assessment instruments; documentation on suspected areas of need and explanation of student needs; justification for needed services; connection to other reports and assessments; and information on interviews with

Table 16-3

Assessment Report Format

- Reason for assessment
- Background information
- Assessment and testing
- Standardized assessments or tests
- Observation in natural setting
- Non-standardized assessment or methods
- Activities within natural setting
- Behaviors observed during assessment
- Information on progress in academic or curricular areas
- Information on classroom assessments and statewide assessments
- Information from others (e.g., parents, teachers, aide, other MDAT members)
- Input from the student
- Impressions
- Summary and conclusions
- Recommendations

Reprinted with permission from Moore, B. J., & Montgomery, J. K. (2018). *Speech-language pathologists in public schools: Making a difference for America's children.* Austin, TX: Pro Ed.

parents and teachers. Reports should be written in a professional manner, using professional terminology, but written so parents understand. (Moore & Montgomery, 2018, p. 116)

A typical assessment report format is outlined in Table 16-3. As mentioned previously, some districts require the assessor to make a qualifying statement related to suspected areas of disability and the assessment results in comparison to the eligibility category/categories considered. Such a statement would identify the eligibility criteria code and then make recommendations based on the assessment results. The following are documentation tips for assessments and assessment reports:

- Document the referring concerns and the reason for the assessment, as well as the purpose of the assessment.
- Remember that protocols are considered student records and will be maintained in the child's special education folder. Notes and impressions made on these documents should be professional and germane to the assessment question.
- Document communicative behaviors during observations, as well as the context and the communicative demands. Ensure that observations occur in more than one setting and that the length of time of the observation is at least 20 to 30 minutes in order to make it meaningful.
- Ensure the use of objective and professional language.
- Ensure the use of appropriate grammar and spelling.
- If using a template, be sure that the report is individualized to this student and no errors occur that contain other students' names or data.
- Describe why certain assessment instruments were selected as each pertains to the individual student. Describe the parameters of dynamic or portfolio assessments if used. The use of standardized measures in a non-standardized manner is strongly discouraged.
- Be sure to include descriptions of cultural considerations if appropriate (e.g., the use of an interpreter).
- Ensure discussion with other members of the MDAT, so that there is consistency in the reports regarding student behavior and needs. If there are variations in results from different assessors, a discussion in the report is necessary.
- Ensure a summary that contain interpretive information that will allow the reader to follow the conclusions and recommendations.
- Include impressions, conclusions, and recommendations.

The assessment report may be a stand-alone report or may be part of a multidisciplinary report. Remember that this is a most important piece of documentation and will be referred to many times over the course of the student's school career, and potentially beyond. This document will impact the student and lead the team to make educational decisions about the student. Failure to ensure that all pertinent and required aspects of the assessment are included in the assessment report could lead to unintended consequences, such as inappropriate service decisions and legal challenges.

Individualized Education Program Meetings

The documentation requirements for the development of the IEP itself will be discussed in the next section. The IEP meeting is a specialized process that has its own documentation requirements. Several key requirements of IDEA come together at the IEP meeting, so the documentation related to this meeting is an essential part of ensuring that legal requirements are followed and procedural safeguards are ensured. These requirements include the following:

- Provide the parent with adequate Notice of Meeting in writing. Notice requirements are specific and vary from state to state and local regions. Be sure to check with your local agency to ensure timely and appropriate procedures. Also, the Notice of Meeting may or may not comply with PWN requirements. PWN is required for initial evaluations and other types of meetings. Again, refer to local policy. PWN puts the parent on notice that the district is intending some action for the student.

- Hold a meeting to review an initial evaluation and/or any other type of assessment and subsequently follow the processes indicated due to the basis of that assessment.
- Conduct a meeting for the purpose of an annual review or triennial evaluation meeting.
- Convene a meeting for some other defined purpose such as a Manifestation Determination, development of an Individualized Transition Plan, or development of a Behavior Support Plan.
- Convene a meeting at the request of a parent or other team member.
- Ensure parental participation and document parent's questions, input, concerns, and suggestions.
- Ensure that all required members of the IEP team are at all meetings, including the parent, the general education teacher, a special education teacher, and a representative of the LEA, generally an administrator. An individual who can explain testing and curriculum is also required, if the administrator is not able to do so. Other individuals who have a legitimate educational interest may also be in attendance.
- Always have a written report to provide to the parent at the meeting. As often as possible, provide the parents the report in advance so they can come to the meeting prepared to discuss it.

In the section on IEPs, the requirements for the IEP document will be highlighted. The IEP team should prepare a draft IEP document prior to the meeting. Remember that the IEP document will reflect the student's levels of performance and needs and recommend goals and services. The IEP team cannot predetermine services, but specialists and the team certainly should go into meetings with recommendations. Too often, IEP teams do not recommend what they believe is appropriate for a student for fear that the parents will not accept the offer. Lawyers advise that educators remember that the offer of a FAPE must be designed to confer educational benefit (Rowley Standard) in light of the child's circumstances (Endrew F. Standard). This means that the IEP needs to be written to benefit the student and not base the IEP on what it is thought the parent might accept. In order to help with the decision-making process, utilize the service-level decision-making framework in Figure 16-4.

At the meeting, it is critically important the required process is followed. Because IEP meetings can involve many people and many issues, as well as many procedures, many IEP teams find it beneficial to use an agenda and share it with the parents at the beginning of the meeting. In fact, many teams find it beneficial to post the agenda on the wall or make copies for all in attendance. If an agenda is used, it is wise to attach it to the IEP document. See Appendix 16-C for a sample IEP meeting agenda.

The IEP meeting processes and procedures should always follow the same routine (Figure 16-5). An IEP meeting begins with present levels of performance. If assessment was completed, then the assessment report are reviewed and discussed. Otherwise, updated information from teachers and reports on prior goals will then lead to a discussion of needs, goals needed to address the needs, and finally services and programs. Following this process ensures that violations do not occur. The meeting notes should document the process every step of the way.

Meeting notes are not mandated but are strongly encouraged, unless it is against local policy or practice. Meeting notes can serve to document the process, parent questions and responses, discussion, and how decisions were reached. The meeting notes may also document the district's offer of a FAPE. Meeting notes are not intended to be a verbatim transcription of the meeting but can serve to ensure that all parties have a collective recollection of what happened at the meeting. This will also serve as the record in the event of future disputes. For example, if the speech-language pathologist has recommended dismissal and the parent disagrees, the meeting notes can reflect the recommendation, rationale, ensuing discussion, and decision.

The IEP team should decide ahead of the meeting who will take the notes. This can vary from team to team and district to district. In general, it is very difficult to be the person running the meeting, giving a report and updating goals, and also taking the notes. There are several people at the meeting. Decide who will do what before sitting at the table. New staff, whether new to the field or new to the school, should inquire as to the culture and expectations at IEP meetings for all of the processes and procedures.

Therapy Notes/Documentation of Services

Keeping therapy notes is the standard in the speech and hearing field, regardless of the work setting (Moore, 2010). School services are no different. Therapy notes are required to document the services provided and the outcomes realized by the student. In hospital and clinic settings, SOAP (subjective, objective, assessment, plan) notes are the common practice. Although this is not necessarily expected in school settings, the format provides information that is useful should the notes be called into question for legal matters, including due process hearings, parent challenges, and/or an audit by Medicaid. Therapy notes are considered school records. Therapy notes must include information on the goals addressed, description of the activity and student response, and the setting and model of service. These are not intended to be long and cumbersome but must reflect what happened in the session and the student's progress. (Other chapters in this book provide additional information on therapy notes that can be applied to a school

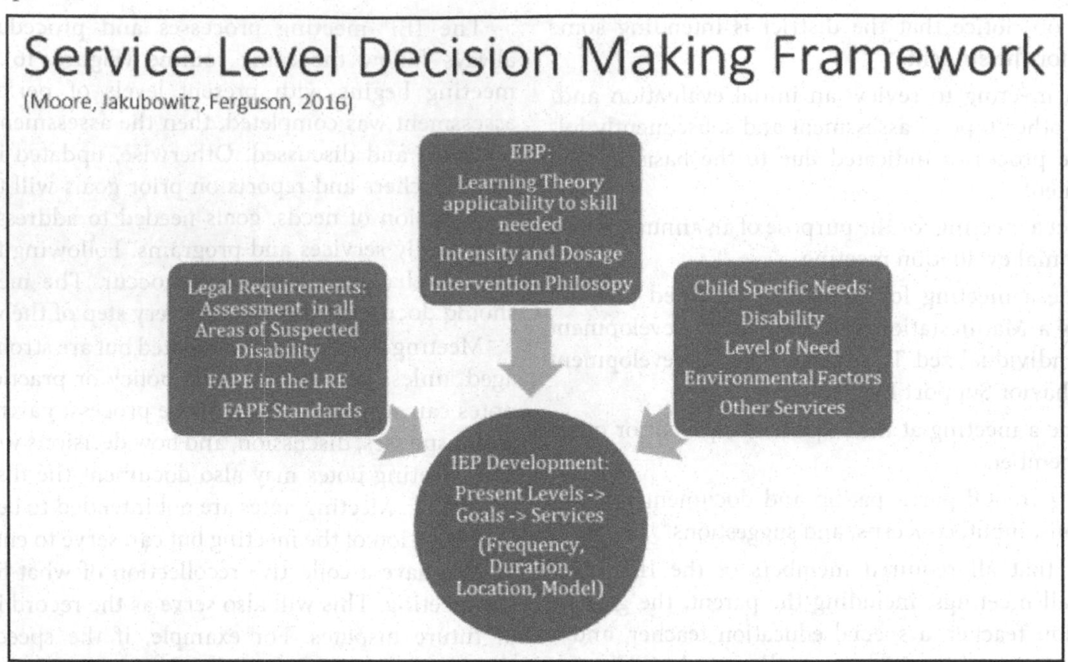

Figure 16-4. Service-level decision-making framework. (Adapted from Moore, B., Jakubowitz, M., and Ferguson, M. (2016, November). *What! I Don't Have Time to Treat 5X a Week!!* Presented at American Speech-Language-Hearing Association Convention, Philadelphia, PA.)

setting.) Parents may ask to see the notes, and the notes will need to be copied and provided to them. Inform administration any time there is a request for records because the district will also need to document the timeliness and compliance with the request. Additionally, such requests may be an indication of an impending dispute.

School Records and Parent Communication

School records are covered by FERPA and include the following:

- Mandatory permanent pupil records: Required by state law, which usually includes identifying information about the pupil, when the student attended the schools in the district, and records of subjects taken, grades, immunizations, and date of graduation or exit
- Mandatory interim pupil records: Held for a stipulated period of time, including health information, special education information, language training records, progress reports, parental restrictions, parent/pupil challenges to records, parent authorizations/prohibitions for student participation in certain programs, and results of standardized tests
- Permitted pupil records: Counselor/teacher rating scales, standardized tests older than 3 years, routine discipline, behavioral reports, discipline notices, attendance records

Medical records are covered under the Health Insurance Portability and Accountability Act (HIPAA). When medical records are requested and received by school districts, they become part of the student's school records, so are governed by FERPA. School-based speech-language pathologists are trained in both FERPA and HIPAA and should treat records with great respect, especially as they are creating them (Moore, 2013).

One common question that speech-language pathologists have is regarding email and personal notes and whether these are considered part of a student record. Email is not considered a student record but may be subpoenaed. The author recently went through this experience, and it was most challenging. If emails are shared or printed and put in the student's file, it definitely becomes a student record. The same is true of personal notes. Although some lawyers may say that personal notes are acceptable, the author advises that it is not wise to think that such notes might not be eventually seen by the parents (Moore, 2012). Always be prudent regarding what is put in writing. Also, it is wise to be cautious. There have been times that an email, unintended for the parents, has been forwarded to them intentionally or unintentionally. If more evidence is

IEP Meeting Process

Determination of Present Levels of Educational Achievement

- **Review evaluation data**
- **Review classroom performance**
- **Review other related information**
- **Consider input from parents, teachers, and specialists**

↓

Determination of Goals and Short-Term Objectives or Benchmarks

- **Based on identified areas of need**
- **Designed to enable the child to progress in the general education curriculum**
- **Must be measurable**

↓

Determination of Program, Placement, and Services

- **Includes services needed in order for goals to be achieved**
- **Designed to confer meaningful educational benefit**

Figure 16-5. The IEP meeting process. (Reprinted with permission from Moore, B. J., & Montgomery, J. K. (2018). *Speech-language pathologists in public schools: Making a difference for America's children*. Austin, TX: Pro Ed.)

needed to be cautious, it should be noted that in California, the California Supreme Court has ruled that when a public employee uses a personal account for district communication, it may be subject to disclosure under the California Public Records Act (*City of San Jose v. Superior Court of Santa Clara County*, 2017; Fagen, Friedman & Fulfrost LLP, 2017). Although this case does not pertain to student records and confidentiality, it does have to do with electronic communication and not limiting access if it applies. Again, caution is wise, even on personal accounts.

Parent communication is critical to any therapeutic relationship, and especially when working with children in schools. Although this chapter contains references to litigation and potential challenges that can and should be addressed by complete documentation, this is not intended to diminish the importance of open communication and actively seeking partnerships with families. Parent involvement is one of the foundation principles and rights of special education. However, keeping documentation of all phone calls, letters, pertinent incidental conversations, and email or other written communication is very important. If there are challenges to the case, be sure to share these records with the district administrator and attorney, if necessary.

Parents may feel like they are not being involved in the IEP process and decision making. Interviews with parents often show their frustration and dismay with the process (Moore & Heisler, 2015). Remembering to consider the feelings of the parent and the importance of parent involvement is key to success. Documenting efforts to do so is also advised.

Individualized Education Program

IEPs are the cornerstone of special education. When a student is identified by the MDAT as a child with a disability, the student is now a member of a protected class in the United States. These children are entitled to specialized services to address their identified needs. Special education is heavily laden with processes and procedures that are developed to ensure that students are afforded their rights and protections. The U.S. Supreme Court ruled that an IEP should be "designed to confer educational benefit" (*Board of Education of Hendrick Hudson Central School District v. Rowley*, 1982). In 2017, the Supreme Court extended the Rowley Standard, ruling that the IEP team must offer an IEP that is "reasonably calculated to enable the child to progress in light of the child's circumstances". (Endrew F. by Joseph F. v Douglas County School District RE-1 [Case #15-827]) Documentation and compliance are the ways that school districts ensure that student needs are met and that the district has evidence of a legally constituted IEP should a legal challenge or a state or federal review of compliance occur. Procedural errors may be determined by a judge to be a denial of an FAPE.

States and LEAs have their own IEP documents, typically in electronic form. The data inputted into the IEP form demonstrates compliance with the requirements of special education. IEP documents are typically prepared as drafts prior to the IEP meeting. At the IEP meeting, the family and the district representatives follow the process described previously and make adjustments to the information. Certain sections can be drafted ahead of time, but others cannot and should not. School districts are prohibited to predetermine placement, so completing the placement and services section prior to the IEP, even in draft form, would be considered predetermination and a denial of the parents' right to participate. Be sure not to complete the services section of the IEP ahead of time. Common documentation errors and recommended practices are identified in Appendix 16-D.

There are many training manuals, templates, and models for IEP writing, yet this continues to be a challenging area. Many speech-language pathologists and other educators complain about the paperwork burden of special education, but these requirements have only increased over the years. Being attentive to writing clear and specific information in assessment reports and on the present levels section of the IEP will help guide the IEP team in its development so that it is clear to the parent and other educators, which also yields education benefit to the student.

The following are documentation tips for IEPs:

- Attend to the accuracy of dates and student information.
- Ensure that there is a clear connection in the record between the assessment, identified areas of need, goals, and services.
- Ensure that baselines on goals are clearly identified.
- Ensure that goals are measurable.
- Report to parents on progress toward goals, and document this information.
- Review progress on goals at the annual review.
- Do not copy information in present levels from one year to another. Each year should provide updated information on the student's status and present levels.
- Do not carry over goals from one year to the next. If the student is not meeting goals, it needs to be revised.
- Call an IEP meeting during the year if goals and services need to be adjusted.

The IEP document tells the student's story and the story of the supports and services received. Appropriate documentation is not only a service to the student, it is a service to the next service provider who reads, and needs to implement, the IEP.

Medicaid

In some states, school districts are allowed to bill for speech-language pathology assessment and treatment services under certain conditions. Medicaid is a federal and state program that provides medical care to families with low incomes. If a state participates in this program, school districts can bill for the provision of speech-language pathology and audiology services, as well as other health services, mental health services, transportation, and psychological assessments. School districts may have a third-party vendor who manages the billing, or they may have a staff person who manages this process and these records. At the IEP meeting, parent permission to bill Medicaid or other insurance must be secured.

The ASHA website provides the following guidance regarding documentation guidelines for Medicaid:

> Documentation is a key component for any speech-language pathologist or audiologist to receive proper reimbursement for services provided. If a service is not fully documented, health care providers may deny reimbursement. In the schools, [speech-language pathologists] and audiologists should follow Medicaid documentation guidelines (ASHA, n.d.-b).

Medicaid requires providers to keep records for each individual receiving services. These records must contain all screening elements. Documentation must also include the following:

- Dates of service
- Who provided the service
- Where the service was provided
- Any required medical documentation
- Medical condition of the recipient
- Length of time required for service
- Third-party billing information (ASHA, n.d.-b)

In schools, an electronic system will be utilized for documentation of services. The speech-language pathologist does not need to identify which students are Medicaid eligible in most states. This is done through the electronic system. What is important is to ensure that the IEP documentation matches the services provided. Many districts find that using the electronic system that is used for Medicaid also is a good way to keep therapy notes for all students on the speech caseload.

Speech-language pathologists should study the manual and guidelines for their state. There are specific regulations related to what service delivery models are allowed for reimbursement and how this is to be documented.

Record retention is also different for Medicaid than it is for education under FERPA. A Medicaid audit may occur up to 7 years later. If records are lost or not able to be located, then the district runs the risk of losing funds for services provided for which the district already received payment. This is one of the benefits of electronic records, but many agencies still require hard copies for records in addition to electronic.

Funds raised through Medicaid billing are intended to go back to the program(s) that generate the funds. The school district is required to have a collaborative consisting of participating members (i.e., those who can bill) and these individuals make a plan for how to expend these dollars for the benefit of the students and the programs that generated the dollars. A collaborative might include nurses, social workers, psychologists, occupational or physical therapists, a community member, and a parent. Licensed personnel who are providing services that are medically necessary are able to bill. Transportation and health care procedures also are billable under certain situations. In order for the services to be eligible for reimbursement, the services must be listed in the IEP. The funds received are intended to supplement, not supplant fund that the district is required to spend on special education and services.

For more information on Medicaid, see the ASHA website (ASHA, n.d.-b).

Conclusion

Documenting compliance with legal requirements is a critical function for school-based speech-language pathologists. School services are anything but free. Failure to document adequately can have several costs, including costing a student inadequate services, costing the school district litigation expenses, and costing the speech-language pathologist to suffer in terms of professional reputation. On the other hand, appropriate documentation leads to ensuring that the student's needs are accurately identified, that parent and student rights are protected, and that those reading the file can follow the rationale for how and why services were provided in the manner described. Clear documentation also provides a legally defensible record, which demonstrates that the student was served as intended under IDEA.

References

American Speech-Language-Hearing Association. (n.d.-a). Cultural competence. Retrieved from http://www.asha.org/PRPSpecificTopic.aspx?folderid=8589935230§ion=Key_Issues

American Speech-Language-Hearing Association. (n.d.-b). Introduction to Medicaid. Retrieved from http://www.asha.org/practice/reimbursement/medicaid/medicaid_intro/

American Speech-Language-Hearing Association. (2010). Roles and responsibilities of speech-language pathologists in schools [Position Statement]. Retrieved from https://www.asha.org/slp/schools/prof-consult/guidelines.htm

Board of Education of Hendrick Hudson Central School District v. Rowley, 458 U.S. 176 (1982).

City of San Jose v. Superior Court of Santa Clara County (S218066, March 2, 2017)

Endrew F. by Joseph F. v Douglas County School District RE-1, 580 U.S. Part 2 (2017)

Every Student Succeeds Act (ESSA), Pub. L. No. 114-95 (2015).

Institute on Education Sciences & National Center on Educational Statistics. (n.d.). Expenditures. Retrieved from https://nces.ed.gov/fastfacts/display.asp?id=66

Fagen, Friedman & Fulfrost LLP. (2017). CA Supreme Court: Personal emails and texts may be subject to PRA requests. Retrieved from https://www.f3law.com/newsflash.php?nf=511

Family Educational Rights and Privacy Act (FERPA), 20 U.S.C. § 1232g; 34 CFR Part 99 (1974).

Fergus, E. (2010). Distinguishing difference from disability: The common causes of racial/ethnic disproportionality in special education. *Equity Alliance at Arizona State University*. Retrieved from http://ea.niusileadscape.org/docs/FINAL_PRODUCTS/LearningCarousel/Distinguishing_Difference_from_Disability.pdf

Gaviria, A., & Tipton, T. (2012). CEP-EL: A comprehensive evaluation process for English learners. San Diego, CA: San Diego Unified School District. Retrieved from https://www.sandiegounified.org/sites/default/files_link/district/files/dept/special_education/ParentServices/CEP-EL%20Manual.pdf

Individuals With Disabilities Education Act of 1990, 20 U.S.C. § 1400 et seq. (1990) (amended 1997).

Individuals With Disabilities Education Improvement Act of 2004, 20 U.S.C. § 1400 *et seq.* (2004).

Lewis, N., Castilleja, N., Moore, B. J., & Rodriguez, B. (2010). Assessment 360: A panoramic framework for assessing English language learners. *ASHA Special Interest Division 14 (Communication Disorders and Sciences in Culturally and Linguistically Diverse Populations) Perspectives, 17*(2), 35–56.

Moore, B. (2010). If it's not documented, it didn't happen. *ASHA Special Interest Division 11 (Administration and Supervision) Perspectives, 20*, 106–112.

Moore, B. (2013). Documentation issues in speech-language pathology and audiology. In R. Lubinski & M. Hudson (Eds.), *Professional issues in speech-language pathology and audiology* (4th ed.). Clifton Park, NY: Cengage/Delmar Publishers.

Moore, B. J. (2012). Five common documentation questions—answered. *The ASHA Leader, 17,* 22–24.

Moore, B. J., & Heisler, L. (2015). Individual education plans: The rule of law and the art of collaboration. Seminar presented at American Speech-Language-Hearing Association Convention, Denver, CO.

Moore, B. J., & Montgomery, J. K. (2018). *Speech-language pathologists in public schools: Making a difference for America's children* (3rd ed.). Austin, TX: Pro Ed.

Munoz, M., White, M., & Horton-Ikard, R. (2014). The identification conundrum: How do we keep bilingual children from being over- or under-identified with speech-language impairments? *The ASHA Leader, 19,* 48–53.

New standards and tiered systems: A perfect fit. (2014). *The Special EDge.* Retrieved from http://www.calstat.org/publications/spedge_publications.php?nl_id=129

Rudebusch, J. (2008). *The source for RTI: Response to intervention.* East Moline, IL: LinguiSystems.

U.S. Department of Education. (2016). Special education—Grants to states. Retrieved from https://www2.ed.gov/programs/osepgts/funding.html

Review Questions

1. Discuss the ways public schools receive funding.
2. What requirements must be met before a student can receive speech and language services in the schools?
3. How are students referred for speech and language services?
4. Discuss the types of records parents have the right to receive.
5. Describe how Medicaid funds are used in public schools.

Activity A

1. Search the website of your local school district for the procedural safeguards for parents under IDEA. Review this document. Discuss with a classmate the following:
   a. If you were a parent of a child with a disability, how easy was it to find this document?
   b. If you were the parent of a child with a disability, how clearly presented is the information about rights, processes, and who to ask for help?
   c. What is your overall impression of the rights and protections afforded to parents and children?
   d. How important is it for speech-language pathologists in schools to know and understand the rights and protections afforded to parents and children?
2. From your practicum assignment, review an assessment and IEP for a student receiving speech and language services. Can you follow the referral process through to the determination of services? Why or why not? Discuss with your master clinician.
3. Develop a graphic of important documentation requirements and how you will ensure that you incorporate these into your practice.

Appendix 16-A

Instructional Support Team Sample Meeting Data Collection Form

INSTRUCTIONAL SUPPORT TEAM (IST)
SAMPLE MEETING DATA COLLECTION FORM

STUDENT: **ID#:** **BIRTHDATE:** **GRADE:** **SCHOOL:** **DATE:**

BACKGROUND INFORMATION	STRENGTHS	PRESENT CONCERNS	STRATEGIES/ACTIONS	RESPONSIBILITY (Who/When)

MEMBERS IN ATTENDANCE:

Parent/Guardian	Date	Student	Date	Teacher	Date	FOLLOW-UP AND ACTIONS
Teacher	Date	Teacher	Data	Teacher/Other Member	Date	
Counselor	Date	Principal/Assistant Principal	Date	IST Member	Date	

Karge & Ramirez, 2016

Reprinted with permission from Karge, B. D., & Ramirez, F. (2016). A father's perspective into the special education referral process [unpublished manuscript].

Appendix 16-B
Evaluation Requirements

Initial and Re-Evaluation Procedures

Sec. 300.304 Evaluation procedures.

(a) Notice. The public agency must provide notice to the parents of a child with a disability, in accordance with Sec. 300.503, that describes any evaluation procedures the agency proposes to conduct.

(b) Conduct of evaluation. In conducting the evaluation, the public agency must:

(1) Use a variety of assessment tools and strategies to gather relevant functional, developmental, and academic information about the child, including information provided by the parent, that may assist in determining:

(i) Whether the child is a child with a disability under Sec. 300.8; and

(ii) The content of the child's IEP, including information related to enabling the child to be involved in and progress in the general education curriculum (or for a preschool child, to participate in appropriate activities);

(2) Not use any single measure or assessment as the sole criterion for determining whether a child is a child with a disability and for determining an appropriate educational program for the child; and

(3) Use technically sound instruments that may assess the relative contribution of cognitive and behavioral factors, in addition to physical or developmental factors.

(c) Other evaluation procedures. Each public agency must ensure that:

(1) Assessments and other evaluation materials used to assess a child under this part:

(i) Are selected and administered so as not to be discriminatory on a racial or cultural basis;

(ii) Are provided and administered in the child's native language or other mode of communication and in the form most likely to yield accurate information on what the child knows and can do academically, developmentally, and functionally, unless it is clearly not feasible to so provide or administer;

(iii) Are used for the purposes for which the assessments or measures are valid and reliable;

(iv) Are administered by trained and knowledgeable personnel; and

(v) Are administered in accordance with any instructions provided by the producer of the assessments.

(2) Assessments and other evaluation materials include those tailored to assess specific areas of educational need and not merely those that are designed to provide a single general intelligence quotient.

(3) Assessments are selected and administered so as best to ensure that if an assessment is administered to a child with impaired sensory, manual, or speaking skills, the assessment results accurately reflect the child's aptitude or achievement level or whatever other factors the test purports to measure, rather than reflecting the child's impaired sensory, manual, or speaking skills (unless those skills are the factors that the test purports to measure).

(4) The child is assessed in all areas related to the suspected disability, including, if appropriate, health, vision, hearing, social and emotional status, general intelligence, academic performance, communicative status, and motor abilities;

(5) Assessments of children with disabilities who transfer from one public agency to another public agency in the same school year are coordinated with those children's prior and subsequent schools, as necessary and as expeditiously as possible, consistent with Sec. 300.301(d)(2) and (e) to ensure prompt completion of full evaluations.

(6) In evaluating each child with a disability under Sec. Sec. 300.304 through 300.306, the evaluation is sufficiently comprehensive to identify all of the child's special education and related services needs, whether or not commonly linked to the disability category in which the child has been classified.

(7) Assessment tools and strategies that provide relevant information that directly assists persons in determining the educational needs of the child are provided.

(Authority: 20 U.S.C. 1414(b)(1)-(3), 1412(a)(6)(B))

C.F.R.: Part 300/D/300.305/a

(a) Review of existing evaluation data. As part of an initial evaluation (if appropriate) and as part of any re-evaluation under this part, the IEP team and other qualified professionals, as appropriate, must:

(1) Review existing evaluation data on the child, including:

(i) Evaluations and information provided by the parents of the child;

(ii) Current classroom-based, local, or State assessments, and classroom-based observations; and

(iii) Observations by teachers and related services providers; and

(2) On the basis of that review, and input from the child's parents, identify what additional data, if any, are needed to determine:

(i) (A) Whether the child is a child with a disability, as defined in Sec. 300.8, and the educational needs of the child; or

(B) In case of a re-evaluation of a child, whether the child continues to have such a disability, and the educational needs of the child;

(ii) The present levels of academic achievement and related developmental needs of the child;

(iii) (A) Whether the child needs special education and related services; or

(B) In the case of a re-evaluation of a child, whether the child continues to need special education and related services; and

(iv) Whether any additions or modifications to the special education and related services are needed to enable the child to meet the measurable annual goals set out in the IEP of the child and to participate, as appropriate, in the general education curriculum.

Adapted from Education, 34 C.F.R. § 300.305, (2012); Individuals With Disabilities Education Improvement Act of 2004, 20 U.S.C. § 1400 et seq. (2004).

Appendix 16-C

Sample Individualized Education Program Meeting Agenda

1. Welcome and introductions
2. Explanation of purpose of meeting and time-ordered agenda
3. Procedural safeguards
4. Review demographic information
5. Present levels, including parents' input and concerns
6. Eligibility: Only if one of the purposes of the meeting is to determine eligibility. If student is not eligible, do not need to complete the rest of the items.
7. Review past goals
8. Determine areas of need based on present levels and reviewing past goals
9. Proposed goals: May need to change depending on discussion at meeting
10. Accommodations/participation in statewide assessments
11. Individual Transition Plan (only for students in high school)
12. Service time recommendation: Based on present levels and proposed goals
13. Extended school year determination (regression and recoupment) and transportation discussion (based on severity of need)
14. District offer of FAPE
15. Read notes back and review IEP for accuracy
16. Obtain signatures of all IEP meeting participants
17. Provide copy of IEP to parents

(B. Nishida, personal communication, March 9, 2017)

Appendix 16-D

Common Individualized Education Program Documentation Errors and Recommended Process and Practices

IEP Requirement	Common Process and Documentation Errors	Recommended Process and Documentation Practice
Parents' concerns/ input	• Failure to solicit parents' concerns regarding their child's education • Soliciting parent input at the end of the meeting • Parent states "no concerns"	• Start the meeting by asking the parents for their concerns regarding their child. If the parents have an issue they would like to address at the meeting, tell them when that will occur as part of the meeting or on the agenda. • Encourage parent input and take time to listen to parent concerns. Be sure these are addressed in the meeting when discussing areas of need. • Document the parents' concerns and disposition.
Present levels of academic achievement and functional performance	• Copying information from prior IEPs • Listing standardized testing scores only • Listing class grades only • Not identifying an area of need that subsequently has a goal or service • Descriptors that blame the student or parents for their behavior or actions • Poor documentation examples: ∘ Mary has a lisp. ∘ Juan uses poor grammar. ∘ Johnny is not motivated to learn. ∘ Chelsea doesn't talk in class because she stutters. ∘ Billy doesn't care about others' feelings.	• Identify key strengths and learning needs identified in recent assessment and classroom performance. Present information using positive language. • Identify the needs that create the basis for goals. • Identify the unique needs of the student. • Good documentation examples: ∘ Mary presents with an [th/s] articulation disorder that frequently impacts the ability of unfamiliar listeners to understand her message (70% of the time). Mary is often reluctant to answer questions in class. ∘ Juan's presents with expressive and receptive syntax disorder which affects his ability to respond at an expected level in his general education classroom. He requires support to access grade-level reading and comprehension that include complex or compound sentences. ∘ Johnny's interaction with peers and adults are restricted to when others engage him. He requires prompting to engage in classroom activity 4 times in a 30-minute period. ∘ Chelsea avoids speaking situations in the classroom and during recess. ∘ Billy is learning about feelings, including emotional states in self and others. He is able to identify two feelings in self and zero in others.

IEP Requirement	Common Process and Documentation Errors	Recommended Process and Documentation Practice
How the disability impacts the student's ability to achieve in the curriculum	• Listing only the student's grades • No observation in the classroom • Poor examples: ∘ Annie can't read. ∘ Jenny can't remember numbers. ∘ Zach is a pleasure to have in class.	• Based on assessment, document how the communication disorder impacts the student's ability to achieve in the classroom. • Good examples: ∘ Annie's auditory processing disorder affects her ability to follow teacher directions. She requires visual support and outlines and benefits from strong routine. ∘ Jenny's number concept and auditory memory deficit impact her math performance. She benefits from manipulatives paired with visuals and writing the numbers to facilitate retention. ∘ Zach's social skills are a benefit to participation in general education setting. His vocabulary deficit causes challenges in reading and during oral presentations.

IEP Requirement	Common Process and Documentation Errors	Recommended Process and Documentation Practice

Goal development	• Writing goals that are not measurable or connected to assessments or present levels of performance
	• No goals in identified areas of need
	• No goals for recommended service(s)
		• Annual goals, including academic and functional goals, must be measurable and designed to:
		  ∘ Meet the child's needs that result from the child's disability to enable the child to be involved in and make progress in the general education curriculum
		  ∘ Meet each of the child's other educational needs that result from the child's disability (300.320 through 300.324)
		• Goals must be a statement of what a student may reasonably be able to accomplish in 1 year.
		• Goals must be based on present levels of academic achievement and functional performance.
		• Goals must follow the following outline:
		  ∘ Who (always the student)
		  ∘ Does what (identify the communicative behavior)
		  ∘ When will it occur (reporting period)
		  ∘ Under what conditions
		  ∘ Measure (performance data)
		• Repeating goals from year to year is not recommended.
		• Need to identify periodic reporting periods throughout the year.
		• Be sure to support outcomes with data at the IEP meeting. Be sure to keep data on goals during treatment.

IEP Requirement	Common Process and Documentation Errors	Recommended Process and Documentation Practice
Accommodations and modifications	• Checking all of the boxes on the IEP document • Having the same accommodations and modifications for each student • Examples of accommodations used for many students without specific identified need: Extra time, testing in a separate location, shortened assignments • Not informing the general education teacher of agreed-upon accommodations/ modifications if the teacher not at the IEP meeting • Writing that the student needs to ask for the accommodation	• Accommodations and modifications must be specific to the student's needs. • Need to document how the accommodation/modification will benefit the student. • Need to document that the teacher has been informed and trained (if necessary) regarding the agreed upon accommodations and modifications.
Offer of FAPE (i.e., services and placement)	• Unclear FAPE offer • Offering multiple services and sites	• FAPE offer is the unique combination of facilities, personnel, location, or equipment. • Must be a clear, single, written offer. • Speech and language service recommendations should be consistent with what is required to implement goals, which were developed based on assessment findings.

17

Outpatient Settings Pediatric

Nancy B. Swigert, MA, CCC-SLP, BCS-S

Intake Forms

When a parent contacts the outpatient center, some information needs to be gathered over the phone to begin the process of determining if services will be covered. The form should contain demographic information such as the following:

- Child's name
- Parents' names and contact information
- Referring physician
- Any medical diagnoses given by the physician
- Reason for referral: What the parent sees as the problem
- Whether any previous services for the disorder were received (and request that a copy of those records be sent to the office)
- Insurance information
- Tentative *International Classification of Diseases, Tenth Revision* (ICD-10) code and Current Procedural Terminology (CPT) code(s); the parents will need this information to check insurance coverage
- Preferred days/times for initial evaluation
- Date/time of evaluation if scheduled

Some clinics will schedule the evaluation at the time of this first phone call, but others will want to wait to schedule until insurance coverage has been determined. See Appendix 17-A for an example of an intake form.

Physician's Order

Adults who are using Medicare Part B must have a physician's order for the services (see Chapter 15). It is highly unusual for any third-party payer for pediatric services to require a written physician's order, but the clinic should be familiar with the requirements of each of the payers.

Determining Whether Services Will Be Covered

Each private insurance policy is unique, with different coverage limitations. However, there are common limitations to coverage of pediatric services, including the following:

- Does not cover disorders considered to be developmental, implying that the child will outgrow the disorder
- Does not cover the service unless it is medically related. This might mean related to chronic middle ear infections or to a medical disorder such as cerebral palsy. Each policy is different in how it defines medically

Swigert, N. B.
Documentation and Reimbursement for Speech-Language Pathologists: Principles and Practice (pp. 319-343).

related or medically necessary. Recall that often private insurance adopts definitions and guidelines developed by Medicare. The definition of medical necessity, even according to Medicare guidelines, is not clear cut. Medicare defines something as medically necessary if the documentation supports that the services are:

- Skilled
- Rehabilitative services (note that for children, this part of the definition does not typically apply because those services are habilitative)
- Provided by clinicians (or qualified professionals when appropriate)
- Provided with the approval of a physician/non-physician provider
- Safe
- Effective (i.e., progress indicates that the care is effective in rehabilitation of function) (Centers for Medicare & Medicaid Services [CMS], 2017)

- Limits the number of visits that will be paid in a calendar year if the disorder is covered

It is the family's responsibility to determine what their insurance covers, although they will often ask the speech-language pathologist to look at their policy or provide information about what services (i.e., CPT codes) will be used. The speech-language pathologist can easily share information about the likely CPT evaluation and treatment codes that will be used but should encourage the family to discuss that information directly with their insurance company. The family might want to obtain in writing what the insurance company says it will cover.

Some insurance companies want to preauthorize the evaluation. Other private insurance companies will reimburse the cost of the evaluation if the disorder is covered; however, many then require preauthorization for treatment.

Due to all of the limitations to coverage for pediatric disorders in private insurance, some pediatric clinics have the parents sign an agreement acknowledging that the insurance may only cover part of the cost or may refuse reimbursement. The insurance company sets the rates of reimbursement, and because the clinic or practice has an agreement with the insurance company, they cannot bill the patient for the remainder of the cost. However, if the insurance company refuses to reimburse at all, the family can then be charged.

Each state has its own Medicaid program. The coverage may be structured like a fee-for-service insurance plan, but more and more Medicaid programs are utilizing a managed care approach. Some will require preapproval be obtained before the evaluation, and most require authorization after the evaluation before treatment is rendered.

New Modifier for Habilitative Services

Beginning in 2017, states may require use of the SZ modifier to indicate that services were habilitative for patients with Affordable Care Act (ACA)-compliant health plans or Medicaid Managed Care or those newly enrolled in Medicaid. At the time of this writing, specific guidelines had not been established. To locate ACA plans operating in your state, find the health insurance market place for your state online. When a patient presents requiring habilitation services and is enrolled in one of the ACA health plans, call the member services representative number on the card to ask whether the plan is an individual or small-group health plan. This is important because ACA-compliant plans only pertain to individual and small-group health insurance products. Having the patient's member ID will help the member representative locate that information. ACA-compliant plans can choose how to operationalize the separate visit limits for habilitation services and may not require use of the SZ modifier. Providers should not assume that they will because a claim could be returned unpaid if the plan is not set up to handle this modifier (Grooms, 2016).

Coverage for Autism

A number of states require health insurance coverage for autism. Those states that have specific or limited coverage generally cover speech-language services through habilitative (i.e., learning a new process), rehabilitative (i.e., relearning a once-known process), or therapeutic (treating through remedial methods) care. This information is reviewed annually, so clinics should check carefully to know what is required to be covered in their state. Some insurance plans (e.g., not based in the state) may be exempt from these requirements (American Speech-Language-Hearing Association [ASHA], n.d.-b).

CMS describes the coverage that state Medicaid plans must provide for individuals under the age of 21 with autism spectrum disorder (ASD). The bulletin from CMS lists four major categories of treatment that are beneficial for children with ASD, specifically services available to individuals with ASD through the federal Medicaid program. The categories are (1) behavioral and communication approaches, (2) dietary approaches, (3) medications, and (4) complementary and alternative medicine. Applied behavior analysis therapy is recognized as one treatment for the child with autism, but the bulletin also identifies other treatments that are available to the ASD population and to others in need of those services (ASHA, 2014).

Case History and Interview Forms

Case history forms, rather than interview forms, are more typically used with the pediatric population. Sending the form to the parents before the initial evaluation and having the family complete the form and mail it back in (or in some settings complete the form online) provides the speech-language pathologist with the opportunity to customize the evaluation. Certain specific testing instruments may be chosen given information provided on the case history form.

A case history form collects demographic information, as well as information about the presenting problem. The form can be basic and generic, used for any type of client. However, case history forms designed for specific disorders can gather more detailed information. The more information that can be obtained before the evaluation begins, the more efficient the speech-language pathologist can be during the evaluation session. The case history form can then also serve as the format for the clinician to interview the parent to fill in any gaps in the information provided. See Appendix 17-B for an example of a generic case history form for pediatric communication disorders and Appendix 17-C for an example of a case history form for dysarthria.

Sometimes a child is referred for one problem, but there may be other deficit areas that have not been identified. In that case, supplemental interview questions can be very helpful. For example, children with speech and language disorders are at risk for phonological awareness/reading disability. A list of interview questions to probe for possible problems can be used at the time of the evaluation or at any time during the course of treatment. See Appendix 17-D for an example of probe questions regarding reading difficulty.

Regardless of the form or format used to gather the information, the speech-language pathologist should be certain to learn the parents' perspective on why the evaluation is needed. Their perspective may be very different than that of the person who made the referral.

Evaluations

Evaluation reports in pediatric outpatient settings may be completed in an electronic health record, typed in a Microsoft Word document, or, less likely, handwritten. Regardless of the format, the speech-language pathologist should find ways to be as efficient as possible in the documentation of the evaluation.

Templates, Standard Paragraphs, and Appendices

If the outpatient setting is not using an electronic health record, the evaluation reports are likely in the form of a Word document. Templates should be developed to help organize the information and to streamline the documentation process. Numerous templates for feeding and swallowing can be found on the ASHA's website (ASHA, n.d.-a). The headers for the template can likely be the same regardless of the age of the client or type of evaluation being completed. The header typically contains the following:

- Demographic information on the client
  - Name
  - Date of birth
  - Age
  - Address
  - Phone
- Parents' information
- Facility-specific identifying information such as case number
- Referral source
- Date of evaluation
- Time of evaluation
  - Time in
  - Time out required if using a timed evaluation code
  - Any additional report-writing time if required with that code
- CPT/procedure code(s)

A generic template can be used that includes the main areas that should be included in each report, including the following:

- Demographics
- Background information
- Reason for referral
- Behavioral observations
- Tests given
- Clinical findings
- Impact on activity and participation
- Hearing screening
- Diagnostic code(s)
- Impressions
- Prognosis
- Personal and environmental factors
- Recommendations
- Frequency and duration

See Appendices 6-B and 6-C for examples of report templates that can be used with pediatrics. Appendix 17-E is an example of a template that may be more appropriate for very young children because it highlights such things as emerging skills and strategies for parents.

A way to further streamline the report-writing process is to develop slightly different templates, based on the disorder or type of client being evaluated. These templates also make it easier for the reader to follow. The basics of each template will be the same, with slight changes based on the disorder. Things like recommendations can be prepopulated, and then any recommendations that are not indicated can be removed. See Appendix 17-F for a report template for Paradoxical Vocal Fold.

The templates can also be gender specific; two templates for the same disorder can have feminine pronouns throughout one and masculine pronouns throughout the other. This saves the speech-language pathologist from having to change the pronoun to the appropriate gender in multiple places.

A bank of recommendations from which to choose can be developed for specific disorders. This saves time for the speech-language pathologist writing the report. These recommendations can be tweaked and modified, skipped if they do not apply, or added as needed. A blank can be left for the child's name. An even more efficient process is to put in the word "child" and then do a find and replace in the Word document to insert the client's name. The pronoun conundrum can be solved by putting he/she, him/her, and his/her in the template and doing a find and replace to insert the appropriate gender pronoun. See Appendix 17-G for an example of a recommendation bank for spelling and written language.

When standardized tests are used, it is helpful to the reader if a description of the test and any specific information about how to interpret scores are included in the report. The speech-language pathologist should not have to create that standard paragraph each time a report is written. The clinic or practice can develop a standard paragraph for each of the tests used in the setting. Appropriate citations should be included. Then, these paragraphs, saved electronically, can be inserted into the report.

If a number of standardized tests are used, it is more efficient for the speech-language pathologist, and easier for the reader of the report, if these standard paragraphs are attached as appendices. When this format is used, the report can often be condensed to a one-page summary, with attached appendices the reader can peruse if more detail is desired. Sometimes it is more efficient to include an appendix if only one standardized assessment was utilized.

Current Procedural Terminology Codes for Evaluations

Most evaluation CPT codes used by speech-language pathologists are not timed (top of Table 17-1). That is, regardless of the amount of time spent with the client, only one CPT code will be billed, and it will be reimbursed at the level that payer has agreed to pay for that service. In situations of private pay, the clinic or practice may establish different rates for different types of evaluations, and the individual will be billed different rates. However, when billing a third-party payer, most contracts are set with one fee per CPT code.

There are multiple codes for evaluations, but four were new CPT codes in 2014:

1. 92521: Evaluation of speech fluency (e.g., stuttering, cluttering)
2. 92522: Evaluation of speech sound production (e.g., articulation, phonological process, apraxia, dysarthria)
3. 92523: Evaluation of speech sound production (e.g., articulation, phonological process, apraxia, dysarthria); with evaluation of language comprehension and expression (e.g., receptive and expressive language)
4. 92524: Behavioral and qualitative analysis of voice and resonance

Some discussion of the difference in 92522 and 92523 is warranted because each includes evaluation of speech sound production, but 92523 also includes evaluation of language comprehension and expression. There is not a code for evaluation of language without an evaluation of speech sound production. The codes were designed that way because more the 50% of the time when language is evaluated, speech sound production is as well. Unless it is blatantly obvious that the child has no deficits in speech sound production, the evaluation typically includes an assessment of that area. If the speech sound production assessment is not completed, the speech-language pathologist can append modifier -52 to indicate less extensive service (Swanson, 2014).

Two codes pertinent only in the pediatric population are developmental screening (96110) and developmental testing (96111). Therefore, the developmental screening code (96110) may or may not be reimbursed by third-party payers. The developmental screening code has a further description (e.g. developmental milestone survey, speech and language delay screen), with scoring and documentation per standardized instrument. The description of the developmental testing code (96111) indicates that multiple areas need to be assessed in order to use the code: "includes assessment of motor, language, social, adaptive, and/or cognitive functioning by standardized developmental instrument(s) with interpretation and report" (McCarty & White, 2011).

However, there are some evaluation codes that are time based (see bottom of Table 17-1). To bill a timed code, the time spent must exceed the halfway point dictated by the code. This is often referred to as the *8-minute rule*, because to use a 15-minute code, you have to spend at least 8 minutes with the client, or more than one-half of the time. In other words:

- 1-hour unit ≥ 31 minutes
- 30-minute unit ≥ 16 minutes
- 15-minute unit ≥ 8 minutes

Table 17-1

Current Procedural Terminology Evaluation Codes

CPT Code	Descriptor
31579	Laryngoscopy, flexible or rigid fiberoptic, with stroboscopy
92511	Nasopharyngoscopy with endoscope (separate procedure)
92512	Nasal function studies (e.g., rhinomanometry)
92520	Laryngeal function studies (i.e., aerodynamic testing and acoustic testing)
92521	Evaluation of speech fluency (e.g., stuttering, cluttering)
92522	Evaluation of speech sound production (e.g., articulation, phonological process, apraxia, dysarthria)
92523	Evaluation of speech sound production (e.g., articulation, phonological process, apraxia, dysarthria); with evaluation of language comprehension and expression (e.g., receptive and expressive language)
92524	Behavioral and qualitative analysis of voice and resonance
92551	Screening test, pure tone, air only
92567	Tympanometry, impedance testing
92597	Evaluation for use and/or fitting of voice prosthetic device to supplement oral speech
92610	Evaluation of oral and pharyngeal swallowing function
92611	Motion fluoroscopic evaluation of swallowing function by cine or video recording
92612	Flexible fiberoptic endoscopic evaluation of swallowing by cine or video recording
92613	FEES: Interpretation and report only
92614	Flexible fiberoptic endoscopic evaluation, laryngeal sensory testing by cine or video recording
92615	Interpretation and report only
92616	Flexible fiberoptic endoscopic evaluation of swallowing and laryngeal sensory testing by cine or video recording
92617	FEESST: Interpretation and report only
96110	Developmental screening (e.g., developmental milestone survey, speech and language delay screen) with scoring and documentation per standardized instrument
96111	Developmental testing (includes assessment of motor, language, social, adaptive, and/or cognitive functioning by standardized developmental instruments) with interpretation and report

Timed Evaluation Codes

CPT Code	Description	Time
92607	Evaluation for prescription of speech-generating device	First hour
92608	Evaluation for prescription of speech-generating device	Each additional 30 minutes
92626	Evaluation of auditory rehabilitation	First hour
92627	Evaluation of auditory rehabilitation	Each additional 15 minutes
96105	Assessment of aphasia, with interpretation and report	Per hour
96125	Standardized cognitive performance testing (e.g., Ross Information Processing Assessment) per hour of a qualified health care professional's time, both face-to-face time administering tests to the patient and time interpreting these test results and preparing the report	Per hour

Abbreviation: FEESST = flexible endoscopic evaluation of swallowing with sensory testing.

Adapted from American Speech-Language-Hearing Association. (n.d.). Medicare CPT coding rules for speech-language pathology services. Retrieved from https://www.asha.org/practice/reimbursement/medicare/SLP_coding_rules/

Some of these timed evaluation codes, prescription of speech-generating device (92607) and auditory rehabilitation (92626), have a base code for the first hour and a different code for the subsequent period of time, either a 15- or 30-minute subsequent period of time. The subsequent units billed may not be counted until the full value of the first unit of time plus one-half of the value of the second unit of time is exceeded.

Two of the timed assessment codes, aphasia (96105) and standardized cognitive performance testing (96125), are per-hour codes. That is, there is not a separate code for the additional time; rather, the speech-language pathologist might bill more than one of that base code. These two codes also allow the inclusion of time spent on interpretation and reporting for billing. Assessment of aphasia would rarely be used with the pediatric population, whereas the standardized cognitive performance testing might indeed be used.

For any of the timed codes that include interpretation and report, the speech-language pathologist's documentation must breakdown the time spent face to face and the time spent on interpretation and report. The evaluation report should include time in and time out, and this amount of time should match the amount of time billed for the evaluation. The time documented in the report must correspond to the number of units billed on the claim.

A few other tips on using evaluation codes follow:

- If the speech-language pathologist is evaluating cognition but is not using standardized testing instruments, then 96125 is not appropriate; 92523 could be used, but speech-language abilities should be the focus.
- 96125 and 92523 can be used on the same date if the speech-language pathologist has completed both a full cognitive evaluation and a full speech sound production and language evaluation. The cognitive evaluation should include standardized testing and take at least 31 minutes, including the time it takes to interpret and write the report. The -59 modifier must be added to CPT 96125 to indicate the evaluations are separate and distinct procedures.
- 92523 can be used for an auditory processing evaluation, but if speech sound production was not also assessed, then modifier -52 should be added to indicate it took less time than typical because all areas described in the code were not assessed. (Swanson, 2014)

Preauthorization for Treatment

Most third-party payers, such as private insurance payers and some state Medicaid plans that are managed care, require the speech-language pathologist to obtain a preauthorization for treatment. Each company may have a slightly different process and different forms that need to be completed. If the facility fails to obtain the preauthorization, the third-party payer is not obligated to reimburse for the services. In order to ensure minimum delay between the evaluation and the beginning of treatment, the speech-language pathologist will need to complete the evaluation report and treatment plan in a timely way, because these documents are sometimes requested along with the other required forms.

Tips for completing documentation for preauthorization for treatment include the following:

- Write goals that are functional and measurable.
- When appropriate, use the term *medically necessary.*
- Talk with representatives of the insurance company for more specific guidelines on the information they will need in order to make the determination.
- Avoid using the terms *educational, developmental, instructional, and learning.*
- Keep reports brief and easy to read (Huntress, 2003).

Treatment Plans

Chapter 7 provided information about the development of treatment plans. Treatment plans should be established in collaboration with the parents, and with the child if age-appropriate to do so, with a focus on function. The treatment plan outlines the long- and short-term goals of the planned intervention.

To increase efficiency when writing treatment plans, goal banks can be developed. A goal bank includes the long- and short-term goals and treatment objectives typically used for a specific disorder. These can be modified and others added, but being able to select goals from the bank greatly reduces the time spent in documentation. The goals can be written with blank spaces for percent accuracy and the method of measurement (Table 17-2). Commercially available therapy resource books often contain goal banks for the disorder addressed (Swigert, 2003, 2005, 2010).

Treatment Notes

Chapter 8 discussed treatment notes. In outpatient settings, it is typical for a treatment note to be written each time the client is seen. However, in pediatric settings, the payers usually don't require that, and there are other, less stringent requirements. Although of course the child would be receiving therapy only if skilled services were needed, there typically is no demand from payers that skilled treatment be documented in progress notes. There may be no need to use the SOAP (subjective, objective, assessment, plan) format. Instead, tallies of correct responses can be kept, along with a few short notations about the child's performance for sessions where something of note occurred. Abbreviated formats for notes may help the speech-language pathologist document during the

Table 17-2

Sample Goals From Apraxia of Speech Goal Bank

Area	Goal	Long or Short Term
Apraxia of Speech (AOS)	Child will communicate in age-appropriate utterances with smooth rhythm and appropriate rate.	Long
AOS	Client will produce vowel sequences on ___ of ___ opportunities with _____ cues over _____ consecutive sessions.	Short
AOS	Client will consistently produce consonants in isolation in ___ of ___ opportunities with _____ cues over ___ consecutive sessions.	Short
AOS	Client will produce consonant-vowel (CV) and vowel-consonant (VC) syllables with _____ cues on ___% of trials over _____ consecutive sessions.	Short
AOS	Client will produce CVC words in response to questions or to name pictures with _____ cues with ___% accuracy over ___ sessions.	Short

treatment session, which is admittedly more difficult with younger children. See Appendix 17-H for an example of a streamlined progress note format.

The treatment note also typically lists the CPT code(s) that were billed for that session. The treatment codes typically used by speech-language pathologists are listed in Table 17-3.

Most of these treatment codes are untimed, and most third-party payers reimburse a flat rate regardless of how long the session was. There are a few timed treatment codes, although certain payers may restrict their use. When using a timed treatment code, keep in mind the 8-minute rule to determine how many units of the code can be billed.

Periodic Written Summaries

Children can be in treatment for long periods of time (if not restricted by the payer). If there is third-party reimbursement, the payer may require periodic reports in order to authorize more visits. If the family is paying privately, they will also appreciate periodic written summaries of the child's progress. There is not a prescribed format for these updates.

Discharge Summaries

Chapter 9 addressed discharge summaries. Completing a discharge summary for any outpatient seen should be standard practice. The document provides a snapshot of the intervention provided and the client's response to the treatment. The discharge summary should be sent to the referring physician, any other physicians treating the child, and any other professionals caring for the child, such as a physical therapist, classroom teacher, or another speech-language pathologist.

Ethics and Reimbursement

The ASHA *Issues in Ethics Statement: Representation of Services for Insurance Reimbursement, Funding, or Private Payment* delineates specific situations related to reimbursement that would be unethical. These were described in Chapter 4, but several warrant highlighting here because these situations arise in pediatric outpatient settings:

- Misrepresenting information to obtain reimbursement or funding, regardless of the motivation of the provider
    - For example, parents may report that their insurance covers therapy for apraxia of speech and ask the speech-language pathologist to use that code, when clearly the child has a phonological disorder and not apraxia.
    - Seeing children in a group but charging each an individual therapy code.
- Scheduling services more frequently or for longer than is reasonably necessary
    - When the child's insurance coverage is running out and they have reached maximum gain from treatment, the family may want to pay privately to continue services. If there is no reason to expect further improvement, it would be unethical to accept payment from the family.

Table 17-3

Speech-Language Pathology Current Procedural Terminology Codes

CPT Code	Description	Notes
92507	Treatment of speech, language, voice, communication, and/or auditory processing disorder; individual	Not timed
92508	Group, two or more individuals	Not timed
92526	Treatment of swallowing dysfunction and/or oral function for feeding	Not timed
92606	Therapeutic service(s) for the use of non–speech-generating device, including programming and modification	Not timed
92609	Therapeutic services for the use of speech-generating device, including programming and modification	Not timed
92630	Auditory rehabilitation; prelingual hearing loss	Not timed
92633	Postlingual hearing loss	Not timed
97532	Development of cognitive skills to improve attention, memory, problem solving (includes compensatory training), direct (one-on-one) patient contact by the provider	Each 15 minutes
97533	Sensory integrative techniques to enhance sensory processing and promote adaptive responses to environmental demands, direct (one-on-one) patient contact by the provider	Each 15 minutes
97535	Self-care/home management training (e.g., activities of daily living and compensatory training, meal preparation, safety procedures, and instructions in use of assistive technology devices/adaptive equipment) direct (one-on-one) contact by provider	Each 15 minutes

Adapted from American Speech-Language-Hearing Association. (n.d.). Medicare CPT coding rules for speech-language pathology services. Retrieved from https://www.asha.org/practice/reimbursement/medicare/SLP_coding_rules/

- Providing professional courtesies or complimentary care for referrals or otherwise discounting care not based on documented need
  - Perhaps the child of a pediatrician who refers many patients needs services. It would be unethical to provide complimentary services to the pediatrician's child.
- Supervision of students or other service providers in a fee-for-service environment. In states that allow speech-language pathologists to bill Medicaid directly and also allow services by speech-language pathology assistants, there are strict rules about supervision (ASHA, 2010).

Appendix 17-I provides an example of a pediatric case seen at a private practice. The child is covered by private insurance.

References

American Speech-Language-Hearing Association. (n.d.-a). Pediatric feeding history and clinical assessment form. (2016). Retrieved from http://www.asha.org/uploadedFiles/Pediatric-Feeding-History-and-Clinical-Assessment-Form.pdf

American Speech-Language-Hearing Association. (n.d.-b). State insurance mandates for autism spectrum disorder. Retrieved from http://www.asha.org/Advocacy/state/State-Insurance-Mandates-Autism/

American Speech-Language-Hearing Association. (2010). Issues in ethics: Representation of services for insurance reimbursement, funding, or private payment. Retrieved from http://www.asha.org/Practice/ethics/Representation-of-Services/

American Speech-Language-Hearing Association. (2014). CMS issues clarification of Medicaid coverage of services to children with autism. Retrieved from http://www.asha.org/News/2014/CMS-Issues-Clarification-of-Medicaid-Coverage-of-Services-to-Children-With-Autism/

Centers for Medicare & Medicaid Services. (2017). Medicare Benefit Policy Manual: Chapter 15—Covered medical and other health services. Retrieved from https://www.cms.gov/Regulations-and-Guidance/Guidance/Manuals/downloads/bp102c15.pdf

Grooms, D. (2016). Get ready for new coding requirements for habilitation services. *ASHA Leader, 21*, 30–31. doi:10.1044/leader.BML.21102016.30

Huntress, L. M. (2003). Managing insurance issues in a small private practice. *Fluency and Fluency Disorders Perspectives, 13*, 20–22.

McCarty, J., & White. S. (2011). New codes available for AAC evaluation, developmental delay testing, preventive services. *ASHA Leader, 16*, 9. doi:10.1044/leader.BML4.16152011.9

Swanson, N. (2014). Bottom line: Cracking the new evaluation codes. *ASHA Leader, 19*, 30–31. doi:10.1044/leader.BML.19032014.30

Swigert, N. B. (2003). *The source for reading fluency.* Austin, TX: LinguiSystems.

Swigert, N. B. (2005). *The source for children's voice disorders.* Austin, TX: LinguiSystems.

Swigert, N. B. (2010). *The source for pediatric dysphagia.* Austin, TX: LinguiSystems.

Review Questions

1. What is the purpose of an intake form?
2. What are some typical limitations that private insurance companies place on coverage for pediatric speech-language services?
3. Explain what a goal bank is and an advantage of developing them.
4. Explain how to use each evaluation code that was new in 2014.
5. Give an example of unethical behavior related to reimbursement.

Activity A

Using Appendix 17-C as an example, develop a case history form specific for one of these disorders:

- Fluency
- Pediatric feeding in infant
- School-aged language disorder
- Apraxia of speech

Activity B

Using the same disorder selected for Activity A, develop examples of long- and short-term goals. See Appendix 17-G for an example.

Appendix 17-A
Pediatric Intake Form

Referral for Speech-Language Pathology Evaluation

Date: ______________________ Time: ______________ Staff member taking call: ______________

Child's name: ____

Parent(s) names and contact information: ____

____

Referring physician: ____

Any medical diagnoses given by the physician (ask for ICD-10): ______________________

Reason for referral (what the parent sees as the problem): ______________________

____

Any previous services for the disorder (request that a copy of those records be sent to the office): ______________

____

Name of insurance company: ______________________ Policy #: ______________

ICD-10 code that may describe communication/feeding/swallowing disorder: ______________

CPT code(s) likely to be used in evaluation: ______________________________

Preferred days/times for initial evaluation: ______________________________

Date/time of evaluation if scheduled: ______________________________

Case history and clinic information mailed/faxed to parent: ______________________

Appendix 17-B
Generic Pediatric Case History Form

Questionnaire for Children With Speech-Language Disorders

Today's date: ____________________

Name: ______________________________ Age : ______________ Birthday: ______________

Address Street: ____

City: __________________________ State: ____________________ Zip Code: ____________

Telephone: ______________________________________ Sex: ________ Male ________ Female

Person completing this form: ____

Relationship to client: ____

Parent #1 name: ____________ Address: ______________________________ Age: ________

Parent occupation: ________________________ Employer: ___________________________

Education completed: ____

Parent #2 name: ____________________ Address: ______________________________ Age: ________

Parent occupation: ______________________________ Employer: ______________________

Education completed: ____

List all children in the family from oldest to youngest:

NAME	AGE	SEX	GRADE IN SCHOOL	GENERAL HEALTH

Does anyone else in the family have speech, language, or hearing problems? ____________________

____

Who referred you for the evaluation? ____

Child's pediatrician or family doctor: ____

Address: ____

Other doctor(s) treating child: ____

Has child had any previous testing or therapy for speech, language, or hearing problems? __________

If so, name of agency and date tested: ____

(Please request that copies of all test results be sent to our office.)

Why is this testing being requested? ____________________

____

____

____

Birth History

Weight of child at birth: ____________ Was child full term? ____________

Were there any unusual factors relating to the pregnancy? ____________________

____

____

Type of birth: _____ Normal _____ Induced _____ Forceps _____ Breech _____ Caesarean

_____ Premature: How much? ____________

Were there any physical deformities or malformations observed at birth (e.g., "blueness," jaundice, abnormal shape of head)? ____________________

____

____

Developmental History

In early childhood, did the child have any feeding problems (e.g., poor control of sucking, food allergies, digestive upsets)? Y N

If yes, please describe: ____________________

____

Give ages of development for the following behaviors:

Sitting unsupported: ____________ Walking: ____________

Eating solid foods: ____________ Self-feeding: ____________

Crawling: ____________ Self-dressing: ____________

Standing alone: ____________ Bladder/bowel control: ____________

Do you feel that the child was late or had difficulty in the development of these behaviors? Y N

Medical History

Date and type of last medical examination: ____________________

List ages for any childhood diseases: ____________________

Were there any complications with any of the above, such as high/persistent fevers, seizures, persistent muscle weakness, etc? ____________________

____

Is the child subject to frequent colds, sore throats? ____________________

Does the child have allergies? ____________________

Does the child tend to breathe with mouth open? ____________________

Has the child had any operations? If so, describe: ____________________

Has the child had tonsils and adenoids removed? If so, when? ____________________

Has the child had any trouble with his/her ears (e.g., ear aches, infection, running ears, evidence of hearing loss)? __________

Has hearing been tested? If so, when? __________ Results: __________

Has your child ever had ear (PE) tubes inserted? If so, when? __________

Does child still have ear (PE) tubes? __________

Has the child ever worn eyeglasses or had any difficulty with eyes? __________

Does the child have any dental problems? __________

Has the child had any special examinations? Explain: __________

Education History

Current school: __________ Address: __________

Grade: __________ Teacher: __________

Did the child attend preschool? __________ From age: __________ to age: __________

At what age did child attend kindergarten? __________

Does the child like school? __________ Does the child like his/her teacher? __________

Describe performance in school (please note strong and weak areas): __________

Does child attend any special classes (e.g., speech therapy, reading, resource room, special classroom)? __________

Daily Behavior

Where does your child usually play? __________

Are there children close to your child's age in the neighborhood? __________

Does child prefer to play alone? __________

Does child prefer to play with older or younger children? __________

Does child have a special friend? __________

List some good things about your child: __________

List some things about your child that are challenging: __________

Does your child have difficulty concentrating? __________

Communication History

Is your child's speech understandable to you? ______________________

To child's friends? __________ **To strangers?** ________ **To other family members?** ________________

List sounds or words that child has trouble saying: ____

____

How does the child compare with siblings in speech development? __________________________________

____

Does child use words in meaningful ways for his/her age? ____

Give example of sentences your child uses by him/herself? (Not ones that are repeated after you): __________

____

____

____

At what age did your child babble? ______________________ **Say first words?** ______________

Put two words together in a sentence? ______________________ **Use three-word sentences?** __________

Does your child seem to understand directions? ____

Does your child prefer to use speech or gestures when communicating? ______________________________

Do you have any further information to share? ____

____

____

____

What questions do you want to be sure we address? ____

____

____

Appendix 17-C
Pediatric Motor Speech Dysarthria Case History

Today's date: ______________

Name: ______________ Age : ______________ Birthday: ______________

Address Street: ______________

City: ______________ State: ______________ Zip Code: ______________

Telephone: ______________ Sex: ______Male ______Female

Person completing this form: ______________

Relationship to client: ______________

Parent #1 name: ______________ Address: ______________ Age: ______________

Parent occupation: ______________ Employer: ______________

Education completed: ______________

Parent #2 name: ______________ Address: ______________ Age: ______________

Parent occupation: ______________ Employer: ______________

Education completed: ______________

List all children in the family from oldest to youngest:

NAME	AGE	SEX	GRADE IN SCHOOL	GENERAL HEALTH

Does anyone else in the family have speech, language, or hearing problems? ______________

____

Who referred you for the evaluation? ______________

Child's pediatrician or family doctor: ______________

Address: ______________

Other doctor(s) treating child: ______________

Has child had any previous testing or therapy for speech, language, or hearing problems? ______________

If so, name of agency and date tested: ______________

(Please request that copies of all test results be sent to our office.)

Why is this testing being requested? ______________

____

How old was the child when the speech problem first started? ______________

What has the doctor said is the cause of the speech problem? ______________________________

What has the doctor said about the disease/reason for the speech problem? ______________________________

(If the child's speech problem has been present since starting to talk, skip the next two questions.)

Did the child's speech change suddenly or over a period of time? ______________________________

Who first noticed the change in your child's speech? ______________________________

Is the speech problem getting worse? Staying the same? Getting any better? ______________________________

Is your child's speech better or worse at certain times of the day? ______________________________

Does your child have any trouble eating: Chewing, forming the bolus with the food, swallowing liquids? ________
____

Does your child cough or choke? ______________________________

Does food or liquid ever come out your child's nose? ______________________________

What bothers you about your child's speech? ______________________________

Does your child seem aware of the speech problem? ______________________________

What seems to bother your child about his or her speech? ______________________________

When does your child have the most trouble being understood?

- ____________ On the phone
- ____________ Talking to strangers
- ____________ In noisy situations
- ____________ Other

Does your child avoid situations because of his or her speech? If so, describe: ______________________________
____

How often does your child communicate with:

- Familiar children: ____________
- Familiar adults: ____________
- Strangers: ____________

How does your child respond when people don't understand? ______________________________
____

Have you found anything that helps people understand your child better (e.g., writing, using gestures, speaking in well-lit room)? ______________________________

Is your child taking any medications? ______________________________

What do you hope we accomplish with therapy? ______________________________
____
____

What questions do you have about the evaluation/your child's speech problem? ______________________________
____
____

Appendix 17-D
Interview Probe Possible Reading Disorder

For All Ages

Is there a history of reading problems in parents or siblings? This family history makes the child at higher risk for reading problems.

Negative answers indicate possible problems.

Preschool (Ages 4 to 5)

- Can your child make up a word to rhyme with another (doesn't have to be a real word) (e.g., run, fun, sun)?
- Does your child know the names of at least 10 letters of the alphabet, such as those in his/her name?
- Does/did the child exhibit a delay in speaking or is/was your child hard for strangers to understand beyond the age of 2½?
- Can your child recite nursery rhymes?

Kindergarten: Beginning of the School Year (Age 5)

- Can your child tell if two words rhyme (e.g., "Do mop and hop rhyme?")?
- Does your child know the names of most letters of the alphabet in upper and lower case?
- Can your child quickly name colors?

Kindergarten: Later in the Year (Ages 5½ to 6)

- Can your child break a word into syllables (e.g., clap each syllable or tell how many syllables in a 2-, 3-, or 4-syllable word)?
- Can your child tell which of three words starts with the same sound as the key word (e.g., "Which word begins with the same sound as cat . . . boy, car, or run?")?
- Can your child tell what the first sound is in a word (e.g., "What's the first sound you hear in the word 'man'?" Child should make the /m/ sound, not say the letter name)?
- Can your child blend the sounds to tell what the word is when you say it one sound at a time (e.g., "m–a–n" . . . .and the child can tell you the word is man)?
- Does your child know all the names of the alphabet letters and most of the sounds they make?

First Grade (Ages 6 to 7)

- Can your child tell how many sounds he/she hears in a two- or three-sound word (e.g., "How many sounds do you hear in 'big'? . . . in 'up'?")?
- Does your child have a reading vocabulary of 300 to 500 words?
- Can your child spell short, easy words?

Second Grade (Ages 7 to 8)

- Can your child break apart and read words with multiple syllables?
- Can your child read second-grade books?
- Does your child sound smooth and fluent when reading aloud?
- When your child tries to spell, does he/she represent all the sounds (e.g., spells burn as brn . . . not br or bun)?

Third Grade (Ages 8 to 9)

- Does your child sound smooth and fluent when reading aloud?
- Can your child figure out the meaning of a word from a prefix, suffix, or root (e.g., knows magician because he/she sees the word "magic" in it)?
- Does your child read for pleasure?
- Can your child tell the main idea of a story he/she has read?

APPENDIX 17-E
Example Early Intervention Report Template

Report of Speech-Language Assessment

Early Childhood Template

Name: ________________ **Gender:** ____________________ **Facility identification number:** ____________

Date of birth: ______________ **Referral Source:** ________________________________

Age: ________ **(Adjusted age:** ________ **)** **Physician(s):** ______________________________

Parent(s): ______________________________________ **Date of evaluation:**

____ **Time in/out:**

Address: ______________________________________ **Telephone:** ______________

Pertinent medical/birth history: ____

State of health: ____

Level of response: ____

Persons present: ____

Sources/measures used (see scores and comments attached)

____ **Behavioral checklist:**

____ **Standardized tests:**

____ **Parent interview:**

____ **Criterion-referenced instrument:**

____ **Observation**

Pure tone hearing screening: ____

Middle ear screening: ____

Concerns reported by caregiver: ____

Priorities stated by caregiver: ____

Strengths observed: ____

Needs observed: ____

Emerging skills: ____

Family resources: ____

Strategies, materials, equipment to support development: ______________________

Comments: ____

____

Parent education: ____

Diagnostic codes: ____

Recommendations: ____

Strategies and activities for parent to implement: ______________________

Speech-language pathologist signature, title, degree(s), credentials

Shared verbally with caregiver: Date: ______________ In Person: ________ Phone Conversation: ____________________

Copy to caregiver: ______________ Mail/Fax/In Person

Copy to Agency: ______________ Name: ______________ Date: ______________ Mail/Fax

Copy to Pediatrician: Name: ______________ Date: ______________ Mail/Fax

Appendix 17-F

Paradoxical Vocal Fold Motion Report Template

Report of Evaluation

Paradoxical Vocal Fold Motion

Name: ______________________________ Telephone: ______________________________

Birthdate: ________________ Age: ______ Physician: ______________________________

Parents: ________________________ Referral Source: ______________________________

Address : ______________________________ Date/time evaluation: ______________________________

______________________________ CPT Code(s): ______________________________

Background and related information: ______________________________

Reason for referral: Client presents with difficulty breathing in the following situations:

Behavioral observations: ______________________________

Clinical findings: Client/parent described "attacks" of difficulty breathing. Client does/does not present with additional symptoms of voice disorder.

Impact on activity and participation: These attacks occur ______________________________ and interfere with ______________________________

Pure tone hearing screening: Pass/fail/deferred (reason): ______________________________

Middle ear screening: Pass/fail/deferred (reason): ______________________________

Diagnosis/diagnostic code(s): Paradoxical vocal fold motion: J 38.5 Laryngeal spasm

Impressions: Symptoms reported are/are not consistent with a diagnosis of paradoxical vocal fold motion.

Prognosis: For client mastering techniques to prevent attacks is excellent/good/fair/poor

Personal and environmental factors:

Recommendations:

1. Therapy for vocal cord dysfunction by speech-language pathologist to reduce tension in extrinsic laryngeal musculature to eliminate paradoxical vocal fold adduction.
2. Consultation with physician re: behavioral and medical management of possible gastroesophageal reflux disorder.

Frequency: 1–2x/week initially

Estimated duration of treatment: 4–6 weeks; 1x/month follow-up for 2–3 months

____

MA, CCC-SLP

Speech-Language Pathologist

CC:

Appendix 17-G

Bank of Recommendation Statements for Written Language/Spelling

1. Child would benefit from individualized instruction to address his/her spelling. Particularly, Child's morphological awareness skills should be addressed. In addition, exposure to multisyllabic words and the rules which govern them would help to improve spelling (e.g., prefixes, suffixes, consonant doubling). This might involve use of the Seeing Stars Program for Reading Fluency and Spelling.
2. Child's written language weaknesses should be addressed to improve his/her use of contextual conventions. In addition, sentence and paragraph construction should be addressed. Child should be taught how to write different types of paragraphs (e.g., descriptive, narrative, persuasive, expository). The skill of proofreading should also be taught. This work can be done with Child using a computer.
3. To help Child complete multiple-step projects, he/she should be exposed to organizational strategies such as staging.
4. To help Child read and comprehend grade-level texts, he/she would benefit from learning skills such as outlining, prereading the questions, and using questions to increase comprehension of the text. There should be some focus on helping Child learn to identify the main idea, draw conclusions, and make inferences. Noting Child's weakness in phonological memory, he/she should be taught strategies to use when he/she is reading and needs to pause to comprehend a word, phrase, or concept.
5. Pending completion of further verbal expressive language testing, more goals may be added in this area. At minimum, Child needs to work on his/her ability to construct a variety of sentence types.
6. Child needs intensive intervention to improve his/her spelling skills. This would include:
   a. Improving his/her sound blending and segmentation skills and achieving a level of automaticity with these
   b. Teaching increased awareness of morphology
   c. Teaching and applying rules
   d. Assessing his/her spelling of the 1,000 most common words used in print and helping him/her to memorize spelling of those words
   e. Enhancing visualization
   f. Helping Child apply these strategies to learn new spelling words
7. Child needs to be taught compensatory strategies for his/her dysgraphia. These might include:
   a. Using a keyboard/computer for much of his/her written work
   b. Learning how to outline for note-taking
   c. Teaching use of abbreviations in note-taking
   d. Using a Franklin Language Master
8. Child needs intervention for his/her written language disorder. This intervention should address:
   a. Increasing Child's metacognitive awareness of the nature and purpose of writing assignments he/she is likely to encounter in school
   b. Teaching Child how to stage a task into its subcomponents and how to sequence the subcomponents
   c. Teaching Child how to gather and develop his/her ideas
   d. Helping Child learn how to orally rehearse before beginning his/her writing assignment
   e. Helping Child use vocabulary and semantics to enrich his/her sentence types in written work
   f. Organizing his/her written work into specific types of text (e.g., descriptive, narrative, persuasive, expository)
   g. Learning how to proof and edit written work
9. At the beginning of the school year, Child's teacher should be apprised of his/her dysgraphia and written language deficits, with specific suggestions on ways to help Child compensate for these disorders.

Appendix 17-H
Example Streamlined Treatment Note

Client's name: ___________________________________ Note: CPT 92507 for each of these sessions

Short-Term Goals	Date 4/26/17	Date 4/28/17	Date 5/2/17	Date 5/4/17	Date 5/9/17	Date 5/11/17	Date 5/16/17	Date 5/18/17
Lakshmi will point to 4–6 body parts named with no cues 90% over 3 sessions.	85% for 3	85% for 3	85% for 4	85% for 4	90% for 4	90% for 5	90% for 5	D/C
Lakshmi will point to item named from choice of 5 common objects with minimal tactile cues 90% over 3 sessions.	90% with only 3	80% with 5	75% with 5	80% with 5 max cues	80% with 4 max cues	85% with 4 mod cues	90% with 4 min cues	90% with 4 min cues
Lakshmi will follow 2-step command with objects with moderate cues with 75% accuracy over 3 sessions.	Did not address	Did not address	Did not address	50% with tactile cues	50% with no cues	65% with no cues	65% with no cues	75% with min cues
Lakshmi will point to pictures named in a book representing actions and objects with no cues 100% over 3 sessions.	Objects only 75%	Objects only 80%	Objects only 90%	Action words 60%	Action words 65%	Did not address	Objects and actions 65%	Objects and actions 80%
Lakshmi will answer simple yes/no questions with head nod or sign with 95% accuracy over 3 sessions.	Signed no 75%; no yes responses	Signed no 80%	Signed yes for first time!	No with sign 80%	Yes 50% max cues	Yes 50% max cues	Yes 60% no cues	Yes 60%; no 75%

Notes: 4/26/17 Session attended by maternal grandmother only

5/2/17 Able to introduce additional body part. Tried action words in books, but she is not ready.

5/11/17 Seems to be getting the idea of "yes."

5/18/17 Goals still appropriate. Making good progress.

____

Signature

Appendix 17-I

4-Year-Old Outpatient With Private Insurance Case Example

Date	Actions	Billed and Coded	Documented
September 25	Child's mother contacts speech-language pathology office to schedule visit. Indicates child is difficult to understand. Asks what CPT codes will likely be used and what ICD-10 codes will describe the problem. Says child has had multiple middle ear infections. Front desk staff inquire about use of language and indicate that might need to be assessed as well. Tells child's mother that the evaluation will likely be three CPT codes: • 92523 Evaluation of speech sound production (e.g., articulation, phonological process, apraxia, dysarthria); with evaluation of language comprehension and expression (e.g., receptive and expressive language) • 92522 Evaluation of speech sound production (e.g., articulation, phonological process, apraxia, dysarthria) AND pure tone screening and impedance testing: 92551 and 92567 Schedules evaluation and asks child's mother to contact her insurance company. ICD-10 code for speech disorder F80.0 ICD 10 code for speech-language disorder F80.1 or F80.2 ICD-10 code for the already diagnosed middle ear disorder. This code was supplied by the pediatrician: H65.06 Acute Serous Otitis Media, Recurrent Bilateral Case history mailed to mother to complete.		Front office staff complete an intake form.

Date	Actions	Billed and Coded	Documented
September 29	Child's mother calls back to say the insurance company has preauthorized the evaluation and 12 visits.		Front desk staff document this insurance information on the intake form. Practice has a contract with this insurance company and has agreed to the rates they set. There is one evaluation rate regardless of which CPT evaluation code is used.
October 3	Completed case history received. Speech-language pathologist assigned for evaluation reviews and selects tests. History indicates possible language delay as well.		
October 5	Evaluation of speech and language completed. Child has moderate articulation disorder, normal receptive language skills, and mild expressive language disorder. Spends 1 hour and 20 minutes with child and 10 minutes reviewing results with child's mother. Pure tone screening and middle ear screening deferred because child is being followed by audiologist and was seen within past 2 weeks. 25 minutes spent scoring tests and writing report. Because 12 visits are authorized for the remainder of the calendar year, the speech-language pathologist recommends seeing child 2x/week for the first 2 weeks (4 visits) and then 1x/week with more intensive home practice to maximize the approved # of visits.	92523 (This is an untimed code and can be billed only once.)	Front desk staff member has child's mother fill out release of info form and sign attendance policy and HIPAA documents. Speech-language pathologist uses pediatric report template the practice has developed for speech-language assessments. Uses standard paragraphs for the tests administered.
October 6	Front desk staff send copies of report and treatment plan to those on the release of info form: Pediatrician, ear-nose-throat, audiologist; preschool teacher.		Speech-language pathologist completes the treatment plan based on goals child's mother agreed to address.
October 10, 12, 17, 19 (4/12 authorized visits)	Child seen for individual sessions with mother participating. Initial articulation targets addressed along with expressive syntactic goals.	92507 for each date	Speech-language pathologist uses a streamlined progress note with percent correct on each treatment objective.
			Provides home practice for child and his mother.

DATE	ACTIONS	BILLED AND CODED	DOCUMENTED
October 26; November 2, 9, 16, 30 (9/12 authorized visits)	Child seen for individual sessions with mother participating. Initial articulation targets addressed along with expressive syntactic goals.	92507 for each date; giving an artic test during a session is not an evaluation.	Uses the streamlined progress note for each date. Provides home practice.
December 7, 14 (11/12)	Child seen for individual sessions with mother participating. Initial articulation targets addressed along with expressive syntactic goals. On December 14, speech-language pathologist administers articulation test to determine current level. Discusses with child's mother that more visits will be needed and tells mother she will prepare summary report of treatment mother can use to request more visits in next calendar year.	92507 each session	Uses the streamlined progress note for each date. Provides home practice. On December 14, adds more information about the results of the testing in the progress note.
December 19 (12th visit)	Language goals have been met. Individual session with mother participating. A lot of time in session spent reviewing the home management program. Front desk staff send copies of discharge summary and new treatment plan to those on the release of info form: Pediatrician, ear-nose-throat, audiologist, preschool teacher. Uses fax cover to explain that more visits are being requested.	92507 each session Although there is a code 97535 Home Management, the best description of the service is still 92507, and two codes cannot be used for the same session.	Speech-language pathologist completes discharge summary along with an updated treatment plan. Detailed home program because there may be a break while mother tries to get more visits authorized in next calendar year.

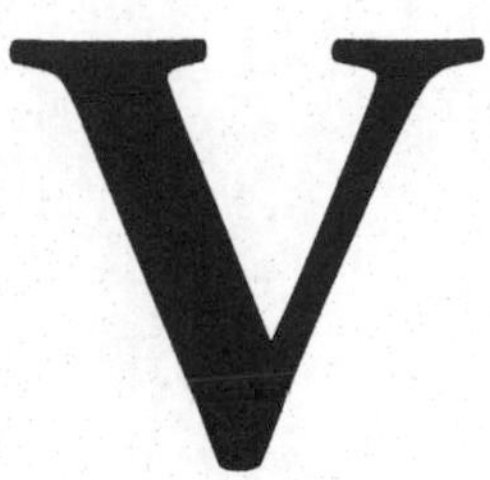

Professional Writing and Presentations

The chapters in Sections I through IV of this book provided the basics of documentation, documentation of different types of services, and documentation and reimbursement in specific settings: Adult, pediatric, health care, and schools. Section V comprises Chapter 18, which includes tips on making your writing reflect positively on you. Formats for letters, fax cover sheets, and emails are discussed. There are also tips on preparing and giving a computer-generated presentations (e.g., PowerPoint) because this is a way that case examples are shared at staff meetings, during rounds, and in continuing education opportunities in work settings.

Also included, following this section, are two appendices:

1. Glossary to help with any terms that might be unfamiliar
2. Abbreviations the speech-language pathologist may encounter in health care and education settings

18

Written Communication and Presentations

Nancy B. Swigert, MA, CCC-SLP, BCS-S

Formats for Written Communication

Most communication occurs electronically, with fewer and fewer occasions when one constructs a letter, prints it, and puts it in the mail. However, cover letters are still needed, even if they are sent as an attachment to an email. Documents should not be faxed without a fax cover sheet, which should look professional. Emails should be constructed with the same format guidelines (e.g., salutations, headers, reference lines, signature) as a printed letter.

Letters

Letters should be sent on letterhead and should be formatted according to standard business letter formats. Business letters have basic sections that should be included (Table 18-1):

- Business letters should be sent on the professional letterhead stationery of the facility.
- The date should be spelled out in full (e.g., April 29, 2017) and typed two to six lines below the letterhead at the right side of the page.
- Reference lines are needed in some letters to indicate what the letter pertains to. If the letter pertains to a client, then the client's name (and perhaps the date of birth or identifying client record number) would appear here.
- The address of the recipient is usually typed three to eight lines below the dateline.
  - Include the title of the person to whom the letter is sent (e.g., Mr., Ms., Dr.). For physicians, use either the title (i.e., Dr. Fizz Iatrist) or the degree (i.e., Fizz Iatrist, MD), but not both.
  - If the person holds a position, include that as well (e.g., Chief, Neurology).
  - The name of the facility
  - Full address of the facility
- Salutation: This is typically "Dear Ms./ Mr./ Dr. _____." If you call the person by his or her first name when talking to him or her, you can use the first name here.
- The body of the message should use paragraphs to organize the information and should ideally be brief. The paragraphs can be in block form (no indentations) or in indented form.

Swigert, N. B.
Documentation and Reimbursement for Speech-Language Pathologists: Principles and Practice (pp. 347-355).

Table 18-1

Formatting Letters

Letter Feature	Example
Date	July 26, 2017
Inside address	Car Diologist, MD 1800 Fayette Lane Lexington, KY 55555 *(Don't use the degree and the title [e.g., Dr. Car Diologist, MD].)*
Reference line	Re: Client's name
Salutation	Dear Dr. Diologist:
Margins	Block or indented; not so narrow as to make it difficult to read
Body of message	Keep it brief
Font	Typically 12-pt font, single-spaced
Closing	"Sincerely," unless you are on a less formal basis with recipient
Signature	Your name, degree, and credentials
Cosignature	Either below or beside
Enclosures	Indicate that something is enclosed; you can specify what (e.g., Enclosure: Report and Treatment Plan)
CC:	Name of person(s) receiving a courtesy copy

MEMORANDUM

To:

From:

Date:

Re:

Body of the message goes here. Organize with:

- *Opening statement explaining the purpose of the memo*
- *Then paragraphs with information related to the topic*
- *Closing paragraph to make clear what the next steps or recommended action is*

Figure 18-1. How to organize a memo.

- The closing on a business letter is usually "Sincerely" unless the recipient is well-known to the sender, in which case a less formal closing can be used. This is typed two lines after the message and flush left.
- Signature: The writer's signature appears here with appropriate degrees and credentials.
- Cosignature: If a cosignature is needed (e.g., another speech-language pathologist is cotreating or supervising), the cosignature can be stacked under the other signature or off to the right.
- The typed signature appears just as the signed signature. Additional titles (e.g., Speech-Language Pathologist, Rehabilitation Department Director) can also be included.
- Enclosed materials should be indicated by noting "Enclosure."
- Courtesy copies are indicated by "cc:" and the name of the person(s) to whom the copies are being sent (The Emily Post Institute, n.d.).

Memorandum

Memo format can be used when information about a problem or issue needs to be shared with one person or multiple individuals (Figure 18-1). They are not typically used when sending a report or other patient information to a provider. A memo has a header that clearly indicates to whom the memo is being sent. The body of the memo should be organized with an opening that explains the purpose of the memo. The following paragraphs provide the information related to the topic. A closing paragraph should make clear what the next steps are related to the issue (The Purdue Online Writing Lab, n.d.).

FAX MEMORANDUM

DATE: ____________________

TO: ____________________ FROM: ____________________

FAX #: ____________________ FAX #: ____________________

PHONE: ____________________

RE: ____________________

NUMBER OF PAGES (INCLUDING COVER): ____________________

MESSAGE: ____________________

CONFIDENTIAL NOTICE: The materials enclosed with this facsimile transmission are private and confidential and are the property of the sender. The information contained in the material is privileged and is intended only for the use of the individual(s) or entity(ies) named above. If you are not the intended recipient, be advised that any unauthorized disclosure, copying, distribution, or the taking of any action in reliance on the contents of this information is strictly prohibited. If you have received this facsimile in error, please immediately notify us by telephone to arrange for the return of the documents

Figure 18-2. Fax cover sheet.

Fax Cover Sheets

There are multiple formats for a fax cover sheet, and the facility will have one that you are expected to use (Figure 18-2). Basically, a fax cover sheet looks like the header of a memo but should also include the following:

- Number of pages, including the cover page (so the recipient can tell if she has received all of the pages)
- Fax number of the recipient
- Contact phone number for the sender in case the recipient has questions
- Confidentiality statement if the information being faxed is protected health information (see Figure 3-1)

Emails

Email correspondence should follow the etiquette for style, form, and content of other written forms of communication. For example, the type of salutation should be the same you would use in a letter. The email subject line is equivalent to the reference line in a letter. Although you cannot sign an email, the typed professional signature should be the same as used on a letter. Email programs allow the user to store different forms of signatures (e.g., professional signature, personal signature without titles) so that the proper format can be used.

Avoiding Common Mistakes in Writing

It is beyond the scope of this chapter to review all rules of punctuation, spelling, grammar, and syntax. There are resources available for more in-depth study of these rules (Goldfarb & Serpanos, 2009; The Purdue Online Writing Lab, n.d.). There are, however, common errors to be avoided in professional writing that should be highlighted (Gateley & Borcherding, 2016). Carefully checking for these mistakes when proofreading will help avoid sending out a document with errors (Appendix 18-A).

- Use of apostrophes: The apostrophe is used for possessives and not for plurals. Also, an apostrophe is often incorrectly used in the word "its." Unless you mean the words "it is," do not use an apostrophe.

Table 18-2

Capitalization

Capitalize	Do Not Capitalize
Trade names of products or medications • Blom-Singer Laryngectomy Tube • Prilosec	Generic or common terms • laryngectomy tube • omeprazole
Specific organizations • The Joint Commission • Lovely Lexington Rehabilitation Hospital	Generic organizations • accrediting agencies • rehabilitation facility
Proper names of disorders/diseases • Parkinson's disease • Down syndrome	Non-specific disorders/diseases • peripheral neuropathy • concussion
Degrees and designations after a name • Nancy Swigert, MA, CCC-SLP • New Rologist, MD	General mention of degrees • certified speech-language pathologist • physician
Names of tests • Western Aphasia Battery • Hodson Assessment of Phonological Patterns	Generic tests • aphasia screening • articulation test
Names of specific departments • Baptist Health Emergency Department • Baptist Health Respiratory Care Department	General mention of departments • an emergency department • respiratory care departments

- Use of commas: If the comma is inserted in the wrong place, it changes the entire meaning of the sentence. The humorous title of the book *Eats, Shoots & Leaves* has on the cover a picture of a panda bear in the process of eating, not firing a weapon. The sentence to describe what the panda is doing should have been, "Eats shoots and leaves" (Truss, 2004). Try reading the sentence aloud and pausing at the comma to see if it makes sense. If not, omit the comma.
- Use of quotation mark: Use quotation marks when documenting the exact words a client said, but if paraphrasing, no quotation marks are needed.
- Consistency in tense: When describing something the client did, use past tense consistently. Do not insert one sentence that has present tense.
- Singular and plural nouns: If referring to a single person, use a singular noun. Sometimes the plural form (e.g., their) is used to avoid gender bias. Using the plural form throughout in those situations can avoid the use of the awkward she/he or s/he.
- Correct use of possessives: If it is a singular noun, the apostrophe goes before the "s."
- Correct capitalization (Table 18-2)

Proofreading and Spell Checking

In an era when software on our computers, tablets, and smartphones performs a spell check for us, the art of proofreading is sorely missed. However, these spell checkers and grammar checkers sometimes fail us. How many times have you sent a text only to see that the "smart" phone has written something entirely different from what you intended when it corrected a typing error for you? Spell checkers in word processing programs don't know some of our professional terminology and sometimes correct something that doesn't need to be corrected. The word "dysphagia" is often mistakenly changed to "dysphasia."

A tip for making the automated spell checker work for you when using Microsoft Word is to use the custom dictionary feature. You can add words to the dictionary that you commonly use. Also, if you typically type a word incorrectly (e.g., cleint for client), you can use the feature to add this to a list of words to autocorrect.

Oral Presentations

Oral presentations might seem an odd topic in a chapter on professional writing, but unless the presenter is giving an off-the-cuff talk, the preparation probably involves writing down at least an outline for the presentation. The more prepared the presenter is, the more effective the presentation. In clinical situations, the speech-language pathologist may be asked to present a case to other speech-language pathologists or in a multidisciplinary setting, which may be grand rounds or a continuing education event. If you are invited to give a case presentation, observe carefully the format used in previous presentations. If you haven't routinely attended the meetings of the group to whom you are going to present, ask the coordinator of the group for information concerning who will be in attendance and the format:

- Length of time you will be expected to talk: Practice your presentation so that you are neither talking too long or not long enough.
- How the information should be organized:
  - Is the patient's name used?
  - How much background information is provided concerning the patient?
  - Are you expected to present information only or to seek input from others in attendance?
- Should any printed materials/handouts be provided?
- Are slides used in the presentation?

Knowing who the audience is will help you gear your remarks to the right level. If you are speaking to other medical professionals, for example, you will not need to explain medical terms such as diagnoses or procedures. However, you might need to explain terms specific for speech-language pathology (e.g., penetration, hyolaryngeal excursion, non-fluent aphasia). If you are speaking to non–medical personnel, such as giving a presentation to kitchen staff regarding dysphagia diets or presenting at a consumer support group, the level of the content will need to be adjusted accordingly.

Preparing the Presentation

Perhaps more important than any tips on presentation style is this: Know your topic. You will be expected to be the expert on the information you are presenting. Spend as much time as possible gathering information on the topic. Take notes or use an outline format to organize the information. This information goes in the body of the talk. After working on the body of the presentation, determine what a good introduction and summary will be. Some speakers like to make speaker notes on cards or in an outline format (Goldfarb & Serpanos, 2009). If you are using slides, the speaker notes will be available to you. Before putting the final touches on the presentation, think about what kind of questions the participants might ask. Decide if you want to include the answers to those questions in the presentation to reduce the number of potential questions. The final step is to practice, practice, practice until you feel comfortable with the content and the timing. Present it to a friend or colleague who can give you tips on the content and your presentation style.

Computer-Generated Slide Presentations

With any presentation, whether slides will be used or not, first determine what your objectives are for the presentation. The content should then be developed to match your objectives. PowerPoint and other slide-generating computer programs are not the presentation. They are just a mode through which the speaker presents the content. The speaker should first follow all guidelines for active, adult learning when preparing a presentation. However, effective use of a computer slide presentation can enhance your presentation. The slides provide added information to your audience, but you should not read everything that is on the slide. There are many resources to guide you in developing an effective PowerPoint presentation:

- Carefully consider the color scheme chosen. Dark background colors with lighter font are often used. A white background with black letters can be hard on the eyes.
- Select a font that is clean, crisp, and easy to read. Some effects, like shadow, can look blurry on the screen.
- Avoid too much information on a slide. A general rule of thumb is 6 x 6: 6 words to a line, 6 lines to a slide.
  - See what your slides look like from the back of the room. Be sure the slides can be read easily from that distance.
- Punctuation is not required, but if you use it, be sure it is accurate.
- Complete sentences are not necessary, and in fact may cause the participants to read the slide rather than listen to the speaker.
- Avoid non-standard abbreviations.
- Always spell check. It is embarrassing to spot a spelling error in the middle of a presentation.
- Highlight one idea or concept per slide.
- One slide per minute of presentation time is generally a good guideline.
- Use images and graphics to illustrate a point.
- Include appropriate citations of others' work.
- Use animations sparingly (Atkinson, 2011; Daffner, 2003; Goldfarb & Serpanos, 2009).

TABLE 18-3

DOS AND DON'TS IN RESUME PREPARATION

DO	DON'T
• Include only accurate, true information • Use headers to help the reader find needed information • Use reverse chronological order • Use readable font type and size (minimum 11-pt font) • Use larger or bold font for headers • Print on heavy-weight (e.g., 22–25 lb.), light-colored paper • If sent as attachment to email or online application program, check to be sure it was received and is readable. Sometimes all formatting is lost when attached or embedded in these programs.	• Include personal information like birthdate or social security number • Include a photograph • Include lots of unnecessary, detailed information • Use fancy fonts or colorful ink

Adapted from Goldfarb, R., & Serpanos, Y. C. (2009). *Professional writing in speech-language pathology and audiology.* San Diego, CA: Plural Publishing Inc.

WRITING FOR JOB SEARCH: RESUMES AND COVER LETTERS

Most applications for jobs are completed online, and each human resources department may use a different software program to gather information on applicants; however, what the prospective employer of a speech-language pathologist wants to see is the resume. The resume is meant to be a brief summary of the person's educational background that reflects skills and experience. For a speech-language pathologist seeking her first job after graduate school, the experience will be the graduate externships she has completed. After she has had a job, the experience will be what is listed as experience, and the graduate externships are no longer applicable, unless the speech-language pathologist gained some unique experience or skill in that setting that was not carried over in the first employment setting. In academic settings, a lengthier version, referred to a *curriculum vitae* (CV), is used (Goldfarb & Serpanos, 2009).

The most common format for a resume is chronological. The most recent activities in each section are listed first. For example, the master's degree is listed before the bachelor's degree and the most recent job experience (or externship) is listed before earlier experiences. Most universities offer assistance to students in preparing resumes. Some dos and don'ts are listed in Table 18-3.

The categories usually included in a resume are the following:

- Education (degrees)
- Certifications/licensures
- Professional experience
- Awards/honors
- Publications
- Professional presentations
- Research
- Professional affiliations
- Skills
- References (Goldfarb & Serpanos, 2009)

Although most employers require an online application, sending a resume with a cover letter directly to the person who has the potential to interview you and offer you a position is a good way to get his or her attention. Sometimes there is a lag between the time you complete the online application and the time it reaches the speech-language pathology department. Contacting the head of the department directly and sending your resume with a cover letter can facilitate the process. The cover letter should be brief but should address why you want to work at that facility, not just a general statement that you are looking for a job. Take the time to find out about the facility to which you are applying and make your letter specific to that facility.

REFERENCES

Atkinson, C. (2011). *Beyond bullet points: Using Microsoft PowerPoint to create presentations that inform, motivate, and inspire.* Cranbury, NJ: Pearson Education Inc.

Daffner, R. H. (2003). On improvement of scientific presentations: Using PowerPoint. *American Journal of Roentgenology, 181*(1), 47–49.

The Emily Post Institute. (n.d.). Effective business letters. Retrieved from http://emilypost.com/advice/effective-business-letters/

Gateley, C. A., & Borcherding, S. (2016). *Documentation manual for occupational therapy: Writing SOAP notes* (4th ed.). Thorofare, NJ: SLACK Incorporated.

Goldfarb, R., & Serpanos, Y. C. (2009). *Professional writing in speech-language pathology and audiology.* San Diego, CA: Plural Publishing Inc.

The Purdue Online Writing Lab (OWL). (n.d.). Retrieved from https://owl.english.purdue.edu/

Truss, L. (2004). *Eats, shoots & leaves: The zero tolerance approach to punctuation.* London, UK: Penguin.

Review Questions

1. What should be included in each section of a business letter?
2. List five common grammatical mistakes made when writing.
3. What are some questions you should ask when someone invites you to give an oral presentation?
4. What are dos and don'ts for preparing an effective slide presentation?
5. List some guidelines for organizing a resume.

Activity A

Find the mistakes (spelling, grammatical, formatting, tone) in the following letters.

1.

Swigert & Associates, Inc.

Dr. Ortho Dontist, M.D.
122 Ankle Way
Broken City, CA 22222

Dear Sir:

Thank you for refferring your client to me for articulation therapy. Its a pleasure, as always to receive a refferral from you. Jon's evaluation revealed a moderate Articulation Disorder, characterized by omission of /s/ in blends, and inability to produce/r/. His speech, is, indeed, difficult to understand.

His parent's have agreed to enroll Jon in therapy twice weekely. I've also let his pediatrician know that he will be starting therapy.

Nancy B. Swigert

CC: Paul Pediatrician

2.

September 25, 2017

Dear Dr. Ologist

RE: Said Abedayo

Enclosed is the report on Saids speech and language skills. Sure appreciate you sending him our way. He is having paticular trouble comprehending the teacher in the class room when, she provides lengthy instructions.

Sincerely,

De'Aron Articulation, M.S., CF-SLP

3.

ReCent Graduate
1111 Student City Drive
University, NC 11111

To whom it may concern:

I heard, you might have an opening, for a speech-language pathologist in the department. My friends' told me that it is a good place to work so I thought I would see if there is a spot. My resume is included for you to look over and then give me a call and we can talk.
Very truly yours,

Notthe Brightest
Speech Therapist
P.S. I will need a supervisor, for my clinical fellowship year

APPENDIX 18-A
Common Mistakes to Avoid in Writing

- Do not use an apostrophe when indicating the plural of something that has been abbreviated.
  - Physical therapist (PT) Physical therapists (PTs)
  - Urinary tract infection (UTI) Urinary tract infections (UTIs)
  - Certified nursing assistant (CNA) Certified nursing assistants (CNAs)
- Do not use an apostrophe when you are indicating a plural.
  - Incorrect: The parent's attended the orientation session.
  - Correct: The parents attended the orientation session.
- Use the apostrophe correctly in it's/its.
  - Incorrect: She read the book in it's entirety.
  - Correct: She read the book in its entirety.
- Use commas correctly.
  - Incorrect: The client, brought in her homework, and she had demonstrated the correct pronunciation.
  - Correct: The client brought in her homework, and she had demonstrated the correct pronunciation.
- Use quotation marks only for direct quotes.
  - Incorrect: The client's mother reports the child "just can't seem to sit still."
  - Correct: The client's mother stated, "Yoshia just can't seem to sit still."
- Keep the tense consistent throughout the note and use past tense if the behavior or event has already happened.
  - Incorrect: Jamari completed the open-ended sentence task with 90% accuracy with only phonemic cues. He answers the simple yes/no questions 100% with no cues.
  - Correct: Jamari completed the open-ended sentence task with 90% accuracy with only phonemic cues. He answered the simple yes/no questions 100% with no cues.
- Use the correct singular and plural pronouns.
  - Incorrect: The client was not able to keep their appointment.
  - Correct: The client was not able to keep his appointment.
  - Incorrect/awkward: The student who needs to work on pragmatics should be cued by his/her teacher to use topic introductions.
  - Correct: Students who need to work on pragmatics should be cued by their teacher to use topic introductions.
- Write possessives correctly.
  - Incorrect: Olivias' mother sat in on the therapy session.
  - Correct: Olivia's mother sat in on the therapy session.
  - Incorrect: During group, all of the patient's spouses were in attendance.
  - Correct: During group, all of the patients' spouses were in attendance.

Glossary

Abuse: Practices that are inconsistent with sound business and fiscal principles that result in unnecessary cost. For example, if one facility routinely performed a videofluoroscopic swallow evaluation on every patient admitted with stroke when most other facilities would only perform the study if there were clinical indications, this could be considered abuse. There is no absolute distinction between fraud and abuse because the circumstances surrounding the event would determine which it was.

Accrediting agency: Non–governmental agency that develops rules and regulations for education and health care facilities. The facilities typically voluntarily decide to see accreditation from one or more of these agencies.

Addendum: After an entry in a chart is complete and authenticated, but while it is still the time of service, the clinician needs to add something to the documentation. This addition is marked as an addendum.

Advance Beneficiary Notice (ABN): A document given to a Medicare beneficiary before providing services that are typically not covered by Medicare.

Advanced practice registered nurse (APRN): Can perform many duties of a physician, with limitations typically set by state law.

Authenticate: Entries in charts should be authenticated by the person making the entry. This is done when the person signs his or her name, degree, and credentials and times and dates the entry.

Centers for Medicare & Medicaid Services (CMS): Regulatory agency located in Baltimore, Maryland, that develops, implements, and enforces the regulations for Medicare and Medicaid services.

Certification: The physician's/non–physician practitioner's approval of the plan of care. Certification requires a dated signature on the plan of care or some other document that indicates approval of the plan of care.

Clearinghouse: A public or private entity, often a billing service, that facilitates processing of health information from one entity to another.

Clinician: A term used in CMS manuals to refer to only a physician, non–physician practitioner, or therapist (but not to an assistant, aide, or any other personnel) providing a service within his or her scope of practice and consistent with state and local law.

Coinsurance: The percentage of the cost of the health care service that the consumer must pay. For example, in an 80/20 policy, the health care plan pays 80% and the consumer pays 20%.

Copay: The amount of money (usually a percentage of the charge) the insured individual is responsible for at each visit.

Deductible: The amount of money the insured individual pays before insurance starts to cover.

Designated instruction and services (DIS): These services are available when they are necessary for the pupil to benefit educationally from his or her instructional program. A child must qualify for an Individualized Education Program (IEP) before qualification for DIS is determined (includes speech-language).

Diagnosis-related group (DRG): Methodology by which Medicare pays acute care hospitals for a patient's stay.

Swigert, N. B.
Documentation and Reimbursement for Speech-Language Pathologists: Principles and Practice (pp. 357-359).

Drug interaction: When more than one drug is taken, the two may interact. The result might be less effective results of the drug(s) or serious side effects.

Electronic health record (EHR): Electronic version of a client's medical chart.

Electronic medical record (EMR): Electronic version of a patient's medical chart. This term is used more specifically in inpatient settings but is virtually the same thing as an EHR.

Exacerbation: Worsening of symptoms or increase in severity of disease.

Fraud: Generally considered to be an intentional deception or misrepresentation of information designed to provide a benefit to someone. For example, knowingly billing for services not rendered would be considered fraud.

Health Maintenance Organization (HMO): One form of a managed care health plan.

History and physical (H&P): A document written, dictated, or entered into the medical record by the admitting or attending physician. It typically contains the reason for the current admission as well as pertinent background medical history.

Hypercholesterolemia: Excess cholesterol in the bloodstream.

Independent Educational Evaluation (IEE): A private assessment at public expense if parents disagree with a school district assessment; request should be dated and in writing.

Late entry: Information that needs to be added to documentation later, not at the time of the service, is entered with the date and time the additional information is added and is marked as a late entry.

Least restrictive environment (LRE): Students should have the opportunity to be educated with non-disabled peers to the greatest extent appropriate.

Likert scale: A five- or seven-point scale used to allow an individual to express how much he or she agrees or disagrees with a statement.

Local coverage determinations (LCDs): Documents produced by Medicare Administrative Contractors (MACs) with more detailed information about what services are or are not covered in that part of the country by Medicare.

Maintenance program: A program established by a therapist that consists of activities and/or mechanisms that will assist a beneficiary in maximizing or maintaining the progress he or she has made during therapy or to prevent or slow further deterioration due to a disease or illness.

Malpractice: Improper or illegal activity, typically by a health care practitioner.

Meaningful use: Part of federal legislation that incentivizes the use of electronic health records, with specific goals to be met in order to receive compensation.

Medically necessary: Treatment that is, as defined by Medicare, skilled, effective, and provided by qualified professionals, with approval of the physician.

Medicare Administrative Contractors (MACs): Insurance companies contracted by CMS to administer the Medicare program for a region.

National coverage determination (NCD): Documents that specify services that are or are not covered by Medicare.

Non–physician practitioner (NPP): Advanced practice registered nurse (APRN) or physician's assistant (PA).

Out-of-pocket limit: The maximum amount the insured individual is responsible to pay within a given period (usually 1 year) before insurance takes over and pays 100%.

Person-first language: Puts the person before the disability in attempt to avoid perceived dehumanization.

Pharmacology: The science of drugs, their use, effects, modes of delivery, etc.

Point-of-care (POC) documentation: Documentation that is completed, usually on a computer, while the clinician is with the client.

Post–acute care settings: Any medical setting in which a patient is seen after a stay in an acute care hospital, including skilled nursing facilities, inpatient rehabilitation hospitals, long-term acute care hospitals, home health agencies, and outpatient settings.

Preauthorization: Obtaining authorization from a third-party payer before providing services to ensure the third party will cover the services.

Preferred Provider Organization (PPO): Type of health insurance plan that allows the patient relative flexibility to select providers.

Prevalence: The proportion of a population who have (or had) a specific characteristic in a given time period; in medicine, typically an illness, a condition, or a risk factor such as depression or smoking. Prevalence is calculated if one has information on the characteristics of the entire population of interest (this is rare in medicine). Prevalence is estimated if one has information on samples of the population of interest.

Prior level of function: The baseline level at which the client was functioning before the need for speech-language services arose.

Protected health information (PHI): Under U.S. law, any information about health status, provision of health care, or payment for health care that is created or collected certain health care providers (covered entities) and can be linked to a specific individual.

Qualified professional: A physical or occupational therapist, speech-language pathologist, physician, nurse practitioner, clinical nurse specialist, or physician's assistant who is licensed or certified by the state to furnish therapy services and who also may appropriately furnish therapy services under Medicare policies.

Regulatory agency: A governmental agency that writes the regulations to implement laws passed by Congress. Examples are CMS and the U.S. Department of Education.

Sanctions: Penalties for breaking laws or regulations.

Sentinel event: Any unanticipated event that results in serious physical or psychological injury.

Subject matter expert: Someone with expertise in an area, typically a clinical area, who consults with the team building an electronic health record.

Third-party payer: Typically an insurance company or a government agency like Medicare or Medicaid that is paying for the health services the client receives.

Transfer: Can mean to transfer a patient from bed to chair or transfer to another facility.

Treatment day: A single calendar day on which treatment, evaluation, and/or re-evaluation is provided. There could be multiple visits, treatment sessions, and encounters on a treatment day.

Utilization data: Data obtained from patient medical records about the type and amount of services rendered.

Visit or treatment session: Begins at the time the patient enters the treatment area (of a building, office, or clinic) and continues until all services (e.g., activities, procedures, services) have been completed for that session and the patient leaves that area to participate in a non–therapy activity.

Abbreviations

A

Ā	before
AAP	American Academy of Pediatrics
ABG	arterial blood gas
a.c.	before meals
A/C	assist control (a mode of ventilation)
ADA diet	American Diabetes Association diet
ADD	attention deficit disorder
ADHD	attention deficit hyperactivity disorder
ADL	activities of daily living
AFib	arterial fibrillation
AIDS	acquired immunodeficiency syndrome
AKA	above-knee amputation
ALS	amyotrophic lateral sclerosis
AMA	against medical advice
AND	allow natural death
A&O	alert and oriented
A/P	anterior-posterior
APC	advanced practice clinician
APRN	advanced practice registered nurse
Apt	appointment
ARDS	adult respiratory distress syndrome
AROM	active range of motion
ASAP	as soon as possible
ASD	autism spectrum disorder
ASHA	American Speech-Language-Hearing Association
AUT	autism spectrum

Swigert, N. B.
Documentation and Reimbursement for Speech-Language Pathologists: Principles and Practice (pp. 361-372).

B

Ⓑ	bilateral
BDAE	Boston Diagnostic Aphasia Examination
b.i.d.	twice per day
BKA	below-knee amputation
BLBS	bilateral breath sounds
bm	bowel movement
BP	blood pressure
BR	bed rest
Bs	bowel sounds
BS	breath sounds
B/S	bedside
bx	biopsy

C

$\bar{c}$	with
C	Celsius; centigrade
C1, C2, etc.	first cervical vertebrae, second cervical vertebrae, etc.
CA	cardiac arrest
CA, ca	carcinoma
CAA	Care Area Assessments
CABG	coronary artery bypass graft (x2, x3, etc., indicates how many arteries replaced)
CAD	coronary artery disease
cal	calorie
cath	catheter
CBC	complete blood count
CC	chief complaint
CCU	coronary care unit
C. dif	*Clostidium difficile*
CHF	congestive heart failure
CHI	closed head injury
cm	centimeter
CMS	Centers for Medicare & Medicaid Services
CN	cranial nerve
CNA	certified nursing assistant
CNS	central nervous system
c/o	complains of
Cont	continue(d)
COPD	chronic obstructive pulmonary disease
COTA	certified occupational therapy assistant
CP	cerebral palsy
CPAP	continuous positive airway pressure (but often used to mean CPAP machine)
CPR	cardiopulmonary resuscitation
CPT	Current Procedural Terminology
CRF	chronic renal failure
CSF	cerebrospinal fluid

CT	computed tomography
CV	cardiovascular
CVA	cerebral vascular accident
CXR	chest x-ray

D

d/c	discontinue
DC	discharge
DHH	deaf/hard of hearing
DIS	designated instruction and services
DJD	degenerative joint disease
DM	diabetes mellitus
DME	durable medical equipment
DNK	do not know
DNKA	did not keep appointment
DNR	do not resuscitate
DNT	did not test
DOA	dead on arrival; date of admission
DOB	date of birth
DOE	dyspnea on exertion
DRG	diagnosis-related group
d/t	due to
DVT	deep vein thrombosis
Dx	diagnosis

E

ECF	extended care facility
ECG, EKG	electrocardiogram
ECHO	echocardiogram
ED	emergency department
EEG	electroencephalogram
EENT	eye, ear, nose, throat
EHR	electronic health record
EMG	electromyogram
EMR	electronic medical record
ENT	ear, nose, throat
EPSDT	Early Periodic Screening, Diagnostic, and Treatment
ESRD	end-stage renal disease
ETOH	ethanol (alcohol)
ext	external, exterior

F

F	Fahrenheit
FAPE	free appropriate public education
FCM	Functional Communication Measure
FCP	family cost participation

FEES fiberoptic endoscopic evaluation of swallowing
FERPA Federal Education Rights & Privacy Act
FH family history
fib fibrillation
FIM Functional Independence Measure
fl fluid
fMRI functional magnetic resonance imaging
FOB foot of bed
FTT failure to thrive
f/u follow-up
FWB full weightbearing
Fx fracture

G

GA gestational age
GB gall bladder
GCS Glasgow Coma Scale
GE gastroenterology
G/E gastroenteritis
gen general
GERD gastroesophageal reflux disease
gest gestation
GI gastrointestinal
gluc glucose
GP general practitioner; general paralysis
GSW gunshot wound
GTT glucose tolerance test
GYN gynecology

H

H_2O water
H hour
H/A headache
HAV hepatitis A virus
Hb. hemoglobin
HBP high blood pressure
HBV hepatitis B virus
h.d. at bedtime
HEENT head, eyes, ear, nose, throat
Hep B hepatitis B
HH home health
HHCoPS Home Health Conditions of Participation
HIPAA Health Insurance Portability & Accountability Act
HIV human immunodeficiency virus
h/o history of
HOB head of bed
HOH hard of hearing
H&P history and physical

HR	heart rate
HS	bedtime
Ht	height
HTN	hypertension
HVD	hypertensive vascular disease
Hx	history
Hz	Hertz (cycles/second)

I

Ⓘ	independent
ICC	Interagency Coordinating Council
ICCU	intensive coronary care unit
ICP	intracranial pressure
ICU	intensive care unit
IDEA	Individuals with Disabilities Education Act
IEE	Independent Educational Evaluation
IEP	Individualized Education Program
IFSP	Individualized Family Service Plan
IM	internal medicine
imp.	impression
incr.	increased/increasing
inf	infusion; inferior
int.	internal
I&O	intake and output
IP	inpatient
IRF	inpatient rehabilitation facility
irreg.	irregular
IV	intravenous(ly)

J

J	joint
jt.	joint

K

K	potassium; kidney

L

Ⓛ	left
L	left; liver; liter; lower; light; lumbar
L2, L3	second, third lumbar vertebrae
Lab	laboratory
lac.	laceration
lat.	lateral
LBW	low birth rate

LE	lower extremities
liq.	liquid
LMN	lower motor neuron
LOC	loss of consciousness; level of consciousness,
LOS	length of stay
LP	lumbar puncture
LPN	licensed practical nurse
LRE	least restrictive environment
LTC	long-term care
LTG	long-term goal
LUE	left upper extremity
Lx	larynx
L&W	living and well

M

Max Ⓐ	maximum assist
MBS	modified barium swallow study
MBSImP	Modified Barium Swallow Impairment Profile
MCA	middle cerebral artery
MD	muscular dystrophy; medical doctor; multiple disabled
MDS	minimum data set
mdnt.	midnight
MDRO	multidrug-resistant organism
med.	medicine
mets.	metastasis
MG	myasthenia gravis
MI	myocardial infarction
MICU	medical intensive care unit
min	minute; minimum; minimal assist or cueing (25% to 50%)
ml	milliliter
mm	millimeter
Mod	moderate; moderate assistance (50% to 75%)
Mod Ⓐ	moderate assist
MRI	magnetic resonance imaging
MRSA	methicillin-resistant *Staphylococcus aureus*
MS	multiple sclerosis
MSW	master's social work
MVA	motor vehicle accident

N

n.	nerve
Na	sodium
NaCl	sodium chloride
NAD	no abnormality detected; no apparent distress
NC	nasal cannula
NEC	not elsewhere classified
neg.	negative
neur.	neurology

NG	nasogastric
NIC	neonatal intensive care
NICU	neonatal intensive care unit
NIHSS	National Institutes of Health Stroke Scale
NKA	no known allergies
NKDA	no known drug allergies
NMES	neuromuscular electrical stimulation
no.	number
NOMS	National Outcomes Measurement System of ASHA
non-STEMI	non-ST elevated myocardial infarction
NOS	not otherwise specified
NPO	nothing by mouth (Latin: nil per os)
NSA	no specific abnormality
NSAID	non-steroidal anti-inflammatory drug
NT	nasotracheal
N&V	nausea and vomiting
NVD	nausea, vomiting, diarrhea
N&W	normal and well
NWB	nonweightbearing
NYD	not yet diagnosed

O

O_2	oxygen
O_2 sat.	oxygen saturation
O	none; without; oral
O x ____	oriented x 1, 2, 3, 4 (time, place, person, situation)
OA	osteoarthritis
OB, OBG	obstetrics
OB/GYN	obstetrics and gynecology
Obs	observation
OBS	organic brain syndrome
O/E	on examination
OG	orogastric
OH	occupational history
OHD	organic heart disease
OHI	other health impaired
oint.	ointment
OM	otitis media
OME	otitis media with effusion
OOB, oob	out of bed
Op.	operation
OP	outpatient
OR	operating room
ot.	ear
OT	occupational therapy
OTC	over-the-counter (pharmaceuticals)
Oto	otolaryngology
OTR/L	Occupational Therapist Registered/Licensed
oz	ounce

P

$\overline{P}$	after
PA	physician's assistant
p&a	percussion and auscultation
PACU	post-anesthesia care unit
PAF	paroxysmal atrial fibrillation
palp.	palpate; palpated; palpable
Path	pathology
PA view	posterior-anterior view (on x-ray)
p/c, pc	after meals
PCA	post-conceptual age; patient-controlled analgesic
pdr.	powder
PE	physical exam; pulmonary embolism
Peds.	pediatrics
PEEP	positive end expiratory pressure
PEG	percutaneous endoscopic gastrostomy
per	by
PET	positron emission tomography
PFT	pulmonary function test
PH	past history
pharm	pharmacy
PHI	protected health information
PHYS.	physical; physiology
PI	present illness; pulmonary insufficiency
PICU	pulmonary intensive care unit; pediatric intensive care unit
plts.	platelets
PM	afternoon; post-mortem
PMH	past medical history
PM&R	physical medicine and rehabilitation
PN	poorly nourished
P&N	psychiatry and neurology
Pna	pneumonia
pneu., pneumo,	pneumonia
PNI	peripheral nerve injury
PNS	peripheral nervous system
PNX	pneumothorax
p.o.	by mouth
POC	plan of care
p.o.d.	postoperative day
pos.	positive
post.	posterior
postop	postoperative
pot., potass.	potassium
P&PD	percussion and postural drainage
PPS	prospective payment system
pre-op	preoperative
prep.	prepare for
p.r.n., PRN	as often as necessary; as needed
prod.	productive
Prog.	prognosis

PROM	passive range of motion
prosth.	prosthesis
PSH	past surgical history
Psych.	psychiatry
pt., Pt.	patient
PT	physical therapy
PTA	prior to admission; physical therapy assistant
PUD	peptic ulcer disease
PVD	peripheral vascular disease
PVT	previous trouble
Px, PX	physical examination

Q

Q	every
q.h.	every hour
q.i.d.	4 times/day
qt.	quart
quad.	quadriplegic

R

Ⓡ	right
r	right
RA	rheumatoid arthritis; right atrium
RACs	Recovery Audit Contractors
rad.	radial
rbc/RBC	red blood cell; red blood count
RCA	right coronary artery
RD	respiratory distress
RDS	respiratory distress syndrome
reg.	regular
rehab.	rehabilitation
resp.	respiratory; respirations
RLE	right lower extremity
RN	registered nurse
RO, R/O	rule out
ROM	range of motion; rupture of membranes; right otitis media
ROS	review of symptoms
RSP	Resource Specialist Program
Rt.	right
RT	radiation therapy; respiratory therapy
RUE	right upper extremity
RUG	Resource Utilization Group
RV	residual volume
Rx	therapy; prescription

S

$\overline{S}$	without
S	sensation; sensitive; serum
Ⓢ	supervision
Sa.	saline
SAI	Specialized Academic Instruction
SBA	stand by assist
s.c.	subcutaneous(ly)
SCD	sudden cardiac death
SCI	spinal cord injury
schiz	schizophrenia
SCU	special care unit
SDC	Special Day Class
sec	second
Sens.	sensory; sensation
sep.	separated
SGA	small for gestational age
SH	social history
SI	stroke index
sib.	sibling
SICU	surgical intensive care unit
SIDS	sudden infant death syndrome
SIMV	synchronized intermittent volume
skel.	skeletal
Sl.	slightly
SL	under the tongue (sublingual)
SLI	speech-language impaired
SLP	speech-language pathology; speech-language pathologist
sm	small
SME	subject matter expert
SMERCs	Supplemental Medical Review Contractors
SNF	skilled nursing facility
SOA	shortness of air
SOAP	subjective, objective, assessment, plan
SOB	shortness of breath
SOC	start of care
S/P, s/p	status post (previous condition)
sp. cd.	spinal cord
spec.	specimen
SPED	special education
sp. fl.	spinal fluid
sp & H	speech and hearing
spin.	spine; spinal
sPO_2	estimated percent saturation oxygen
spont.	spontaneous
s/s	signs and symptoms
SS	social service
ST	speech therapy
stat., STAT	immediately
STD	sexually transmitted disease

STEMI	ST-elevation myocardial infarction
STG	short-term goal
subcut.	subcutaneous
subling.	sublingual
sup.	superior
supin.	supination
surg.	surgery; surgical
Sx	symptoms
sys.	system
Syst.	systolic
Sz	seizure

T

T	temperature
T&A	tonsils and adenoids; tonsillectomy and adenoidectomy
tab.	tablet
TAH	total abdominal hysterectomy
TB	tuberculosis
TBI	traumatic brain injury
tbsp.	tablespoon
TEDs	thromboembolic disease stockings
TEE	transesophageal echocardiogram
temp	temperature
therap.	therapy; therapeutic
THR	total hip replacement
TIA	transient ischemic attack
TID	3 times/day
TKR	total knee replacement
TNM	tumor, nodes, and metastases
TO	telephone order
tPA	tissue plasminogen activator
TPN	total parenteral nutrition
TPR	temperature, pulse, respiration
tr	trace
trach	tracheostomy
tsp.	teaspoon
TV	tidal volume
Tx	treatment, traction

U

UA	urinalysis
UCD, UCHD	usual childhood diseases
UG	upward gaze
UMN	upper motor neuron
Unilat	unilateral
u/o	under observation
Ur.	urine
URD	upper respiratory disease
URI	upper respiratory infection

Urol.	urology
u/s, US	ultrasound
UTI	urinary tract infection

V

V	vein
VA	visual acuity
Vag	vagina; vaginal
VC, vit. cap	vital capacity
vent.	ventilator
vert.	vertical
VF	visual fields; ventricular fibrillation
VFSE	videofluoroscopic swallowing exam
VFSS	videofluoroscopic swallowing study
via	by way of
vit.	vitamin
VO	verbal order
VRE	vancomycin-resistant enterococci
VS, V.S.	vital signs

W

W	white
w, wk	week
WAB	Western Aphasia Battery
WBC	white blood cell count
W/C, wh.ch.	wheelchair
WFL	within functional limits
w/n	within
WNL	within normal limits
wt.	weight
w/u	workup

X

x	times
XRMT	intensity-modulated radiation therapy

Y

y.o.	years old
yrs.	years

Z

ZPICS	Zone Program Integrity Contractors

Financial Disclosures

Denise M. Ambrosi has no financial or proprietary interest in the material presented herein.

Renee Kinder has no financial or proprietary interest in the material presented herein.

Daniel Meninger has no financial or proprietary interest in the material presented herein.

Dr. Barbara J. Moore has no financial or proprietary interest in the material presented herein.

Karyn Lewis Searcy has no financial or proprietary interest in the material presented herein.

Rebecca Skrine has no financial or proprietary interest in the material presented herein.

Nancy B. Swigert has no financial or proprietary interest in the material presented herein.

Lynne C. Brady Wagner has no financial or proprietary interest in the material presented herein.

Index

Printed in the United States
by Baker & Taylor Publisher Services